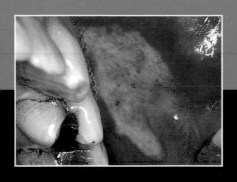
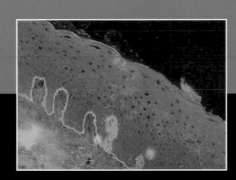
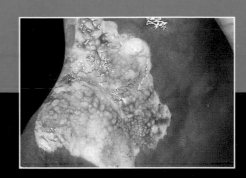

Tyldesley's Oral Medicine

Fifth Edition

Anne Field and Lesley Longman

OXFORD

OXFORD MEDICAL PUBLICATIONS

Tyldesley's oral medicine

Specialist advisers

David Casson
Consultant in paediatric gastroenterology, Liverpool Childrens' Hospital, Liverpool, UK

John Cooper
Consultant in oral and maxillofacial surgery, University Hospital Aintree, Liverpool, UK

Patrick Chu
Consultant haematologist, Royal Liverpool and Broadgreen University Hospital Trust, Liverpool, UK

Mark Davies
Consultant anaesthetist, Liverpool University Dental Hospital and Royal Liverpool and Broadgreen University Hospital Trust, Liverpool, UK

Luke Dawson
Clinical lecturer in oral surgery, Liverpool University Dental Hospital, Liverpool, UK

John Field
Professor of molecular oncology, The University of Liverpool, UK

John Hamburger
Senior lecturer and honorary consultant in oral medicine, The University of Birmingham School of Dentistry, UK

Eileen Manning
Consultant in clinical chemistry, Royal Liverpool and Broadgreen University Hospital Trust, Liverpool, UK

Michael Martin
Senior lecturer and honorary consultant in oral microbiology, Liverpool University Dental Hospital, Liverpool, UK

Shevaun Mendelsohn
Consultant dermatologist, Countess of Chester Hospital, Chester, UK

Paul Nixon
Consultant in oral and maxillofacial radiology, Liverpool University Dental Hospital, Liverpool, UK

Simon Rogers
Consultant in oral and maxillofacial surgery and honorary reader, University Hospital Aintree, Liverpool, UK

Jane Setterfield
Senior lecturer/honorary consultant in dermatology, Kings College, London, UK

Eileen Theil
Clinical lecturer in periodontology, Liverpool University Dental Hospital, Liverpool, UK

Emma Varga
Associate specialist in oral surgery and lecturer in oral medicine, Liverpool University Dental Hospital, Liverpool, UK

Julia Woolgar
Senior lecturer and honorary consultant in oral pathology, Liverpool University Dental Hospital, Liverpool, UK

Joanna Zakrzewska
Senior lecturer and honorary consultant, Barts and the London, Queen Mary's School of Medicine and Dentistry, London, UK

Tyldesley's oral medicine, 5th edition

Anne Field

Senior Lecturer & Honorary Consultant in Oral Medicine,
Department of Clinical Dental Sciences,
Liverpool University Dental Hospital,
Pembroke Place,
Liverpool, UK

Lesley Longman

Consultant & Honorary Senior Lecturer in Restorative Dentistry,
Department of Clinical Dental Sciences,
Liverpool University Dental Hospital,
Pembroke Place,
Liverpool, UK

in collaboration with
William R. Tyldesley

Former Dean of Dental Studies,
University of Liverpool,
UK

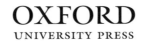

OXFORD
UNIVERSITY PRESS

OXFORD

UNIVERSITY PRESS

Great Clarendon Street, Oxford OX2 6DP

Oxford University Press is a department of the University of Oxford.
If furthers the University's objective of excellence in research, scholarship,
and education by publishing worldwide in

Oxford New York

Auckland Bangkok Buenos Aires Cape Town Chennai
Dar es Salaam Delhi Hong Kong Istanbul Karachi Kolkata
Kuala Lumpur Madrid Melbourne Mexico City Mumbai Nairobi
Sao Paulo Shanghai Taipei Tokyo Toronto

Oxford is a registered trade mark of Oxford University Press
in the UK and in certain other countries

Published in the United States
by Oxford University Press Inc., New York

© Oxford University Press 2003

The moral rights of the author have been asserted

Database right Oxford University Press (maker)

First edition published 1980
Second edition published 1985
Third edition published 1989
Fourth edition published 1995
Fifth edition published 2003

A catalogue record for this title is available from the British Library.

Library of Congress Cataloging in Publication Data
(Data available)

ISBN 0 19 263147 0

10 9 8 7 6 5 4 3 2 1

Typeset by EXPO Holdings, Malaysia
Printed in Great Britain
on acid-free paper by
Butler & Tanner Ltd., Frome, Somerset

Preface to Fifth Edition

The 5th Edition of *Tyldesley's Oral Medicine* has been thoroughly updated in line with current teaching practices. It continues to serve as a comprehensive textbook of oral medicine, not only for undergraduate dental students, but also for continuing medical and dental education. The emphasis throughout the book is on clinical presentation, investigation and management of orofacial diseases. A new author, Lesley Longman, demonstrates the invaluable contribution made by specialists in other disciplines to multi-disciplinary clinics, in which complementary skills and experience combine to improve the quality of patient care in oral medicine.

Specialist advisors, each with their own area of expertise, have made a significant contribution to the book and ensured that recent advances in clinical practice have been incorporated into the text.

High-quality, colour illustrations are included to add interest and demonstrate significant points; no attempt has been made to illustrate all the lesions and conditions described in the text, these will be found in the comprehensive range of oral medicine colour atlases currently available.

This edition has undergone major revision in terms of layout and content. The chapters on facial pain, psychogenic orofacial problems, salivary gland disorders and oral carcinoma have been significantly extended. A section on renal disease has also been added, together with a chapter on medical emergencies in dentistry. Case studies, demonstrating oral medicine conditions, have been introduced at the beginning of each relevant chapter, with a discussion of their differential diagnosis and management options at the end of the chapter. These are included to promote self-directed and active learning but we hope that they will also promote discussion and debate. A number of projects have also been added at the end of chapters with the purpose of encouraging students to consult other reference sources and 'on-line' information.

Tyldesley's Oral Medicine has become firmly established as the textbook of choice for successive generations of dental students and practitioners and we hope that this completely revised edition will accurately reflect current clinical practice and ideas in the rapidly changing discipline of oral medicine.

Anne Field would like to dedicate this book to the memory of her late father, John Elton Costley, and Lesley Longman to the memory of her late mother, Patricia McLoughlin.

Acknowledgements

The authors are grateful for the support and encouragement of their families during the preparation of this completely revised edition of *Tyldesley's oral medicine*.

Our specialist advisers have made an invaluable contribution to the book and we are indebted to them for their patience, knowledge, and encouragement during the preparation of this new edition. Thanks are also due to colleagues who have contributed illustrative materials and to our enthusiastic junior staff who have read draft chapters of the book and made helpful suggestions for improvement.

Finally, we would like to thank Mrs Jan Vicary for her excellent typing and word-processing skills during the many months we have been rewriting the fifth edition of the book.

Contents

List of abbreviations x

1 The oral mucosa 1

2 Principles of oral medicine: assessment and investigation of patients 11

3 Therapy 23

4 Infections of the gingivae and oral mucosa 29

5 Oral ulceration 49

6 Diseases of the lips and tongue and disturbances of taste and halitosis 61

7 Swellings of the face and neck 75

8 Salivary glands and saliva 81

9 Inflammatory overgrowths, developmental and benign lesions, and pigmentation of the oral mucosa 99

10 Precancerous lesions and conditions. Oral carcinoma and carcinogenesis 109

11 Mucocutaneous disease and connective tissue disorders 123

12 Gastrointestinal disease 141

13 Blood and nutrition, endocrine disturbances, and renal disease 151

14 Immunodeficiency, hypersensitivity, autoimmunity, and oral reactions to drug therapy 165

15 Facial pain and neurological disturbances 173

16 Temporomandibular disorders 191

17 Psychogenic orofacial problems 203

18 Disorders of the teeth and bone 217

19 Medical emergencies in dentistry 229

Appendix 239

Suggestions for further reading and reference sources 240

Index 241

List of abbreviations

5-IIT	5-hydroxytryptamine (also known as serotonin)
ACE	angiotension-converting enzyme
ACTH	adrenocorticotrophic hormone
AIDS	acquired immune deficiency syndrome
ANA	antinuclear antibody
ANUG	acute necrotizing ulcerative gingivitis
ASA	American Society of Anesthesiologists
AZT	azidothymidine
BMS	burning mouth syndrome
BNF	British National Formulary
BP	bullous pemphigoid
CAPD	continuous ambulatory peritoneal dialysis
CBT	cognitive behavioural therapy
CD	Crohn's disease
CMC	chronic mucocutaneous candidosis
CO	centric occlusion
CR	centric relation
CRF	chronic renal failure
CRP	C-reactive protein
CRST or CREST	C, calcification; R, Raynaud's phenomenon; E, oesophageal dysfunction; S, sclerodactyly; T, telangiectasia (syndrome)
CT	computerized tomography
DLE	discoid lupus erythematosus
DM	diabetes mellitus
DPT	dental panoramic tomograph
EB	epidermolysis bullosa
EBV	Epstein–Barr virus
EDTA	ethylenediamine tetraacetic acid
EM	erythema multiforme
EMG	electromyography
ENT	ear, nose, and throat
ESR	erythrocyte sedimentation rate
FAPA	(periodic) fever, aphthous ulcers, pharyngitis, and cervical adenitis (syndrome)
FBC	full blood count
FISH	fluorescent *in situ* hybridization
FNA	fine needle aspirate (biopsy)
FTA (abs)	fluorescent *Treponema* antibody absorbed (test)
GFT	glomerular filtration rate
GORD	gastro-oesophageal reflux disease
GP	general practitioner
γGT	γ glutaryl transferase
GTN	glyceryl trinitrate
GUM	genitourinary medicine
HAD	Hospital Anxiety and Depression (scale)
Hb	haemoglobin
HHV-8	herpes virus 8
HIV	human immunodeficiency virus
HLA	human leukocyte antigen
HPV	human papillomaviruses
HSV	herpes simplex virus
HU	herpetiform ulceration
IBD	inflammatory bowel disease
IBS	irritable bowel syndrome
IMF	immunofluorescence
INR	international normalized ratio
LDE	Lichenoid drug eruption
LE	lupus erythematosus
MAGIC	mouth and genital ulcers with inflamed cartilage (syndrome)
MALT	mucosa-associated lymphoid tissue
MCV	mean corpuscular volume
MiRAS	minor recurrent aphthous stomatitis
MjRAS	major recurrent aphthous stomatitis
MMP	mucous membrane pemphigoid
MRI	magnetic resonance imaging
MRS	Melkersson–Rosenthal syndrome
MRTA	magnetic resonance tomographic angiography
MS	multiple sclerosis
NRL	natural rubber latex
NSAID	nonsteroidal anti-inflammatory drug
NSU	non-specific urethritis
OFG	orofacial granulomatosis
OSCC	oral squamous cell carcinoma
OSF	oral submucous fibrosis

OTC	over the counter	SV40	simian virus 40
PAS	periodic acid–Schiff (reagent)	TMJ	temporomandibular joint
PCR	polymerase chain reaction	TMPDS	temporomandibular pain dysfunction syndrome
PPK	palmoplantar keratoderma		
PTA	polymyxin E, tobramycin, and amphotericin (lozenges)	TNFα	tissue necrosis factor alpha
		TPHA	*Treponema pallidum* haemagluttination assay
PTH	parathormone		
RAS	recurrent aphthous stomatitis	TPI	*Treponema pallidum* immobilization (test)
RNP	ribonucleoprotein	TPMT	thiopurine methyltransferase
RT-PCR	reverse transcriptase polymerase chain reaction	TSG	tumour suppressor gene
		UC	ulcerative colitis
SCC	squamous cell carcinoma	USG-FNA	ultrasound-guided fine needle aspiration
SLE	systemic lupus erythematosus	VDRL	Venereal Disease Reference Laboratory (test)
SNP	single nucleotide polymorphism		
SPF	sun protection factor	VVG	vulvovaginal gingival (syndrome)
SS	Sjögren's syndrome	VZV	varicella zoster virus
SSRI	selective serotonin reuptake inhibitor	WCC	white cell count

1

The oral mucosa

Normal oral mucosa
- Structure
- Function
- Age changes

Abnormal oral mucosa

The oral mucosa in generalized disease

The periodontium in generalized disease

The oral mucosa

Normal oral mucosa

Structure

In its basic structure the oral mucous membrane resembles other lining mucous membranes, for example, those of the vagina or the oesophagus. Within the mouth, however, there is a wider range of epithelial thickness than that seen at other mucosal sites. These variations depend largely on differences in the degree of keratinization shown by the mucosae in different areas of the mouth. Some of the reactions of the oral mucous membrane resemble those of the skin, presumably because of its position in the transition area between the gastrointestinal tract and the skin. As a result of this, diseases of both mucous membranes and skin may produce lesions in the mouth. The oral mucosa, however, characteristically behaves as a mucous membrane. Its behaviour in disease processes perhaps most closely resembles that of the vaginal mucosa.

> The epithelium covering the oral mucosa shows a wider variation in thickness and in its pattern of keratinization than mucous membranes at other sites.

The oral mucous membrane consists both anatomically and functionally of two layers: one (the corium or lamina propria) essentially of mesodermal origin and one epithelial (Fig. 1.1). When considering variations of structure, the behaviour of the

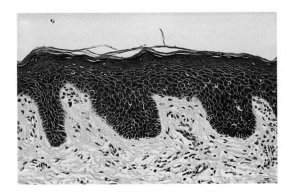

Fig. 1.1 A section of normal mucous membrane from the hard palate with a keratinized surface layer of epithelium overlying the corium.

corium must be taken into account even though the major changes may appear to be within the epithelial layer.

The oral epithelium

The keratinocytes are the main cell component of the oral epithelium but other cell types include melanocytes, Langerhans cells, and Merkel cells.

THE KERATINOCYTES

In normal mucous membrane the integrity of the epithelium is maintained by the division of keratinocytes in the basal layer. As each cell divides one resulting cell remains effectively *in situ*, while one migrates towards the surface, undergoing various structural modifications as it passes through the epithelium (Fig. 1.2). These modifications, which are dependent on the process of keratinization, vary according to the precise site of the mucosa involved and result in the production of a surface layer of cells that are either fully, partially, or non-keratinized and which are shed into the oral cavity at a rate dependent on the rate of mitosis in the basal layer. For each dividing cell, one cell is lost from the surface and, thus, the integrity and dimensions of the epithelial layer are maintained. The rate of turnover of these cells, that is, the 'transit time', for a keratinocyte in the basal layer to reach the surface in various human epithelia has been determined by a number of techniques. The rate in human skin is generally quoted as being of the order of 50 to 70 days and that in the gingival epithelium much the same, but that in the buccal epithelium is much faster—of the order of 25 days.

The epithelium of the oral mucosa shows wide variations in the extent of the keratinization process. In the fully keratinized situation, the rather cubical cells formed by mitosis at or near the basal layer migrate towards the surface, becoming more polyhedral and sharing intercellular attachments, which have given the name 'prickle cell layer' (or stratum spinosum) to this zone. In the light microscope these intercellular 'prickles' appear as single attachments of the cell walls, but by electron microscopy these intercellular junctions (referred to as desmosomes) are seen to be of much greater complexity. It is probable that the desmosomes act in a mechanical manner to give strength to the epithelium. In several diseases marked by epithelial fragility the desmosome attachments are lost or impaired. It should perhaps be added that similar, one-sided structures, hemidesmosomes, attach the

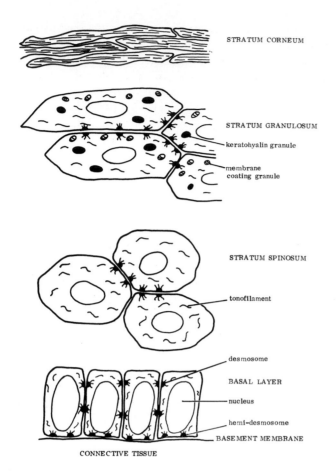

Fig. 1.2 Diagram of a keratinizing squamous epithelium. Compare with Fig. 1.1.

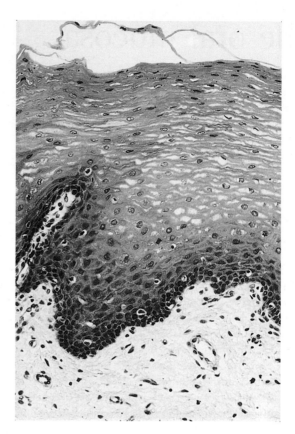

Fig. 1.3 A section of normal buccal mucosa. Compare with the keratinized palatal mucosa shown in Fig. 1.1.

plasma membrane of the basal keratinocytes to the lamina lucida of the basement membrane complex. As the cells of the stratum spinosum migrate to the surface they begin to flatten and granular structures (keratohyalin granules) appear within them. These granules give the characteristic appearance to the 'stratum granulosum' in keratinized epithelia. Finally, at or near the surface, the epithelial cells lose their detailed inner structure, the nuclei degenerate, the keratohyalin granules fragment and disappear, and the insoluble protein complexes mentioned above fill the cell, now fully keratinized (Fig. 1.2). At this stage the desmosomes have effectively degenerated also and the flattened cells ('squames') are eventually lost into the oral cavity. As has been pointed out, each keratinized cell lost in this way must be matched by a dividing cell in the proliferating compartment of the epithelium in order for stability to be maintained. This process of renewal applies only to fully keratinized epithelium—as seen, for instance, in the mucous membrane overlying the hard palate—and is usually referred to as orthokeratinization. In other areas (as in some parts of the buccal mucosa and the floor of the mouth), this process of keratinization does not take place, keratohyalin granules are not formed, and nuclei and organelles (although somewhat effete) can be seen in the surface layers

(Fig. 1.3). In an intermediate form (parakeratotic epithelium), nuclei may still be seen in the surface layers and keratohyalin is sparse or absent. For the purpose of understanding the clinical significance of these differences in keratinization, they should be regarded as being part of a spectrum ranging from complete non-keratinization at one extreme, through varying degrees of parakeratinization, to full orthokeratinization at the other.

The distribution of these differing epithelia in the normal oral mucosa has a close relationship with the function of the tissues at the site. In normal mucosa, non-keratinized or parakeratinized epithelium is seen on the buccal mucosa, the floor of the mouth, and the ventral surface of the tongue, whereas orthokeratinized epithelium is seen on the hard palate and parts of the gingivae. The dorsal surface of the tongue is also orthokeratinized, but differs from the other oral mucosal surfaces in that there are a number of specialized structures present, predominantly the papillae. There are four types of lingual papillae: anteriorly the filiform and fungiform; posteriorly foliate and vallate papillae. The filiform and fungiform papillae are of clinical significance in that their atrophy is often an early sign of mucosal abnormality.

> There are four types of lingual papillae: anteriorly the filiform and fungiform; posteriorly foliate and vallate papillae.

There is currently a great deal of research concerning genetic abnormalities of keratinization, particularly disturbances in the genes coding for specific keratinsthat are responsible for diseases, such as epidermolysis bullosa (Chapter 11). In addition, cell adhesion and the molecules associated with it (for example, cadherins and integrins) are of great importance in disorders of the skin and mucous membranes. In the pemphigus group of immunobullous diseases, there is faulty adhesion between keratinocytes due to the development of autoantibodies against desmoglein I and III, which are members of the cadherin family of adhesion molecules (Chapter 11).

THE MELANOCYTES

The melanocytes appear in, or very close to, the basal layer and on electron microscopy show granular structures (melanosomes) that are the precursors of melanin—the black pigment that modifies the colour of both skin and mucous membranes. These cells, like the Langherhans cells, are dendritic with cytoplasmic prolongations extending between the cells of basal and suprabasal areas of the keratinocytes. Melanocytes synthesize but do not retain melanin; it is transferred by the dendritic processes to adjacent keratinocytes. The melanotic pigmentation of oral mucosa, like that of the skin, shows great racial variation. However, this does not depend on variation of the numbers of melanocytes but on the number and activity of the melanosomes within them. The epithelia of all races contain approximately the same number of melanocytes. It is the rate of production of melanin and its distribution that are different. It is known that hormonal influences are important in the stimulation of melanocyte activity, although the precise mechanisms remain obscure. In some circumstances the melanocytes may be stimulated to produce excess melanin by a wide range of non-hormonal stimulae (Chapter 9).

> Melanocytes synthesize but do not retain melanin. It is transferred by the dendritic processes to adjacent keratinocytes.

LANGERHANS CELLS

The Langerhans cells were first identified in 1860, and for a long time were something of a mystery. There is a substantial number of these cells present near the basal complex of the oral epithelium, with dendritic processes extending between the keratinocytes and with recognizable ultrastructural features. Over the last 3–4 decades research has shown that these cells have an immunological function, acting as peripheral scavenging cells of the immune system, rather like macrophages but lacking their ability to phagocytose effectively. It would seem that at least one function of these cells is to act as antigen-presenting cells and stimulate the activation of T lymphocytes against them. Langerhans cells are therefore considered to be immunologically competent dendritic cells, similar to those found in the peripheral lymphatic system. Their origin appears to be the bone marrow and not the epithelium.

Keratinocytes and Langerhans cells play an important part in the immunosurveillance of the oral epithelium, and both secrete and respond to immunologically active cytokines, including the interleukins and interferons. The concept of localized mucosal immunity is currently under investigation with regard to both its function in maintaining the integrity of normal tissue and its role in mucosal disease. The pathogenesis of lichen planus is not yet fully understood, but probably involves a cell-mediated immune response to an external agent, in which Langerhans cells and keratinocytes release cytokines and adhesion molecules to which T lymphocytes can bind. Subsequent activation of cytoxic lymphocytes is thought to be responsible for damage to the basal cells, which is a characteristic feature of this condition.

> Langerhans cells are immunologically competent dentritic cells.

The corium

The corium (lamina propria) of the oral mucous membrane is separated from the submucosal layer, by a zone of gradual transition rather than a clear boundary. In the corium and submucosa lie the minor salivary glands and sebaceous glands of the oral cavity. These are widely variable in distribution, the mucous glands being most frequent in the mucosa of the lips and posterior palate, whilst the sebaceous glands are mostly concentrated in the buccal mucosa where they may appear as yellow spots, known as Fordyce's spots. The submucosal tissue components are also widely variable: blood vessels, fat, and fibrous tissue being present in differing proportions according to the precise site. Within the corium and submucous tissues are scattered cells of the leukocyte series in varying proportions and concentrations. During disease processes these may alter radically, both in number and in type, depending on the basic nature of the pathological process involved.

> Fordyce's spots are the sebaceous glands of the oral mucosa. They are frequently mistaken for pathological lesions but are completely normal.

The basement membrane

Lying between the epithelium and corium of the oral mucous membrane is a complex multilayered structure, the basement membrane. On ultrastructural study it is seen that the components of the basal zone are much finer than suggested by light microscopy and that, rather than a single membrane, a number of layers are visible, including the lamina lucida and the lamina densa. In the basement membrane, anchoring fibres attach the lamina densa to the underlying tissue and hemidesmosomes attach the basal cells of the epithelium to the lamina lucida. Below the level of the hemidesmosomes is the subbasal dense plate, through which anchoring filaments connect the lamina lucida to the lamina densa. Autoantibodies to components of the lamina lucida have been identified in bullous pemphigoid, which is an immunobullous skin disease (Chapter 11).

Function

Although the oral mucous membrane has several functions, sensory and secretory among them, its main purpose is probably that

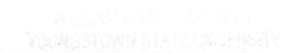

of acting as a barrier. It protects the deeper structures from mechanical insults, such as masticatory trauma and also prevents the entry of micro-organisms and some toxic substances. The oral mucosa has an extensive sensory innervation that can discriminate touch and temperature. Taste buds are also located in oral epithelium. In considering the protective function of the oral mucosa, it is also necessary to discuss other factors, in particular the role of saliva (Chapter 8). The oral mucosa is constantly bathed by saliva, which not only maintains the physiological environment necessary for the maintenance of epithelial integrity but also includes several protective, antibacterial components. A number of these have been described, but perhaps the most important are the secretory immunoglobulins, predominantly of the IgA class, that are found in saliva and that attach to sites on the epithelial surface.

In spite of this barrier function of the oral mucosa, there is a degree of permeability that, apart from its theoretical and scientific interest, is also of clinical significance. During local therapy with mouthwashes and similar preparations, drugs may be transported across the oral mucosa and may exert effects similar to those resulting from systemic therapy. This is an important factor when considering the use of high-concentration steroid mouthwashes for ulcerative lesions of the oral mucosa. The permeability of the oral mucosa is utilized in the treatment of angina by glyceryl trinitrate. In these circumstances rapid absorption of the drug throughout the oral mucosa is an obvious advantage.

The oral mucosa has an important barrier function.

Although the full significance of the role of saliva in maintaining the health of the oral mucosa is, as yet, not fully understood, there can be no doubt that a free salivary flow is an essential part of the oral environment. If the flow is diminished, either by degenerative changes in the salivary glands or by the action of drugs, soreness and atrophic changes in some areas of the oral mucosa rapidly follow. The tongue is perhaps most markedly affected in this way. In some conditions (for example, Sjögren's syndrome—Chapter 8), it is difficult to distinguish between primary mucosal changes and those secondary to diminished salivary flow, but on a clinical basis it is reasonable to accept that atrophic changes in the oral epithelium are regularly associated with dryness of the mouth. The main immunologically active component of saliva is IgA, which is present in a much higher ratio to other immunoglobins, than in the serum.

A further component to be considered as part of the normal healthy oral environment is the microbial flora of the mouth. A wide range of micro-organisms may be present in the oral cavity, living in a commensal relationship with the host. When this relationship is upset by a change in the local or generalized conditions, the commensal micro-organisms may become pathogenic. Oral candidosis is an example of this, although the precise change in the host leading to clinical infection is not easy to identify. The aetiological factors for some common oral infections are discussed in Chapter 4.

A wide range of micro-organisms may be present in the oral cavity, existing in a commensal relationship with the host.

Age changes

Changes occur in the oral mucosa of healthy individuals with increasing age. Reductions in overall epithelial thickness, flexibility of the collagen fibres, innervation, blood supply, and permeability of the mucosa have been described. It has generally been assumed that changes of this kind occur with comparative suddenness at a late age, but recent evidence implies that, at least in the case of the epithelium of the tongue, a continuous trend towards atrophy occurs throughout adult life. The clinical significance of this observation is that sudden changes in the structure of the oral mucosa, such as depapillation of the tongue, should never be considered as being due to age alone without full investigation and the elimination of other factors such as haematological and nutritional disorders (see Chapter 13).

Age changes may also affect the function of salivary glands. It has been shown that gradually increasing degrees of atrophy and fibrosis affect the secretory units of both the submandibular and the labial salivary glands throughout life, even in the absence of disease processes that might be associated with such change.

Abnormal oral mucosa

Many oral lesions represent the end result of breakdown or abnormality of the normal structuring of the epithelium. Variation in the rate of keratin formation, disproportion between the different layers of the cells, breakdown of the normal intercellular bonds of the prickle cells, splitting of the epithelium from the connective tissue, and many other similar abnormalities may occur in different diseases. For instance, in a number of mucosal abnormalities hyperkeratosis occurs (Fig. 1.4). This may arise as a result of abnormal irritation of the mucosa or apparently spontaneously in some conditions. In other lesions, atrophy of the epithelium may occur. This represents a thinning of the normal epithelial layer, perhaps to only a few layers of cells, often accompanied by incomplete keratinization (Fig. 1.5). Such

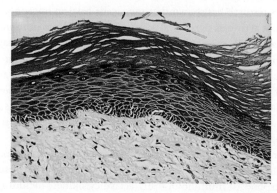

Fig. 1.4 Hyperkeratotic epithelium in an alveolar mucosal lesion.

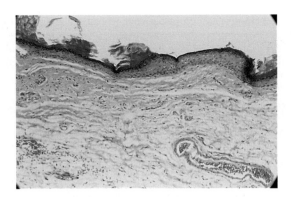

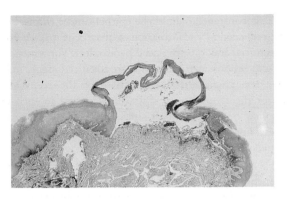

Fig. 1.5 Atrophic epithelium from the dorsum of the tongue—the normal complex structure is entirely lost.

Fig. 1.7 A subepithelial bulla formed by the separation of the entire epithelial layer (including the basal cell layer) from the underlying corium.

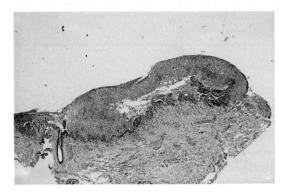

Fig. 1.6 An intra-epithelial bulla formed as a result of loss of intracellular cohesion in the prickle cell layer.

epithelium is easily lost following a minor degree of trauma and thus atrophic lesions of the mucosa readily become ulcerated. Many of the 'so-called' erosive lesions are of this type. It should be remembered that ulceration is in itself a quite unspecific process and implies only the loss of epithelium from the mucosal surface followed by inflammatory changes in exposed connective tissue. Bullae or blisters of the mucosa may occur in one of two ways, either by degeneration of the cells and of the intercellular links in the prickle cell layer of the epithelium (Fig. 1.6) or by separation of the whole of the epithelium from the underlying corium (Fig. 1.7). Frequently, there are also changes in the supporting tissues and, in some cases, the visible epithelial changes may be secondary to changes in the underlying corium that affect the nutrition and metabolism of the epithelium. The greatest practical significance of this fact is, perhaps, the necessity, when taking a biopsy of lesions of the oral mucosa, to include a representative thickness of corium in the tissue removed for microscopic examination. In many cases, a biopsy consisting largely of epithelium alone is virtually useless for diagnosis.

The integrity of the oral mucosa is maintained by a complex of interacting factors superimposed on the localized stabilizing mechanisms discussed above. The general hormonal status of the patient and a number of nutritional and metabolic factors are involved in maintaining the cell metabolism and the ordered structure of the mucous membranes. The role of iron metabolism in the maintenance of the structure of the oral mucosa has been the subject of much investigation. It is certainly the case that iron deficiency, even when relatively mild in clinical terms, can result in generalized oral epithelial atrophy and loss of the papillary pattern of the lingual mucosa. It seems that other deficiencies that might affect iron metabolism and erythrocyte production, such as folate and vitamin B_{12} deficiencies, may also contribute to this destabilization of the oral epithelium. This will be discussed at greater length in Chapter 13. If any single factor is disturbed, then sequential changes occur and clinically significant abnormalities of the oral mucosa may follow. It is often difficult to decide which of the various possible factors are involved in initiating these changes—these may evidently occur either as a primary manifestation of localized mucosal abnormality or as a secondary effect of generalized disease processes. It is the role of oral physicians to assess the possible aetiological factors associated with mucosal lesions of this kind and to ensure appropriate investigations and (if needs be) management.

The reactions of the oral mucosa are not exclusively those of a mucous membrane. As has been pointed out, a number of diseases of the skin also find expression in oral lesions. This is not entirely surprising on anatomical grounds since the larger part of the oral mucosa is derived from an embryonic invagination that carries inwards some of the precursor epithelial cells from which both facial skin and oral mucosa are developed. As might be expected, the lesions of oral mucosa and skin that occur in these mucocutaneous diseases are often superficially different, although the basic histological changes seen in the tissues are similar. Such differences are seen in the primary lesions and, presumably, depend on the differences between the structure of the mouth and that of the skin. Quite often secondary changes also occur in oral lesions. The continually damp environment of the mouth, in combination with repeated mild trauma of the tissues by teeth and foodstuffs, and the presence of a wide range of microbial flora further modify the nature of the lesions produced in a number of diseases. For instance, should the epithelium be thinned by atrophy or weakened by the formation of blisters, it is likely to be lost and the initial lesion be replaced by an ulcer. For reasons such as these, oral lesions, particularly at an advanced stage, may show features less characteristic than those of the equivalent skin lesions of the same disease. Clinical diagnosis in such circumstances may be quite difficult since only areas of ulceration of a relatively non-specific nature may be present rather than fully developed specific lesions.

Histopathological changes

It may be helpful to recall some of the terms used to describe changes seen on histological study of the oral mucosa.

- *Hyperkeratosis*: an increase in the thickness of the keratin layer of the epithelium, or the presence of such a layer in a site where none would normally be expected (Fig. 1.4). Hyperorthokeratosis is the term used to specify a thickened, completely keratinized layer, whereas in hyperparakeratosis there is incomplete keratinization with nuclei remaining in the surface cells.

- *Acanthosis*: an increase in thickness of the prickle cell layer of the epithelium. This may or may not be accompanied by hyperkeratosis.

- *Atrophy*: a decrease in the thickness of the epithelium (Fig. 1.5).

- *Oedema*: the collection of fluid in or between the prickle cells, intra- or intercellular, the two forms often occurring simultaneously. Oedema may also occur between the epithelium and the corium in the region of the basal complex.

- *Acantholysis*: loss of the intercellular attachments in the prickle cell layer leading to separation of the cells. When associated with intercellular oedema this leads to the production of intra-epithelial bullae or blisters (Fig. 1.6).

- *Atypia*: a term used to describe variations in the maturation of the epithelial cells that may be associated with malignancy or premalignant potential. Such features as abnormal mitoses and lack of normal structure of the epithelium are taken into account in the assessment of atypia.

The oral mucosa in generalized disease

Oral lesions may occur in a wide variety of generalized diseases. This fact is important, not only because of the need to treat the often painful oral lesions, but also in view of their significance in providing a diagnostic indicator. The mouth is readily available for inspection (and for biopsy) and oral lesions may appear early

Table 1.1 Interrelationships between generalized and oral disease

- In one group of conditions the oral lesions are similar in aetiology and histology to those found elsewhere in the body, being modified only by the oral environment. Many of the oral lesions of skin diseases fall into this group as well as those in some gastrointestinal conditions. These are discussed in Chapters 11 and 12.

- A second group of oral lesions results from changes in the metabolism of the tissue under the influence of abnormalities of nutrition, endocrine, and other factors (Chapter 13). These abnormalities themselves are the result of some distant pathological process. The oral lesions associated with malabsorption fall into this group.

- In this group both oral and more generalized lesions result from a systemic (and different) abnormality. Sjögren's syndrome, a manifestation of a generalized autoimmune disease resulting in *salivary gland hypofunction*, is an example of such an association. This is further discussed in Chapter 8.

in some diseases. Thus, a number of important conditions may be first diagnosed following the proper evaluation of oral lesions. The relationship between generalized and oral disease is a very complex one, but it may be helpful to identify three types of such interrelationships (Table 1.1).

Classification of the oral–general disease relationships is difficult and may result in oversimplification. It is evident that more than one form of association might occur in a single case. For instance, a patient with a disease of the lower gastrointestinal tract might well produce primary lesions of the disease on the oral mucosa, as well as secondary mucosal change consequent to malabsorption.

The periodontium in generalized disease

Although gingival changes may occur in some generalized conditions, the gingivae are usually not particularly good diagnostic indicators of the disease process involved—the changes are often clinically non-specific. The histological changes in abnormal gingivae are also often very difficult to interpret. A pre-existing inflammatory cell infiltrate and, often, secondary inflammatory features confuse the picture and make gingival biopsies much less useful than might be expected. If the alternative exists between taking a gingival biopsy or one from another area (for example, the buccal mucosa), the gingival site is best avoided.

A few systemic conditions have been described in which clinically recognizable gingival changes occur. For instance, in Wegener's granulomatosis, an uncommon vasculitic disease with widespread systemic implications, a quite characteristic gingival picture has been described although it certainly does not occur in all cases. In Wegener's granulomatosis, the gingival lesion may be an initial sign of the disease. Clinically, the gingival surface appears granular and flecked with yellow, an appearance resembling that of 'over-ripe strawberries'. The prognosis of Wegener's granulomatosis, if untreated, is poor and therefore early recognition of the gingival lesion is important.

> In Wegener's granulomatosis, the gingival lesion may be an initial sign of the disease. Clinically, the gingival surface appears granular and flecked with yellow, an appearance resembling that of 'over-ripe strawberries'.

Such specific and recognizable changes are rare compared to the non-specific gingival changes that may occur in other disease processes and that represent an accentuation or modification of the widespread changes of chronic periodontal disease occurring in a large proportion of the population. For example, patients with severe, untreated diabetes mellitus may develop a rapidly destructive periodontal disease. In the mucocutaneous diseases, such as lichen planus and pemphigoid, the gingival changes are the result of a 'collision' lesion between the generalized condition and pre-existing or superimposed changes of chronic gingivitis. The non-specific nature of the resulting gingival changes is illustrated by the adoption of the term 'desquamative gingivitis', used to describe the reaction of the gingivae in both these and other conditions (Fig. 1.8). Gingival lesions in diseases of the skin are discussed in Chapter 11 and endocrine-induced changes in Chapter 13.

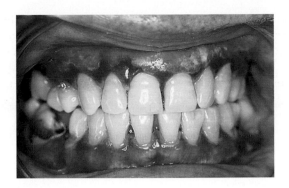

Fig. 1.8 'Desquamative gingivitis'. The definitive diagnosis was of lichen planus.

Projects

1. Discuss the functions of the basement membrane in the oral epithelium.

2. Describe the different zones within the basement membrane. Which proteins are known to become target antigens in the acquired blistering diseases? (see Chapter 11).

2

Principles of oral medicine: assessment and investigation of patients

The speciality of oral medicine

Patient assessment
- History taking
- The examination

Investigations
- Blood examination
- Clinical chemistry
- Immunological tests
- Endocrine function
- Urinalysis
- Biopsy
- Microbiological investigations
- Imaging techniques

Diagnosis

Principles of oral medicine: assessment and investigation of patients

The speciality of oral medicine

Oral medicine is generally understood as being the study and non-surgical treatment of the diseases affecting the orofacial tissues, especially the oral mucous membrane, but also other associated tissues and structures such as the salivary glands, bone, and the facial tissues. Oral medicine is predominantly an out-patient speciality. The boundaries of oral medicine are poorly defined. For instance, the investigation of facial pain and other neurological disturbances may be considered to be in the field of oral medicine or of oral surgery. It is the responsibility of the general dental practitioner to diagnose and manage some of these conditions. Others are often better treated in specialist clinics, but the general dental practitioner, to a very great extent, bears the responsibility for the recognition of oral disease at an early stage.

Definition of oral medicine

Oral medicine is that area of special competence concerned with the health of and with diseases involving the oral and panoral structures. It includes those principles of medicine that relate to the mouth, as well as research in biological, pathological, and clinical spheres. Oral medicine includes the diagnosis and medical management of diseases specific to the orofacial tissues and of oral manifestations of systemic diseases. It further includes the management of behavioural disorders and the oral and dental treatment of medically compromised patients.

Proposed by the World Workshop on
Oral Medicine, held in Chicago, USA, 1998

The development of the discipline of oral medicine has depended largely on the adoption of an analytical approach based on the application of fundamental principles. It follows that the practice of oral medicine as a speciality depends largely on the availability of diagnostic facilities, often greater than those available to the general dental or medical practitioner. Perhaps the most important role of those working in the field of oral medicine is in the recognition of changes in the oral cavity resulting from generalized disease processes. Many oral lesions that, in the past, were considered to be of entirely local origin are now known to be associated with systemic abnormalities. For this reason specialists in oral medicine have a close working relationship with a large number of medical and surgical specialities. The most potent factor in the expansion of the scope of oral medicine was the change of emphasis from the purely descriptive to the investigative. The modern concept of the subject implies a recognition of basic aetiological factors, of the histopathological and molecular changes occurring in the involved tissues, and of the significance of such matters as the general medical status of patients. The challenge for the future of the speciality is to develop evidence-based management protocols.

Patient assessment

History taking

The basis of any investigation is a careful and detailed clinical history and examination. The patient should be allowed to describe their complaint(s) and concerns in their own words. It is, however, often necessary to ask the patient for more precise or detailed information. The specific questions asked will depend upon the presenting complaint and this will be addressed in the appropriate chapters. Regardless of the orofacial condition that the patient has, it is important that the clinician, when questioning the patient, does not try to influence the patient's response. In addition, the patients must not feel as if they are being hurried. Sensitivity may be especially required for some conditions. As with all patient care, confidentiality is of the utmost importance.

It is of great importance to obtain details of the medical history of the patient and of any current or recent drug therapy. Similarly, the patient should be asked at this stage about their use of alcohol and tobacco. Some people are poor historians with regard to their medical history and it is therefore often necessary to ask the patient's general medical practitioner to fill in the details. This is particularly relevant when a patient has a chronic condition that has been managed by several specialists. The correspondence that the general medical practitioner has concerning such a patient can give great insight into the patient's complaint and care. In the hospital environment, the request for and careful reading through of the patient's general hospital case sheet can be, by far, the most productive method of assessment in complicated cases. When dealing with the past medical history it is necessary to use direct questioning on some points. As an example, soft-tissue lesions of the mouth may be associated with skin rashes, eye and genital lesions. The connection with mouth lesions may seem quite tenuous to the patient who may very well fail to volunteer information on these points unless directly asked.

Patient assessment: sources of helpful information

- Hospital case notes
- Résumé of medical and social history from general medical practitioner
- Correspondence from other clinicians involved in caring for the patient

The examination

When examining the mouth, the whole of the oral mucosa must be carefully examined. All removable appliances should be taken out. The practitioner should approach the examination of the patient in a systematic manner to ensure that all the relevant tissues have been seen. The lips and cheeks must be gently retracted to display the full extent of the sulci and the tongue gently held with the aid of a gauze napkin, and extended forward and to each side. Care must be taken that the whole of the floor of the mouth and undersurface of the tongue is seen. The posterior part of the tongue, tonsillar fauces, soft palate, and part of the pharynx are exposed by gentle pressure on the tongue and helped by phonation of 'ah' by the patient. This examination of the oral mucosa must be combined with a careful assessment of the other dental structures, facial skeleton, salivary glands, and soft tissues of the face and neck. A search for palpable lymph nodes should be made, remembering that normal lymph nodes are not detectable by simple palpation. Swellings of the lymph nodes are further discussed in Chapter 7. The assessment of neurological abnormalities is discussed in Chapter 15. Practitioners should be familiar with the tests required to assess gross function of the cranial nerves, in particular the fifth and seventh cranial nerves.

The extraoral examination may be extended to include the general appearance and demeanour of the patient. The eyes, scalp, neck, hands, and the skin of the face and arms should usually be inspected to obtain significant information (Table 2.1). Each of these visually accessible areas can demonstrate signs that alert the practitioner to possible underlying systemic disease.

The intraoral examination should take place with an adequate light source. Sometimes tissues require drying to enable thorough visualization—this is particularly relevant to teeth. Occasionally, in patients with a 'parchment' dry oral mucosa, it is helpful to allow the patient to rinse with water before continuing with the intraoral examination—this will help lubricate the soft tissues and prevent your gloves or mirror sticking to and traumatizing

Table 2.1 Useful information from extraoral examination

Observation	Information (examples of associated conditions)
General demeanour, appearance, and manner	Wasted, undernourished, cachectic appearance (e.g. malnutrition, eating disorder, underlying malignancy); low mood, anxiety, agitation (e.g. depression)
Breathlessness	Cardiorespiratory problems
Face	Shape and symmetry (masseteric hypertrophy, craniofacial syndromes); Cushingoid appearance (e.g. corticosteroid therapy); neurological deficits (e.g. Bell's palsy, cranial tumours); cyanosis (e.g.cardiorespiratory disease); pallor (e.g. anxious, unwell, anaemic)
Scalp and facial hair	Scant hair (e.g. ectodermal dysplasia)
Eyes	Conjunctival scarring (e.g. pemphigoid, keratoconjunctivitis sicca); pale sclera (anaemia); yellow sclera (jaundice); exophthalmia (hyperthyroidism); xanthomas of periocular skin (hypercholesterolaemia)
Neck	Enlarged lymph nodes (oral infection, neoplasms); goitre
Hands	Raynaud's phenomenon; koilonychia and other lesions of the nails; fingers: joint swelling and acquired disfigurement (rheumatoid arthritis); Hebden's nodules (osteoarthrosis); palmar keratosis (Papillon–Lefèvre syndrome); 'liver palms'; tobacco staining; finger clubbing (chronic cardiorespiratory problems, including infective endocarditis)
Wrists	Purple papules consistent with lichen planus
Skin	Petechiae or ecchymoses (e.g. blood dyscrasia); cyanosis (cardiac or pulmonary insufficiency); jaundice; pigmentation (possible endocrine problems)

the tissues. Conversely, in some patients with copious viscous saliva, a mucolytic mouthwash may be helpful prior to intraoral examination.

It is essential that case note entries are:
- legible
- contemporaneous
- dated
- signed

It is of paramount importance that all the details of the history and examination of the patient are comprehensively recorded in the patient's records. It is often helpful to make a sketch of some lesions in the case notes. This will indicate the shape and position of the lesion and help clinicians at future appointments. A topogram of the oral cavity (Fig. 2.1) is particularly useful for this purpose. A well taken clinical photograph can also provide a valuable record of an orofacial lesion. It will also be useful for teaching and essential if a case report is to be submitted for

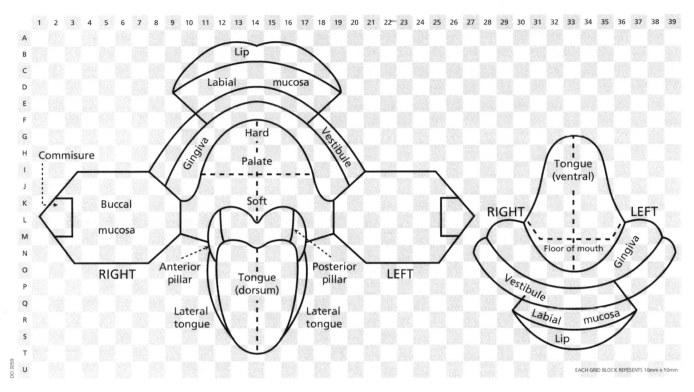

Fig. 2.1 A topogram of the oral cavity. (Reproduced with the permission of Zila Europe.)

publication. The patient should be informed as to why photographs are required and the patient's permission is always required. It is essential to obtain written consent if it is envisaged that the photograph will be used in a publication.

Investigations

A large number of diagnostic tests and procedures must be available to those working in the field of oral medicine. Table 2.2 lists many of the investigations and diagnostic tests used; however, this list is not exhaustive. The advantages of close association with specialized departments, such as those of clinical immunology, haematology, microbiology, clinical chemistry, gastroenterology, and dermatology, are evident, and virtually all centres in which oral medicine clinics are successfully conducted enjoy such associations. Although the range of investigations carried out in the oral medicine clinic itself may be wide, it is evident that, in many instances, it is proper to refer the patient to a colleague in some other speciality for subsequent investigation following initial diagnosis in the oral medicine clinic. Some units will have special interest or expertise in certain diseases and may be able to offer sophisticated investigations and integrated multidisciplinary care that is not routinely available in all oral medicine clinics.

The importance of taking a patient's temperature when there is a disseminated infection should not go unmentioned. This will indicate if there are any systemic effects from the infection.

Special investigations will be discussed subsequently, in the appropriate chapters and in relation to the subject of the investigation. However, it is helpful to present an overview of the tests in this section. It should be remembered that very few special investigations provide a definitive diagnosis. It is more usual for the results of several investigations to be combined with the clinical history and presentation before a definitive diagnosis can be

Table 2.2 What to consider in patients assessment

History	Investigations
Complaint and history	Haematology
Full medical history	Clinical Chemistry
Specific questions	Immunology
Skin involvement	Endocrine studies
Eye problems	Urinalysis
Genital symptoms	Biopsy
Gut problems	Microbiology
Drug history	Imaging
Social history (lifestyle)	Plain radiographs
Tobacco	Salivary gland imaging
Alcohol	CT scan
	MR scan
	Ultrasound
Clinical examination	Blood pressure
Extra-oral	Body Temperature
Intra-oral	Biochemistry

made—this is exemplified by the diagnostic criteria for Sjögren's syndrome. The most common laboratory investigation requested in the oral medicine clinic is a screening procedure for possible blood abnormalities. In view of its widespread application this merits preliminary discussion.

Blood examination

The assessment of oral medicine patients often involves haematological, biochemical, and serological investigations. These tests may be done either as screening tests to help in the diagnosis of some unidentified condition or to confirm a diagnosis by the application of specific tests. In the first instance it may be helpful for the reader to categorize tests generically—according to the department that performs the investigation.

Haematology

As a screening procedure for possible haematological abnormality, a haemoglobin estimation, white cell count, and blood film examination were once considered to be sufficient. Oral signs and symptoms may, however, accompany relatively minor changes in the blood and oral lesions may occur early in patients with haematological abnormalities, well before these are shown up by the simple examination of peripheral blood. A significant lowering of serum or red cell folate levels or (less frequently) lowered serum B_{12} levels may occur in the absence of any detectable change in the peripheral erythrocytes, particularly in patients with stomatitis and recurrent ulceration. It therefore follows that the simple full blood count is an insufficient procedure for the initial investigation of such patients. Haematology reports (and also those of other investigations) should be interpreted with the aid of the normal values of the laboratory involved. The figures quoted in Table 2.3 must be regarded as a guideline only, particularly in relation to borderline values. In the case of borderline results of clinical

Table 2.3 Representative laboratory normal values for haematological tests

Test	Normal value*
Haemoglobin	12.5–17.5 g/dl (male); 11.5–16.0 g/dl (female)
Mean Cell Volume	80–95 fl
ESR	0–15 mm/h
Red cell count	4–6×10^{12}/l (males); 4–5×10^{12}/l (females)
White blood cell count	4–10×10^9/l
Haematocrit	40–50 l/l (males): 34–47 l/l (females)
Platelets	150–400×10^9/l
Serum Folate	1.5–5.5 µg/l
Red cell Folate	125–600 µg/l
Serum B_{12}	170–590 µg/l

* All results should be compared to the normal values of the testing laboratory.

significance it is recommended that a second sample should be taken if at all possible, laboratory figures are subject to some degree of variation. It must be repeated that such results should always be interpreted in the light of the age of the patient and the normal values given by the laboratory involved.

In Table 2.4 the meanings of some of the terms used to describe variations from normal in the size and shape of erythrocytes are given, together with an indication of some of the conditions in which these forms may occur.

Haematological investigations are helpful in the diagnosis of the following conditions:

Leukopenias	Anaemias
Thrombocytopenias	Infectious mononucleosis
Myelomas	Polycythaemias
	Leukaemias

Table 2.4 Variation in size and shape of erythrocytes

Description	Erythrocyte characteristics	Seen in
Hypochromic	Pale staining	Iron deficiency anaemia
Hyperchromic	Dense staining	Pernicious anaemia
Microcytic	Small	Iron deficiency anaemia
Macrocytic	Large (10–12 µ)	Pernicious anaemia
Megalocytic	Very large (12–25 µ)	Pernicious anaemia
Anisocytosis	Much variation in size	Most anaemias
Poikilocytosis	Much variation in shape	Most anaemias
Spherocytic	Spherical	Congenital haemolytic anaemias
Target cell (leptocytes)	Concentrically stained	Any chronic anaemia
Erythroblast	Nucleated	Denotes excessive erythropoiesis
Normoblast	Normal size	After haemorrhage, very severe anaemias and leukaemias
Microblast	Small	Pernicious anaemia, carcinoma stomach, after total gastrectomy
Megaloblast	Large	
Reticulocyte	Reticulated when stained with vital stains	If higher than 1% in adults—an active marrow response to a demand for erythrocytes

A significant proportion of patients attending the oral medicine clinic will require full haematological screening. It is suggested that the following groups warrant this extended screening procedure (see also Chapter 13):

• patients with recurrent apthous stomatitis

Table 2.5 Useful biochemical investigations

Investigation	Description
Glucose	Raised in diabetes mellitus, Cushing's syndrome
	Hypoglycaemia occurs most commonly in diabetic patients and may occur in severe liver disease
Urea	Raised in dehydration, renal failure
Creatinine	Raised in renal failure
Electrolytes	
Sodium	Elevated in dehydration
	Low in conditions causing overhydration, e.g. cardiac failure
Potassium	Raised in renal failure, diabetic ketoacidosis
	Hyperkalaemia is commonly artefactual due to haemolysis, delayed specimens, or ethylenediamine tetraacetic acid (EDTA) contamination
	Hyperkalaemia is a medical emergency and must be corrected immediately
	Hypokalaemia is commonly due to diuretics or gastrointestinal losses of potassium
Calcium	High in primary hyperparathyroidism, malignancy, vitamin D excess
	Low in rickets, osteomalacia, hypoparathyroidism
Phosphate	High in renal failure
	Low in rickets / osteomalacia
Alkaline phosphatase	Raised in conditions with increased bone turnover such as Paget's disease, rickets/osteomalacia
	Also raised in liver disease, particularly cholestasis
Total protein	Raised in dehydration, liver disease, myeloma, connective tissue diseases, and sarcoidosis
	Reduced in overhydration, enteropathy, renal failure
Albumin	Raised in dehydration
	Reduced when there is an acute phase response, e.g. inflammation, postoperatively, carcinoma
	Also raised in severe liver disease, malabsorption, nephrotic syndrome, connective tissue diseases
Ferritin	Raised in liver disease, haemachromatosis, leukaemia
	Reduced in iron deficiency anaemia
Liver enzymes	Disturbed in liver disease, some drug therapies
	Enzyme-inducing drugs, e.g. carbamazepine, phenytoin, phenobarbitone, cause a mild elevation in alkaline phosphatase and γ glutaryl transferase (γGT)

- patients with a persistently sore and/or dry mouth.
- patients with oral lesions with an atypical history or unusually resistant to treatment;
- patients complaining of a sore or burning mouth or tongue, or abnormal taste sensation, even though no mucosal changes can be seen;
- all patients with persistent orofacial candidosis.
- Patients showing abnormalities following an initial screening (ie haemoglobin and full blood count) .

Since these groups constitute a significant proportion of patients attending the oral medicine clinic, the above screen is almost a routine procedure in this environment.

Clinical chemistry

There are several biochemical investigations that are frequently requested for patients presenting with oral medicine problems and several of these are given in Table 2.5.

Plasma glucose measurements are required to diagnose diabetes mellitus (DM) and in the monitoring of this serious condition. The diagnostic criteria for the diagnosis of DM were altered in 1999 and are as follows: symptoms plus random plasma glucose >11.1 mmol/l; repeated random blood glucose >11.1 mmol/l in asymptomatic individuals; or fasting plasma glucose >7.0 mmol/l. Formal glucose tolerance tests are now performed less frequently than previously and are required only in complicated patients.

Immunological tests

A wide range of immunological tests is available to assist in the diagnosis of diseases affecting the oral cavity and many such tests form an essential part of the diagnostic processes of the oral medicine clinic. Table 2.6 highlights some of the tests that may be requested. Many immunologically based tests are now matters of routine. Others are only available in specialist centres.

Table 2.6 Useful immunological tests

Autoantibodies
Rheumatoid factor
Antinuclear factor
SS-A, SS-B antibodies
Parietal cell antibody
Anti-gliaden
Anti-endomysial
Epithelial intercellular cement
Epithelial basement membrane
C1 esterase inhibitor (reduced in hereditary angioedema)
Viral antibodies
HIV
Epstein–Barr virus
C-reactive protein (raised in inflammation and malignancy)

Haematological screening protocol

When a screening procedure is decided upon, a reasonable scheme of investigation is as follows:

1. Full blood count and film examination. From this, evident anaemias are demonstrated by variations in red cell morphology and lowered haemoglobin values. Abnormalities of the white cells and platelet numbers are also shown. Haematological indices such as the red and white blood cell counts, the mean corpuscular haemoglobin, mean corpuscular volume, the haematocrit and platelet count are important and abnormal values may indicate underlying systemic disease.

2. Estimation of serum ferritin as a measure of full body iron status. This test has almost entirely replaced the estimations of serum iron, total iron binding capacity, and saturation formerly used as a screening test, although these are still used in the investigation of complex iron-deficiency states.

3. Serum B_{12}, folate and red cell folate estimations. These are valuable indicators of malabsorption and, hence, of gastrointestinal diseases of many kinds. The red cell folate level is a relatively stable indicator of folate deficiency, whereas the serum folate levels are more labile and indicate the current status. It has been shown that these may show independent clinically significant variation in patients presenting with oral signs and symptoms. Coeliac disease is an example of a gastrointestinal disease that can result in malabsorption of haematinics. Low folate levels may also be due to anticonvulsant drug therapy, pregnancy, and alcoholism.

A vitamin B_{12} deficiency should be suspected if there is a macrocytosis—indicated by a raised mean corpuscular volume and packed cell volume.

4. As an additional test an erythrocyte sedimentation rate (ESR) measurement is useful as a non-specific guide to underlying pathological processes—alternatively measurement of C-reactive protein (CRP) may be used as a similar marker for pre-existing disease (see Clinical Immunology). The ESR is raised in pregnancy, chronic inflammatory conditions, acute infection, giant cell arteritis, and neoplasia.

The assay of circulating autoantibodies is an important procedure in the oral medicine clinic. Some autoantibodies are closely associated with specific disease processes—for instance, gastric parietal cell antibodies with pernicious anaemia. In other autoimmune diseases, however, a wide range of autoantibodies may be produced. For this reason it is usual to carry out a range of autoantibody tests rather than a single one.

Direct immunofluorescent techniques, for the detection of immunoglobulins and other immunologically active proteins fixed within tissue, have acquired great importance in the diagnosis of oral mucosal lesions—particularly those associated with skin diseases and connective tissue disease. The principle of the technique depends on the fact that antibodies combined with fluorescein retain both their immunological activity and the property of the fluorescein to fluoresce under ultraviolet light. The antibodies can, therefore, be located at the exact site of combination with their antigenic antagonists by microscopic observation under ultraviolet illumination. A wide range of highly specific antibodies to the various immunoglobulins and complement components is available and can be used to demonstrate the type and site of bound complexes. In some conditions the results may be highly specific and diagnostic (in pemphigus and pemphigoid, for example). In other conditions (such as lichen planus) they are not clear. The findings in a number of conditions are discussed in Chapter 11. The special requirements for the taking of biopsy material for this technique are mentioned later in this chapter.

Endocrine function

Endocrine disorders are important in oral medicine for the following reasons.

- Patients may present with a complaint that leads to the diagnosis of an endocrine disturbance. An example is a patient with oral dysaesthesia or xerostomia who upon investigation is found to be an undiagnosed diabetic.

- Poorly controlled hormonal imbalances may lead to orofacial disease.
- Therapy of orofacial disease may lead to hormonal imbalances. An example of this is the use of systemic steroids to treat severe ulceration or bullous disease—long-term therapy will induce adrenal suppression and predisposes towards diabetes and osteoporosis.
- Concurrent endocrine disease or hormone replacement therapy may influence the management of the patient.

Examples of hormone studies that may be requested in oral medicine are thyroid function tests and parathormone, growth hormone, and cortisol levels.

Urinalysis

Urinalysis, which can be done quickly and cost-effectively, is used to identify the presence of glucose, blood, proteins, ketones, and bile products. This can alert the clinician to the possibility of underlying systemic disease and, therefore, further investigations will be required. Urine samples are usually collected from the midstream flow—avoiding the urine flow at the beginning and end of micturition.

Biopsy

> A biopsy involves the removal of part or all of a lesion so that it can be examined by histopathological techniques.

Many lesions may be diagnosed only after examination of an appropriate biopsy specimen of the affected tissue. This is so, not only in cases of suspected neoplasia, but, for example, also in the differential diagnosis of white patches that may occur in the oral mucosa and of the bullous, ulcerative, and desquamative lesions in the mouth. Many bone conditions are, similarly, diagnosed by examination of a biopsy sample. It is generally agreed that, in the case of suspected or possible malignancy of the oral mucosa, biopsy is mandatory and, with simple precautions, is unlikely to cause dissemination of tumour cells. There are several methods of obtaining biopsies and these will be dealt with under the following headings: excisional, incisional, and fine needle aspiration. The decision to take an excisional or incisional biopsy will depend upon the nature of the lesion, its size, and location.

> Prior to biopsy the patient should be informed about:
> - the reasons for the procedure
> - what to expect
> - any discomfort
> - possible complications
>
> A patient information leaflet is a helpful aid in obtaining informed consent.

Biopsy techniques

- Incisional
- Excisional
- Fine needle aspiration

Excisional biopsy

If the lesion in question is small, it may be best to remove it entirely by local excision, including a small area of normal tissue. The specimen may then be sectioned and its histology reviewed to determine whether further treatment will be needed. The biopsy is far better taken with the knife than with the cutting diathermy, which may cause considerable distortion of the tissues. After its removal, the biopsy specimen should be placed with the minimum of delay into a fixative, 10 per cent formol saline being the most universally used. Full clinical details should always be given to the pathologist who is to examine the specimen.

Excision biopsy is particularly useful for the diagnosis of single small ulcers and small, localized, soft-tissue swellings. In these cases it is possible to combine primary treatment with biopsy.

Incisional biopsy

This is the removal of a section of a lesion for histological study without any attempt being made to remove the whole of the lesion. In taking such a biopsy of the oral soft tissues, the aim should be to include within one specimen, if possible, a clinically typical area of the lesion and also the edge of the lesion. If the choice must be made between the two possibilities, the clinically typical area should be chosen—a large area of normal tissue beyond the lesion is quite unnecessary. The specimen should be big enough to allow the pathologist to make a diagnosis, as too small a biopsy is difficult to handle and to orientate for sectioning.

The technique for biopsy of a lesion of the oral epithelium is to make a wedge-shaped cut into the chosen area, to complete the triangle by a third cut, and to then take off the epithelial layer, together with a thickness of corium, by sliding the knife below and parallel with the surface. Even if it is the epithelium that is of particular interest, it is essential that a sufficient layer of corium should be included in order that the subepithelial reactions may be seen. If the biopsy is of a lump, then the wedge section must be taken into the swelling, making sure that any capsular tissue is cut through and that a representative area of the lesion proper is obtained.

Anaesthesia for the biopsy should be obtained by the injection of local anaesthetic as far from the biopsy site as consistent with obtaining a satisfactory result. It is clearly unwise to inject directly into an area of doubtful malignancy and, quite apart from any question of dissemination of neoplastic cells, there is a danger of distortion of the histological picture if the area is infiltrated by anaesthetic. The biopsy site may be closed by one or two sutures.

If the specimen is a thin one, as is often the case with biopsies of the oral mucosa, it is often most convenient to lay it flat on a piece of card or a swab before placing into the fixative. The tissue practically always adheres to this backing, and curling and distortion of the specimen is prevented. Multiple biopsies may be required of large mucosal lesions or in cases with widespread oral lesions that are clinically dissimilar.

Frozen sections for rapid diagnosis are rarely required in oral medicine. Very often the histological sections require careful and detailed study, this being difficult with frozen tissue specimens. Rapid reporting of frozen sections in the urgent situation is possible, for instance, during surgery when it is essential to identify malignancy, but this is not a situation relevant to the regular practice of oral medicine. The major use of frozen sections in oral medicine is in immunofluorescent diagnostic techniques.

Biopsy for immunofluorescence

Antigen–antibody complexes in tissues can be identified by various staining and labelling techniques. Fluorescein is a commonly used label. Direct immunofluorescent studies of biopsy material have become an essential part of the diagnostic procedure for immunobullous oral lesions (as discussed earlier in this chapter and in the appropriate later chapters). In the case of non-bullous and non-erosive lesions there are no particular problems. The specimen is taken from the lesional tissue with some marginal clinically normal tissue if convenient. In the case of bullous or erosive lesions, however, the situation is quite different in that the most characteristic immunological findings are likely to be in the clinically normal tissue adjacent to the lesion. When bulla formation or erosion has occurred, the biopsy technique of the lesion itself becomes very difficult and the results (largely because of secondary infection and similar factors) become much more difficult to interpret.

It is essential when taking biopsy specimens for immunofluorescent studies that the laboratory should be pre-warned so that the fresh, unfixed tissue is passed on directly for immediate processing (or for deep frozen storage). It can be safely transported in a polythene bag or placed on an ice tray. Prior to taking a biopsy the practitioner should decide what type of biopsy is required and what is going to happen to the biopsy specimen. This will prevent unnecessary repeat biopsies.

> Both direct and indirect immunofluorescent studies are of value in the diagnosis of immunobullous diseases (for example, pemphigus and pemphigoid).

Fine needle aspiration (FNA) biopsy

Soft-tissue lesions can be collected for microscopic examination using a needle aspirate. This technique is also useful for collecting fluid contents of a lesion, particularly pus or cystic fluid. A 20/21 gauge needle is employed for sampling tissue and ultrasound can be used to guide the positioning of the needle in an attempt to ensure that the biopsy is taken from the centre of the lesion. Sometimes it is not possible to obtain a definitive diagnosis from a FNA biopsy. Often there is enough information to differentiate between malignant and benign. An experienced cytologist is required to interpret the sample and it should be remembered that the specimen harvested may not always be representative of the lesion.

Microbiological investigations

Not all orofacial infections require the services of a diagnostic microbiology laboratory. However, when such services are required, the clinician needs to be aware of the range of services available and the type of specimen required. Laboratories can look for the following evidence of infection.

1. Viable organisms. Micro-organisms can sometimes be seen microscopically from a direct smear but usually the specimen is cultured. This will then allow the organisms in the culture to be identified and undergo sensitivity testing to antimicrobial agents. For culture and sensitivity testing an aspirate of pus is preferable to a swab. The latter may be contaminated with normal oral flora and the putative pathogens are less likely to survive the journey to the laboratory.

2. Microbial products. It is possible to detect the presence of micro-organisms by the products that they produce, such as toxins, or by identifying their DNA. The application of molecular techniques to identify genetic material has allowed for the identification of micro-organisms without the need for culture. Gene amplification using the polymerase chain reaction (PCR) and *in situ* hybridization techniques allows for the rapid identification of organisms. This is particularly beneficial for organisms that are hazardous or not easily grown in the laboratory. Hepatitis C is identified in this manner.

3. Antibody detection. The presence of circulating antibodies in the serum, cerebrospinal fluid (CSF), or in saliva may be indicative of infection. Serological techniques are often employed for viral infections such as hepatitis B.

Bacteriology

If a bacterial aetiology is suspected for a lesion, both direct smears and swabs for culture and identification may be taken. Direct smears from the gingival crevice may be of some value in the identification of the fusobacteria and spirochaetes in acute ulcerative gingivitis—although their use is limited. In many instances only normal oral flora will be reported. This is the case, for example, in viral infections. In these circumstances, however, as in many other oral mucosal diseases, the balance of the oral flora is soon disturbed by the onset of abnormal environmental conditions.

Specimens for the identification of micro-organisms

> When a collection of pus is present an aspirate should ideally be taken.

Mycology

Candida may be recognized on direct smears, by culture, and, if an estimate of density of organisms is required, by imprint culture or an oral rinse. They survive well on a dry swab or when placed in an appropriate transport medium. It must be remembered that in some forms of candidosis, where the organisms are within the tissues (as in chronic hyperplastic candidosis; see Chapters 4 and 6), there may be very little growth from a swab. They are best identified by histological methods. Susceptibility testing to various antifungal agents can be undertaken, but the reproducibility of some tests, particularly those relating to azoles, are questionable.

Virology

Virus identification remains a lengthy and relatively difficult process. Confirmation may be given by direct electron microscopy in the few centres where this is available. Tissue culture, antigen detection, and identification of genetic material are commonly employed techniques.

Serum antibody studies can also form the basis for the diagnosis of viral infections. In herpes simplex the baseline level of antibodies in any individual before clinical infection is variable, depending on the past history and the degree of the immune response. At the time of an active clinical infection these levels are raised considerably. If pairs of sera from the patient, taken at an interval (of about 10 days in this case), can be compared, a significant rise in titre confirms the diagnosis. Quite clearly, this is not a particularly useful technique, except in retrospect, since, in the case of primary herpetic stomatitis, the lesions will have gone into remission before the confirmation of the diagnosis is available.

Bacteria and viruses can be identified rapidly using molecular techniques such as polymerase chain reaction (PCR) or fluorescent *in situ* hybridization (FISH).

Imaging techniques

Plain film radiography is the most common imaging technique used in dental practice. The various views are shown in Table 2.7. The value of plain radiography lies in the simplicity of the method and also the fact that it is widely available. The disadvantages are that ionizing radiation is used and imaging of soft-tissue lesions is often unsatisfactory for most diagnostic purposes. In areas of complex bony anatomy the superimposition of adjacent structures on the region of interest can often limit the diagnostic value of the image. This problem is reduced by the technique of tomography which uses movement of the X-ray tube and film to produce a slice through the patient with blurring of the neighbouring structures. The dental panoramic tomograph (DPT) or panoramic view uses this principle.

When imaging bony swellings, two views should be taken that are at right angles to each other.

Digital radiography uses conventional radiographic techniques, but the film is replaced with a sensor that transmits the image to a computer. These systems allow some manipulation of image to be carried out, which can enhance the image quality. Whilst the equipment is expensive, this technique has grown in popularity over recent years. The advantages include the use of a lower dose of radiation than for conventional films, the elimination of film processing, and the immediate visualization of an image on a visual display unit. Table 2.8 lists further specialized imaging techniques that may be useful in oral medicine.

Contrast studies. The appearance of certain soft-tissue structures visualized by using ionizing radiation can be enhanced by altering the radiodensity of a patient's tissues by the introduction of contrast media. The temporomandibular joint space and salivary glands are particularly amenable to this technique. The imaging of these structures will be discussed in greater detail in the appropriate chapters.

Contrast studies are successful in imaging:
- salivary glands (sialography)
- joints (arthrography)
- blood vessels (angiography)
- gastrointestinal tract (barium swallow, meal, and enema)

Radioisotope studies. Certain tissues will preferentially concentrate specific compounds. This can be exploited for imaging if the chemical is labelled with a radioactive compound. This technique will allow functional studies to be carried out over time. For example salivary function of the major glands can be assessed by their entrapment and release of technetium (^{99m}Tc) which is carried in ionic form as pertechnetate. This radioisotope emits gamma rays but the short half-life of ^{99m}Tc (6.5 hours) minimizes

Table 2.7 Radiographic views

Extraoral views	Intraoral views
Panoramic (dental panoramic tomograph, DPT)	Periapical
	Bitewing
Lateral views	Occlusal
Oblique lateral	
True lateral	
Occipitomental	
Posterior–anterior mandible	
Submentovertex	

Table 2.8 Specialized imaging techniques

Utilizing ionizing radiation	Not using ionizing radiation
Digital radiography	Ultrasound
Contrast studies	Magnetic resonance imaging (MRI)
Radioisotope studies	
Computerized tomography (CT)	

the exposure of the patient to radiation. Bone may also be investigated in a similar manner using methylene diphosphonate as the carrier for the radioisotope. In this manner the activity of bone tumours and mandibular condylar growth and infection may be studied. The disadvantage of radioisotope studies is that they subject the whole body to radiation and are time-consuming to perform.

Computerized tomography (CT) uses a sophisticated X-ray machine with a ring of X-ray detectors around the patient. A computer then generates an image that represents a slice through the patient. Manipulation of the data by computer allows the image to be adjusted to highlight bone or soft tissue. Computerized tomography is of value when investigating intracranial lesions, soft- and hard-tissue tumours of the head and neck, facial fractures, and osteomyelitis. It will show if there is involvement of adjacent structures. CT scans are expensive and use high doses of radiation. Metallic objects can cause streak artefacts that obscure information. Thus, extra- and intracoronal restorations and implants can be problematic.

Ultrasound uses a very high-frequency pulsed ultrasound beam that is emitted from a transducer that is placed against the skin. The same transducer picks up the reflected beam and an *echo picture* image is produced. Ultrasound is safe and is useful for evaluating vascular disorders and soft-tissue swellings of the neck and face, including salivary glands and lymph nodes. It is ideal for differentiating between solid and cystic masses. Ultrasound can be used in conjunction with fine needle aspiration to ensure correct positioning of the biopsy needle. Similarly, ultrasound may be used to locate salivary calculi that are to be broken up with a sialolithotripter. The disadvantages of ultrasound in the head and neck region is that its use is restricted to superficial structures because bone will absorb the sound waves.

Magnetic resonance imaging (MRI) utilizes the behaviour of protons in a magnetic field to produce images. This technique is valuable in assessing intracranial lesions, lesions of the salivary glands, sinuses, and pharynx, and also of the temporomandibular joint. MRI produces excellent differentiation between soft tissues, hard tissues, and normal and abnormal tissues, but gives poor hard-tissue detail. This imaging technique is more tissue-sensitive than CT and does not use ionizing radiation. MRI is expensive and is contraindicated in patients with certain types of surgical clips, cardiac pacemakers, and cochlear implants (which contain magnetic elements). Patients who have claustrophobia are also unsuitable for MRI because they are unlikely to enter into the tunnel formed by the core of the magnet.

Since oral medicine represents the whole field of medicine as related to the oral cavity, it is evident that as wide a range of investigations must be applied as in other specialities of medicine. It would, quite clearly, be impossible to even briefly outline these in the present context. The major investigative procedures have been outlined above. Others are discussed in the appropriate later chapters.

Diagnosis

The diagnosis may be obvious from the history and examination of the patient. Further investigations may not be required and the clinician may make a *definitive* diagnosis.

The clinician may have a strong suspicion of the diagnosis but cannot confirm this until further information is returned, such as a biopsy or blood results. In this situation the practitioner can make a *provisional*, *clinical*, or *working* diagnosis and may start therapy for the suspected condition. It is not uncommon, however, that after examination there remains more than one possible diagnosis. These conditions make up the *differential* diagnoses. In this situation the clinician needs to assess the likelihood of each differential diagnosis, taking into account the patient's age, gender, and race, the presenting symptoms, the medical and drug history, and the classical features of the various possible diagnoses. This is a skill that becomes defined with experience and requires logical thought and knowledge of the various conditions.

Projects

1. Identify the medical and surgical disciplines that specialists in oral medicine may liaise closely with and give reasons why these relationships are necessary.

2. The participation of an oral medicine specialist in some multidisciplinary (joint) clinics may benefit patient management. What joint clinics do you think would be advisable and list the orofacial conditions that could be managed on these clinics?

3

Therapy

Principles of therapy

Topical therapy

- Covering agents
- Topical antiseptics
- Topical analgesics
- Topical antibiotics
- Topical corticosteroids

Creams and ointments

Systemic therapy

- Systemic corticosteroids
- Azathioprine
- Other systemic drugs used in oral medicine

Limitations of therapy

Appendix). If the treatment is not unduly prolonged, there is minimal trouble from overgrowth of resistant organisms in the mouth, although a candidal infection may occur and must be appropriately dealt with.

Many of the authors' patients have oral lesions that are persistent and severe. In such cases, the prolonged use of antibiotic-based mouthwashes is clinically justified, particularly in the chlortetracycline–triamcinolone combination (see Appendix) that is used in such conditions as pemphigus and major erosive lichen planus.

> Tetracycline mouthwash may be made by the patient dissolving the contents of one 250 mg capsule in 10 ml of water to give a 2 per cent solution—use as a mouthwash, three times daily.

Topical corticosteroids

One of the most important factors to be considered when using topical steroids is the degree of suppression of adrenal function that may occur when these drugs are administered. The degree of adrenal suppression varies not only from steroid to steroid and according to the method of use, but there is also considerable individual variation. For instance, a dose of systemic prednisolone that may apparently cause no side-effects in one patient may render another markedly Cushingoid. It is the authors' practice to use high-concentration, locally applied steroids to replace systemic medication wherever possible. Excessive use of topical steroid preparations can, however, result in a significant amount of systemic absorption. Application of more potent topical steroids also increases the likelihood of a superimposed oral candidiasis and some oral physicians advocate the concomitant use of a prophylactic, topical antifungal agent.

Steroid mouthwashes

Steroid mouthwashes can be made by the patient dissolving soluble betamethasone or prednisolone tablets in 10–15 ml of water. Steroid mouthwashes should not be swallowed and patients should be monitored for side-effects, as for systemic steroids, because of the risks of systemic absorption.

Alternatively, a triamcinolone mouthwash, often in a chlortetracycline base can be used, at a total dosage that can be varied according to the severity of the condition. Mouthwashes containing levels of triamcinolone varying from 0.75–1.5 mg to 3–6 mg daily are most commonly used. At the higher end of this wide dose-range there is almost certain to be significant systemic absorption, and patients must be carefully monitored for the onset of corticosteroid side-effects. The concentration of steroid in the mouthwash can be easily varied, however, and should be carefully titrated against the clinical response (see Appendix for formulation).

> Betamethasone rinse: dissolve a soluble betamethasone sodium phosphate (0.5 mg) tablet in 10 ml of H_2O and hold in mouth for 3 minutes, before spitting out. Use three times daily, if required. Do not swallow.

Table 3.1 Examples of steroid sprays that can be used for ulcerative oral lesions

Beclometasone dipropionate spray delivering a 50 micrograms metered dose.
Budesonide spray delivering a 100 micrograms metred dose.

Steroid sprays

Steroid sprays or inhalers such as beclomethasone or budesonide can be used for treating one or two isolated ulcers or erosions, particularly if they occur in the anterior part of the mouth which is accessible (Table 3.1).

Intralesional steroids

Intralesional injections of depot preparations of suitable steroids, often used by dermatologists to produce localized high concentrations of the active drug, may be used to treat oral lesions. In general, they do not appear to be as effective in oral medicine practice and are only occasionally used. Intralesional steroid injections have been used for treating swollen lips in patients with orofacial granulomatosis (OFG) (see Chapter 12).

Steroid pastes

Triamcinolone acetonide (0.1 per cent) is available in an adhesive paste and can be applied to aphthous ulcers 2–4 times daily. It is most effectively used at night, when salivary flow decreases and the patient is not eating. Other topical steroids (for example, fluocinonide or clobetasol) mixed with Orabase® (equal proportions) can be used for isolated, ulcerative lesions, particularly those in the anterior part of the mouth (see Chapter 5).

Steroid lozenges

Lozenges (pellets) containing 0.1 per cent hydrocortisone can be used for recurrent aphthous stomatitis (RAS). This steroid is likely to be most effective if used in the prodromal phase of ulceration—it should be placed on (or near) the ulcer and allowed to dissolve. The use of steroid lozenges in ulcer-free periods, albeit at a reduced frequency, has been recommended by some oral physicians for RAS. Whether or not this reduces the occurrence of new aphthae has yet to be proven (see Chapter 5).

Creams and ointments

Creams and ointment are used as vehicles for active ingredients, such as antimicrobial agents and steroid preparations. They may be used to treat a number of conditions seen in the oral medicine clinic that affect the lips (for example, angular cheilitis) and perioral tissues.

Creams are emulsions of oil and water and are usually well absorbed into skin. Generally, creams are cosmetically more acceptable than ointments because they are less greasy and therefore suitable for use on the face. Creams usually contain preservatives (for example, chlorocresol and parabens) unless their active ingredient has sufficient intrinsic antimicrobial activity. Preservatives may cause sensitization and ultimately an allergic contact dermatitis.

Ointments are greasy preparations that are insoluble in water. They are particularly useful for treating chronic, dry skin conditions and are less easily washed off than creams.

Systemic therapy

Systemic therapy with non-specific immunomodulating drugs such as steroids and azathioprine, together with substances such as thalidomide, are increasingly being used for severe ulcerative and erosive oral conditions. These drugs have significant side-effects, however, and patients require careful assessment and monitoring under hospital supervision (see below).

Systemic corticosteroids

The use of systemic corticosteroids for the treatment of oral mucosal lesions is justifiable if topical therapy has failed. Prednisolone has predominantly glucocorticoid activity and is the corticosteroid most commonly taken orally for long-term disease suppression. Oral lesions, such as major aphthae or erosive lichen planus, may need to be managed by a short (2–6 week) reducing course of prednisolone. Other intractable and severe cases may justify and necessitate long-term prednisolone therapy, with its associated disadvantages and side-effects. In many of these cases the oral lesions are part of a widespread and more generalized condition, such as pemphigus or Behçet's syndrome. Scrutiny of a patient's medical history is essential before commencing corticosteroid therapy and it is essential that regular monitoring is carried out to detect any side-effects. Monitoring should include measurements of blood pressure, weight, and blood glucose estimations. Steroid treatment warning cards should be issued to patients and carried by them at all times.

> Steroid treatment warning cards should be issued to patients and carried by them at all times.

Baseline measurements of blood pressure, fasting blood glucose, and weight are checked before commencing therapy and a chest radiograph may be indicated in some cases. Patients should be made aware of the potential adverse effects of the medication (Table 3.2) and the need for regular monitoring. In addition, corticosteroids should not be stopped abruptly. Patients who are taking systemic corticosteroids may be at risk from a hypotensive adrenal crisis if they undergo dental or maxillofacial procedures, particularly under general anaesthesia, and consideration should be given to providing them with additional 'steroid cover'. There are, however, no evidence-based protocols currently available to indicate which patients undergoing dental treatment should be given additional 'steroid cover'. Neither is there any clear indication of the optimum dose and time of delivery. There is evidence that adrenal

Table 3.2 Complications of systemic corticosteroid therapy

Suppression of adrenal function
Hypertension
Sodium and water retention
Potassium loss
Diabetes
Osteoporosis
Mental disturbances (psychoses, mood changes, euphoria)
Muscle wasting
Fat redistribution
Peptic ulceration
Cushing's syndrome
Susceptibility to infections (candidosis, bacterial and viral infections)
Growth suppression in children
Neoplasms, e.g. lymphomas

suppression is reduced if corticosteroids are given once a day (in the morning) and possibly on alternate days.

Fifty per cent of patients on long-term corticosteroids develop osteoporosis and bone loss is greatest in the first 3–6 months of steroid therapy. Preventive therapy, for example, disodium etidronate (Didronel PMO®), should therefore be commenced at the outset of steroid therapy (prednisolone 5 mg or more per day) that is likely to last for more than 3 months. A baseline bone density scan should ideally be organized for adult patients. If the patient is found to have osteoporosis prior to treatment with steroids, more potent bisphosphonates (for example, alendronate or risedronate) may be required and the patient may need to be referred to a metabolic bone disease clinic.

> Patients on prednisolone ≥5mg/day (or equivalent) for more than 3 months should be given prophylactic bisphosphonates.

Azathioprine

Steroid-sparing drugs such as azathioprine may be given to minimize the long-term effects of systemic steroids. Azathioprine is a cytotoxic immunosuppressant with potentially serious side-effects. It should not be prescribed unless adequate monitoring is available throughout the duration of therapy (see drug data sheet). Patients are at risk of developing bone marrow suppression, particularly if they have a deficiency of thiopurine methyltransferase (TPMT), a cytoplasmic enzyme involved in the metabolism of azathioprine. Patients can now be tested for TPMT deficiency.

Other systemic drugs used in oral medicine

Other systemic drugs currently used in oral medicine include dapsone, ciclosporin, colchicine, thalidomide, and mycophenolate. The indications for and monitoring of side-effects associated with these drugs are discussed in the relevant chapters throughout this book. There is also increasing interest in the use of anti-TNF (tissue necrosis factor) alpha therapy for severe inflammatory disease (for example, Behçets disease). These drugs are used on a limited basis only for severe oral disease and have no place in the non-specialist practice of oral medicine.

Limitations of therapy

There is a paucity of objective evidence concerning the effectiveness of a number of current therapeutic regimens for oral medicine conditions and there is clearly a need for the development of evidence-based management protocols. Clinicians should also be aware, particularly when prescribing topical formulations of drugs such as steroid mouthrinses or sprays, that most are not licensed for use in oral conditions and dosage schedules are therefore not established. Patients should be made aware that they are being give a drug outside its licensed indication as that they cannot give informed consent for treatment without this knowledge.

Project

1. Visit your local pharmacy and enquire which therapies are available to buy over the counter (OTC) for mouth ulcers. What advice would the pharmacist give to someone seeking information about mouth ulcers?

4

Infections of the gingivae and oral mucosa

Bacterial infections
- Acute necrotizing ulcerative gingivitis
- Syphilis
- Gonorrhoea
- Non-specific urethritis
- Tuberculosis

Fungal infections
- Oral candidosis

Viral infections
- Herpes simplex virus infections
- Varicella zoster virus infections
- Epstein–Barr virus infections
- Coxsackievirus infections
- Paramyxovirus infections
- Human papillomavirus infections
- Human immunodeficiency virus and AIDS

Infections of the gingivae and oral mucosa

Problem cases

Case 4.1

A 28-year-old lady attends your dental practice for her 6-monthly examination. You notice that she has a healing 'cold sore' (herpes labialis) on her lower lip. On closer questioning this patient reports that she suffers from 'cold sores' every 2–3 months and that they are becoming a 'real nuisance'. She is particularly affected when on holiday abroad and exposed to the sun.

Q1   What advice would you give this lady?

Q2   Does the lesion on her lip present a hazard to members of the dental team?

Case 4.2

A 21-year-old fully dentate man presents at your dental practice complaining of a sore mouth and throat of 6 weeks duration. A pharmacist recommended that he use anaesthetic throat lozenges and a chlorhexidine rinse but these have not helped. The patient appears well and reports no relevant medical history. Extraoral examination reveals no lymphadenopathy. Intraorally, his oral mucosa appears erythematous and there is evidence of extensive white flecks on the soft palate and both buccal mucosae. These can easily be wiped off with a gauze napkin. You make a clinical diagnosis of pseudomembranous candidosis. There are no other abnormalities of the oral mucosa or gingivae.

Q1   How would you manage this patient?

Introduction

It is possible to demonstrate a wide range of potentially pathogenic organisms in the normal mouth. Many of these are present in relatively high numbers, but in spite of this the oral mucosa shows a remarkably low susceptibility to primary infection. This is probably due, at least in part, to the activity of saliva, from which a number of antibacterial substances may be demonstrated. IgA is in the saliva and it has been suggested that, as well as a possible direct effect of this on the oral micro-organisms, a complex may be formed between the immunoglobulin and the oral epithelium itself resulting in a protective surface coating on the mucosa. There is also a further mechanical protective activity of saliva in that foreign material, including micro-organisms, is washed from the oral cavity to the stomach where bacteria are destroyed by gastric fluids.

These local factors, however, represent no more than a first line of defence for the patient against invasion by potential pathogens, and depend for their effectiveness on the integrity of the immune and other generalized protective responses of the host. If the balance between the host and the commensal micro-organisms is disturbed by some factor that impairs the immune defences then opportunistic organisms may begin to act in a pathogenic manner. This is a result of their increase in numbers that exceeds a minimum infectious dose. It is in such a way that many cases of oral candidosis and acute necrotizing ulcerative gingivitis are thought to occur. Apart from infections of the oral mucosa brought about by a disturbance of a normal host–commensal relationship there are others, particularly those of viral origin, that represent the first response of the patient to the infective agent. Even in some of these (orofacial herpes infections are an example) there may be complex immunological changes in the patient that are of great significance in understanding the clinical course of the disease. The importance of primary and secondary immune deficiencies in relation to oral infections is discussed in Chapter 14.

The role of bacteria in the pathogenesis of caries, non-specific gingivitis, and periodontitis is outside the scope of this chapter and readers should refer to specialist texts on these subjects.

In previous editions of this book, streptococcal stomatitis was included as a bacterial infection possibly affecting the oral mucosa. There would seem to be no doubt that there is a readily available reservoir of streptococci in the oral cavity that might be expected to respond to a disturbance in the host–commensal relationship by behaving in a pathogenic manner. It is equally evident that a generalized infection of the mouth and oropharynx might occur as a result of invasion by exogenous cocci. In spite of this, it is by no means clear that a true streptococcal stomatitis does, in fact, exist, although until relatively recently it was generally accepted as a clinical entity. The confusion may have arisen because of the similarity between the symptoms ascribed to a streptococcal stomatitis and those caused by mild viral infections. The symptoms of streptococcal stomatitis were generally described as a generalized erythema of the oral mucosa together with a marked gingivitis, submandibular lymphadenitis, and a mild degree of malaise and fever.

Bacterial infections

Acute necrotizing ulcerative gingivitis (ANUG)

Acute necrotizing ulcerative gingivitis (ANUG) was, until recently, relatively common, but is currently much less so in developed countries. ANUG does still occur in smokers and immunocompromised patients, particularly in those with human immunodeficiency virus (HIV) infection. When irreversible periodontal desctruction has occurred the condition is now more appropriately termed 'acute necrotizing ulcerative periodontitis'. Throughout this section, the term ANUG will be used to describe both conditions. The exact cause of ANUG is not known, but there is no doubt that during an attack there is a proliferation of spirochaetes and fusiform bacteria. There is also a proliferation of obligate anaerobic, non-sporulative rods. These rods are thought to be important and probably more significant than the spirochaetes. Although there are many theoretical speculations about the exact aetiology of ANUG, there is no doubt that, for practical purposes, elimination of the overgrowth of the micro-organisms is coincident with clinical remission of the disease.

Clinical features

The clinical features of ANUG are soreness and bleeding of the gingivae, together with the development of crater-like ulcers, due to the necrosis of the gingival papillae (Fig. 4.1). This ulceration subsequently spreads along the gingival margin. Patients develop a marked halitosis, which has a characteristic odour (Table 4.1). In a few patients with ANUG there are fever, malaise, and lymphadenitis. Most, however, are young adults and, in the more usual, uncomplicated case, the patient is initially perfectly healthy.

Any patient, for whom predisposing factors cannot be identified, should be suspected of suffering from an underlying systemic disorder and, in view of the possibility of a blood dyscrasia in such patients, haematological examination should be undertaken. One of the greatest clinical problems in the management

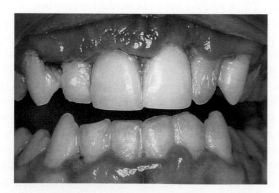

Fig. 4.1 Acute necrotizing ulcerative gingivitis, showing destruction of the gingival papillae.

Table 4.1 Clinical features of acute necrotizing ulcerative gingivitis (ANUG)

Soreness and bleeding of the gingivae
Necrosis of the gingival papillae
Halitosis

of ANUG is that of recurrence. It is evident that the patient with poor oral hygiene or with gingival contours distorted by a previous attack may, because of these local factors, be susceptible to recurrent infection, particularly if predisposing factors still persist.

Predisposing factors

The influence of poor oral hygiene in the initiation of ANUG has been often stressed, but there is no doubt that there are some patients whose standard of hygiene must be considered by normal criteria to be good. The most common predisposing factors other than systemic ones are tobacco smoking and psychological stress, although it is by no means easy to see how these factors operate. Nicotine causes vasoconstriction of blood vessels with a consequent reduction of blood supply to the tissues and increased susceptibility to infection and damage.

Decreased host resistance or depressed immune responses are important systemic factors predisposing to ANUG. A chronic necrotizing gingivitis is associated with HIV infection.

In normal healthy patients with ANUG, spread of the infection from the gingival margins is relatively rare. In a patient weakened by debilitating disease the infection may spread to surrounding tissues. An example of the spread of ANUG in the debilitated patient is seen in cancrum oris (noma) a condition now virtually unknown in Europe.

Diagnosis of ANUG

The clinical diagnosis of ANUG may be confirmed by the demonstration of a fusospirochaetal complex in a Gram-stained deep gingival smear. Bacteria cultured in ANUG include, *Treponema vincentii*, *denticola*, and *macrodentium*; *Prevotella intermedia*; *Porphyromonas gingivalis*; and *Fusobacterium nucleatum*.

Management of ANUG

The initial treatment of ANUG comprises supragingival plaque control, and the use of a systemic antibiotic, such as metronidazole. Smokers should be advised to refrain from smoking. Patients with ANUG present with varying degrees of gingival discomfort, but in most cases it is not feasible to carry out a scale and polish at the initial visit. Gentle debridement of the gingival tissues should be done and the patient given instructions to use a chlorhexidine mouthrinse and attempt gentle toothbrushing. ANUG responds rapidly to the use of penicillin, and a number of other antibiotics, but metronidazole is the usual drug of choice. A dose of 200 mg, three times daily, for 3 days is sufficient in most cases to reduce the symptoms dramatically in 24 hours.

However, if resolution does not occur, an underlying condition should be suspected and appropriate investigations undertaken. When prescribing metronidazole patients should be warned to avoid alcohol. Metronidazole is similar in its effects to disulfiram and blocks the normal metabolic pathway of alcohol elimination. In some patients, side-effects such as nausea, hypotension, and flushing may follow if alcohol is taken during treatment. The teratogenic effects of metronidazole are uncertain and it is therefore not recommended in early pregnancy. Once the acute phase has resolved, periodontal treatment should commence, together with smoking cessation advice.

- Metronidazole is the antibiotic of choice for the initial management of ANUG.
- Patients should be warned not to take alcohol whilst taking metronidazole.
- Metronidazole is best avoided during pregnancy.

Syphilis

Syphilis is a sexually transmitted disease and the causative bacterial agent is *Treponema pallidum*. This gains entry to the body via mucous membranes and minute abrasions in the skin. There is a popular misconception that syphilis is a rare disease but it is a common infection in Russia and the Far East and its incidence worldwide is increasing. Outbreaks of cases continue to be reported in the UK and oral lesions of syphilis may be seen in the oral medicine clinic. Early diagnosis is essential as the long-term effects of untreated syphilis are serious and potentially life-threatening.

Clinical features of syphilis

Primary lesions of syphilis may appear on any part of the oral mucosa and must always be considered in the differential diagnosis of oral ulceration. As in the case of the genital lesion the oral primary lesion (chancre) appears following a period of 2–3 weeks after infection. Usually the chancre presents as a painless indurated swelling, dark red in colour and with a glazed surface (Fig. 4.2), from which large numbers of *Treponema pallidum* can be

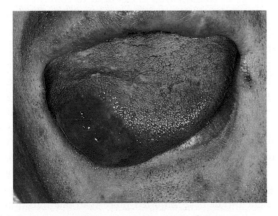

Fig. 4.2 Primary syphilitic lesion (chancre) of the tongue.

isolated and demonstrated on dark-ground microscopy. Chancres are most likely to be found in the relatively soft and unrestricted tissues of the tongue, cheeks, or lips, but where they occur on the palate or gingivae the morphology of the lesions may be modified, and they may appear as more diffuse structures. Whatever the site, size, or shape of the chancre, however, the heavy infection of the surface is consistent, thus providing both a convenient means of diagnosis and a considerable hazard to the unsuspecting diagnostician particularly if gloves are not worn. At the time of the primary lesion there is a nontender enlargement of the cervical lymph nodes affecting the submental, submandibular, pre- and post-auricular, and occipital groups—the so-called 'syphilitic collar'.

This disappearance of the primary lesion, usually after a period of some 2 weeks, marks the widespread dissemination of the micro-organisms and the onset of the second stage of the disease, which may last for many years. The oral symptoms most often described at this stage of the disease are mucous patches (appearing as grey-white ulcers covered by a thick slough) and 'snail track' ulcers. In view, however, of the protean nature of the skin lesions produced during this stage of the disease, it would seem at least a reasonable possibility that there may be an equivalent variation in the form of oral lesions. If this is so, it would seem more than likely that secondary syphilitic ulcers may often pass unrecognized or be mistaken for some less significant non-specific lesion and, for this reason, serological tests for syphilis should be part of the investigation of oral ulceration of unknown origin. In this second stage lymph nodes may again be palpable as non-tender, discrete structures.

In the tertiary stage of syphilis two major forms of oral involvement may occur. The first of these, syphilitic leukoplakia, will be dealt with in detail in Chapter 10 together with other leukoplakias. In the inadequately treated or untreated cases, which are now seen very rarely, leukoplakia of the whole of the oral mucosa but especially of the tongue is an important complication, the more so because malignant transformation can occur. The second type of oral involvement in the tertiary stage is the development of a 'gumma'. This is essentially a chronic granuloma, often in the palatal tissues, that eventually breaks down with the consequent production of a tissue defect. The untreated patient at this stage is likely to have other more widespread lesions, especially of the nervous system, but the micro-organisms are by no means as readily demonstrated as in the earlier stages of the disease. As well as these most commonly described manifestations of late syphilis, a number of other oral changes have been described, including a fibrosing glossitis. Osteomyelitis affecting the jaw is a rare complication of syphilis. A wide range of clinical presentations of tertiary syphilis is possible and this fact emphasizes the wisdom of including serological tests for the disease in the investigation of unusual oral conditions. Even if the patient is of an advanced age when the condition is diagnosed and although no systemic effects are obvious, treatment is indicated. Symptoms such as mental confusion that might be attributed to

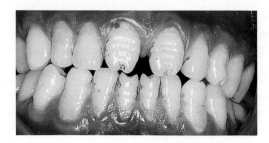

Fig. 4.3 Hutchinson's incisors in congenital syphilis.

senile changes may be, in fact, the result of the syphilitic infection and may respond to antibiotic treatment even at a late stage.

Treponema pallidum crosses the placental barrier and causes congenital syphilis in the fetus. The dental abnormalities mainly affect the permanent dentition, as the deciduous teeth are generally well developed by the time their tooth germs are invaded by the spirochaetes. The first permanent molars ('Mulberry' or 'Moon's' molars) and upper central incisors ('Hutchinson's' incisors) are usually involved in congenital syphilis (Fig. 4.3).

The diagnosis of syphilis

The diagnosis of syphilis is generally based on the results of serological tests. *Treponema pallidum* cannot be cultured *in vitro*—it is propagated in animals to allow organisms to be prepared for serological tests. Current serological tests include the Venereal Disease Reference Laboratory (VDRL) test, the *Treponema pallidum* haemagglutination assay (TPHA), the fluorescent *Treponema* antibody absorbed test (FTA (abs)), and the *Treponema pallidum* immobilization (TPI) test (Table 4.2).

The treatment of syphilis

Penicillin is the treatment of choice and is given in high doses. In primary syphilis the course of antibiotics is up to 1 month but in late (or latent) syphilis this is for up to 12 weeks. Patients who are allergic to penicillin can be prescribed erythromycin or tetracycline.

Gonorrhoea

Primary oral lesions of gonorrhoea are relatively rare. They are the result of transmission of the organism (*Neisseria gonorrhoea*) by direct mucosal contact.

Table 4.2 Serological tests currently used to diagnose syphilis

Test	Abbreviation
Venereal Disease Reference Laboratory test	VDRL
Treponema pallidum haemagglutination assay	TPHA
Fluorescent *Treponema* antibody absorbed test	FTA
Treponema pallidum immobilization test	TPI

Clinical features

Lesions appear predominantly in the pharynx and are invariably a result of orogenital sexual contact.

Diffuse erythematous and ulcerative oral lesions, tonsillitis, a purulent gingivitis, and other oral manifestations have been described. Patients demonstrated to have oral lesions are very few relative to the very large number known to have genital gonorrhoea. The systemic disturbances described as being associated with such oral lesions vary from mild to severe febrile symptoms, and the degree of oral discomfort reported is equally variable, with some patients complaining of difficulty swallowing. Submandibular lymphadenopathy may be present. It is likely that, in most cases, the nature of the infection is not initially suspected on clinical grounds, but becomes clear only as a result of bacteriological examination. The true incidence of oral gonorrhoeal infections probably remains unrecognized because of the relatively non-specific nature of the lesions.

> Clinical features of oral gonorrhoea include diffuse vesicular, erythematous, and ulcerative oral lesions and a purulent gingivitis. Tonsillar involvement may also be a feature.

A diffuse form of gonorrhoea spread by haematogenous routes may very occasionally affect the oral mucosa, although the predominant manifestations are on the skin. Ulcers, haemorrhagic lesions, and other manifestations of hypersensitivity to the disseminating micro-organisms have been described. Occasional patients with gonococcal infective arthritis of the temporomandibular joints have also been reported. The symptoms are similar to those of other types of infective arthritis—pain, swelling, and trismus. In most described cases the diagnosis has depended on bacteriological study of fluid aspirated from the affected joint.

> Gonorrhoea in the orofacial area is likely to be underdiagnosed.

Diagnosis of gonorrhoea

Microbiological confirmation is essential to confirm the clinical suspicion. Examination of a Gram-stained smear of the oral lesions may show Gram-negative diplococci. Microbiological swabs should always be taken for culture and sensitivity.

Treatment of gonorrhoea

As in urogenital gonorrhoea, the treatment is by high doses of antibiotics. Varying regimes have been described, varying from a single, high-dose intramuscular injection of procaine penicillin to oral amoxycillin (or ampicillin) to short courses of oral tetracycline or co-trimoxazole. The patient should be referred to a specialist in genitourinary medicine (GUM) for full assessment. As in all sexually transmitted diseases, it should be remembered that the patient might have acquired more than one infection at the same time.

Non-specific urethritis

Non-specific urethritis (NSU) is probably the most common sexually transmitted disease and in most cases *Chlamydia* species may be isolated from the urethra. The symptoms include a burning sensation on micturition and there may be a purulent discharge in males. Chlamydia infection may be asymptomatic, particularly in females. Microbiological tests are essential to confirm the diagnosis and the majority of cases respond to tetracycline therapy in normal doses over a week or two, even though no microbial agent can be demonstrated. Reiter's syndrome is predominantly seen in young males and may follow infection with gonorrhoea, chlamydia, or enteric bacteria. In this condition there may be polyarthritis, which can affect the temporomandibular joint, urethritis, uveitis (or conjunctivitis), and macular lesions on the palms and soles. Oral lesions tend to be erythematous and often resemble erythema migrans with a whitish border. This appearance has been described as a 'circinate' stomatitis.

> Reiter's syndrome predominantly affects young males and can present as a polyarthritis, urethritis, uveitis, and macular lesions on the palms and soles. Oral lesions have also been reported and include a 'circinate' stomatitis.

Tuberculosis

The genus *Mycobacterium* includes pathogenic and non-pathogenic species. *M. tuberculosis* and *M. bovis* are equally pathogenic for man. Tuberculosis is a worldwide endemic disease with up to one-third of the world's population being affected. There is a resurgence of respiratory pulmonary disease associated with immunodeficiency, malnutrition, and non-compliance with drug regimes, particularly as an AIDS-related phenomenon. The pathogenesis, clinical features, diagnosis, and treatment of pulmonary tuberculosis are outside the scope of this book.

Primary oral involvement with tuberculosis may, however, occur, albeit rarely, and should always be considered in the differential diagnosis of oral ulceration. The oral mucosa is more commonly involved by becoming secondarily infected by the sputum in cases of active pulmonary disease. Tuberculous lymphadenitis frequently affects the cervical lymph nodes. Initially, a firm but mobile lymphadenopathy is palpable. Sinus and abscess formation occur later with cervical lymph nodes becoming fixed (see Chapter 7).

Clinical features of oral tuberculosis

Oral lesions of tuberculosis usually present as painful ulceration. The classical description of a tuberculous ulcer is of an irregular lesion with undermined borders and covered by a grey slough. Ulceration commonly affects the tongue but other areas of the oral mucosa may be involved, particularly towards the posterior parts of the mouth. It should be added that a few lesions have been described in which the presentation of tuberculosis of the oral mucosa is quite different from the ulcers described above.

These lesions, presenting as white patches or granulating lesions, have been described both as primary lesions and as lesions secondary to pulmonary infection.

The diagnosis of oral tuberculosis

A tuberculous origin should be considered in the differential diagnosis of persistent oral ulceration of unknown aetiology. Definitive diagnosis of such a lesion invariably follows biopsy, with histopathological examination of formalin-fixed tissue, showing non-caseating granulomata. The number of acid–alcohol-fast bacilli present in the biopsy specimen may, however, be small and their demonstration by Ziehl–Nielsen staining, or by immunofluorescent techniques, can be difficult. Fresh tissue may be needed to culture mycobacteria on Lowestein medium, but this can take 6–8 weeks. If there is clinical suspicion of a tuberculous ulcer when the patient first presents then the initial biopsy can be divided and half sent for culture.

Management

Patients with oral tuberculosis should be fully investigated for pulmonary or other lesions and it would be expected that measures such as a chest radiograph would be taken at the first moment of suspicion. The treatment of tuberculosis is outside the province of oral medicine and the appropriate action to be taken would involve referral of the patient to a chest physician (or specialist in infectious diseases). It should be reiterated that the increase of tuberculosis is closely related to geographical areas affected by the HIV epidemic.

Fungal infections

Oral Candidosis

Candida spp are fungi that have a wide distribution and that frequently form part of the commensal flora of the human body. Swabs taken from the skin, gut, vagina, or mouth of an apparently healthy individual all may show the presence of *Candida* species and, in particular, *Candida albicans*. The oral carriage rate of oral candidal species is about 40 per cent of the normal population. Table 4.3 shows candidal species that have been isolated from oral lesions. Of these, *C. albicans* is the most frequent.

Table 4.3 Candidal species involved in oral candidosis

*C. albicans**
C. tropicalis
C. pseudotropicalis
C. glabrata
C. krusei
C. parapsilosis

* The most frequently isolated species.

Predisposing factors for oral candidosis

It has long been recognized that disease due to a proliferation of this micro-organism is a mark of lowered resistance or of metabolic change in the patient. The onset of candidosis should therefore lead to a search for the underlying cause. The significance of primary and secondary immune deficiency in relation to candidal infections is described in Chapter 14. It is pointed out that, although primary immune deficiencies are relatively rare, secondary deficiencies are much more common. Clinical situations commonly leading to a lowering of the immune defences and hence to oral candidosis are shown in Table 4.4.

It should be remembered that the onset of candidosis in an adult patient represents a change implying a relaxation of the normal immune defences. It does not imply an infection by 'foreign' candidal strains. Although, in the present context, it is evident that the oral conditions involving *Candida* are those more fully discussed, it must be remembered that candidal lesions may involve other areas and, indeed, may become widespread and disseminated in a few debilitated patients. The condition septicaemic candidaemia may involve the lungs, myocardium, and other vital organs, and is always a disease of very poor prognosis. Apart from such widespread infections, however, infection of the skin, hair follicles, and nails is relatively common. Local tissue trauma may be a significant predisposing feature and, in the case of candidal paronychia, circulatory disturbances and diabetes are commonly the precipitating factors. There is some difference of opinion as to the incidence of *Candida* in the vagina. Most investigations have shown a relatively low incidence in non-pregnant patients, but a high one (of the order of 50 per cent) in patients during late pregnancy. Not all these patients by any means show evidence of clinical infection, but it is evident that this vaginal population of *Candida* must act as a reservoir for infection, particularly of the new-born baby.

C. albicans normally exists in the oral cavity in the form of rather large yeast-like cells (blastospores) that occasionally elon-

Table 4.4 Predisposing factors for oral candidosis

Factor	Description
Physiological	Old age, infancy, pregnancy
Local tissue trauma	Mucosal irritation, dental appliances, poor oral hygiene
Antibiotic therapy	Broad spectrum (local or systemic)
Corticosteroid therapy	Topical, systemic, and inhalers
Malnutrition	Haematinic deficiencies—high-carbohydrate diet
Immune defects	AIDS
Endocrine disorders	Diabetes mellitus, Addison's disease, hypothyroidism
Malignancies	Leukaemias, aganulocytosis
Salivary gland hypofunction	Irradiation, Sjögren's syndrome, xerogenic drugs

Table 4.5 The laboratory diagnosis of oral candidosis

Oral lesion	Investigation*			
	Swab	Smear	Oral rinse	Biopsy
Pseudomembranous	+	±	+	−
Erythematous	+	±	+	−
Hyperplastic	±	±	−	+
Angular cheilitis	+	+	−	−
Candida-associated denture stomatitis (palate and denture)	+	+	+	

* +, Useful; −, inappropriate; ±, may be helpful.

gate to form germ tubes (pseudohyphae). In the inactive state the yeast form is predominant, but when pathological activity occurs the hyphal form is much more evident. These pseudohyphae can be seen, not only superficially on the oral mucosa, but also penetrate the epithelium, as far as the stratum granulosum. The mechanism by which *Candida* exert a pathological effect on tissues is not known, although it has been demonstrated that proteases and extracellular proteins may be produced by the micro-organisms and that these can induce skin lesions in the absence of the organisms themselves.

Laboratory investigations for the diagnosis of oral candidosis

Appropriate laboratory tests are outlined in Table 4.5 and have already been discussed in Chapter 2. A swab, moistened with sterile saline if necessary, is wiped along the surface of the lesion and placed in a suitable transport medium. The sample should be sent promptly to the microbiology laboratory for culture and sensitivity. A smear of the lesion may also be useful and foam pads are used in some centres to sample oral lesions for *Candida* species. An oral rinse, with a phosphate-buffered saline solution, will determine the presence of *Candida* species and also provide the clinician with a quantitative assessment of the candidal count. This helps to differentiate between commensalism and opportunistic infections. Biopsy of oral leukoplakia is essential and will demonstrate *Candida*-associated lesions, such as chronic hyperplastic candidosis (candidal leukoplakia).

Haematological tests including a full blood count, estimations of serum ferritin, vitamin B_{12}, folate (and red cell folate), and a blood glucose test should be undertaken for all cases of persistent oral candidosis, particularly if an underlying systemic condition is suspected. Oral candidosis associated with HIV infection is discussed later in this chapter.

Clinical classification of oral candidosis

The clinical presentation of oral candidosis is variable. The original classification of oral candidosis by Lehner in the 1960s recognized two major groups: acute (pseudomembranous and

Table 4.6 The classification of oral candidosis

Primary oral candidoses (group 1)
Acute: pseudomembranous, erythematous
Chronic: pseudomembranous, erythematous, hyperplastic
Candida-associated lesions: *Candida*-associated denture-induced stomatitis, angular cheilitis, median rhomboid glossitis
Secondary oral candidoses (group 2)
Oral manifestations of systemic mucocutaneous candidosis

atrophic) and chronic (atrophic and hyperplastic). It is, however, now recognized that this original classification had limitations, and the currently accepted one (Table 4.6) is based on clinically relevant terminology. Pseudomembranous candidosis can be 'acute' but, particularly in immunocompromised patients, is often 'chronic'. 'Atrophic' is not an entirely appropriate term in the context of oral candidosis as the mucosa may appear red as a result of either atrophy or increased vascularity, and this differentation is difficult to make clinically. Angular cheilitis, denture stomatitis, and 'median rhomboid glossitis' may be a result of combined bacterial and fungal aetiology and are therefore classified as '*Candida*-associated' lesions. Systemic mucocutaneous candidosis frequently has oral manifestations and these are classified as 'secondary oral candidiases' (see Table 4.6).

Antifungal agents used to treat oral candidosis

Topical and systemic antifungal agents suitable for the treatment of oral candidosis are summarized in Table 4.7.

The polyene antifungal agents, nystatin and amphotericin B, are well established and relatively free from side-effects when used locally. They are available in various forms, such as lozenges, pastilles, creams, and suspensions. Unfortunately, patient compliance is often poor with these preparations, which may take a while to dissolve in the mouth (for example, pastilles and lozenges) and have a 'distinctive' taste. Microbial resistance to polyene antifungals is, however, uncommon. The newer azoles have very useful properties, although resistance is rather more commonly met and may be problematic in the future, particularly in the immunocompromised patient. (*C. krusei* and and *C. glabrata* are usually resistant to fluconazole.) The locally active agent, miconazole is available as an oral gel or cream. As well as its antifungal activity, it has a limited antibacterial effect. The systemically acting azoles, itraconazole, fluconazole, and ketoconazole, are of value in generalized and systemic candidal infections. There may be changes in liver function, particularly with ketoconazole, and patients on these drugs must be carefully monitored. Systemic therapy is generally not necessary in the majority of patients suffering from oral candidosis but in some conditions, such as chronic hyperplastic candidosis, its use is becoming widespread and is often very effective. Azoles have an unfavourable pharmacokinetic interaction with a number of drugs including anticoagulants (for example, warfarin), terfenadine, ciclosporin,

Table 4.7 The treatment of primary oral candidoses in immunocompetent patients

Topical therapy	Systemic therapy
Pseudomembranous, erythematous hyperplastic candidosis	
Amphotericin lozenges (10 mg)	Fluconazole, 50–100 mg daily for 2–3 weeks
or	*or*
Nystatin pastilles (100 000 units)	Itraconazole 150 mg daily for 2 weeks
Dissolve slowly in mouth, after meals; use 4 times daily; usual course is 1–4 weeks.	
Candida-*associated denture stomatitis**	
Amphotericin or nystatin (as above)—remove dentures	Systemic therapy is occasionally required (as above)
If compliance poor:	
Miconazole gel applied to palatal surface of denture 4 times daily for 1–4 weeks	
Miconazole lacquer[†]	
Chlorhexidine 0.2% rinse, 4 times daily (do not use with nystatin)	
Candida-*associated angular cheilitis**	
Nystatin cream; apply to corners of mouth 3–4 times daily, until resolution	Systemic therapy may be required
If microbial report not available or in case of mixed infection:[‡]	
Miconazole cream (or gel); apply 3–4 times daily to angles	

* Intraoral reservoirs of *Candida* should be eliminated from patients with angular cheilitis and denture stomatitis.

[†] Miconazole lacquer (Dumicoat, 50 mg/g) can be applied to fitting surface of upper denture after thorough cleansing and drying—see manufacturers' instructions.

[‡] If *Staphylococcus aureus* only isolated, fusidic acid cream is required (see Table 6.5 for further details).

statins, cisapride, and astemizole. Chlorhexidine solution has antibacterial and anticandidal effects.

Pseudomembranous candidosis

Until recently, this condition, colloquially known as 'thrush', was almost always described as 'acute' pseudomembranous candidosis, according to Lehner's original classification, even though many lesions were manifestly chronic in nature. Reconsideration of the oral lesions of candidosis in HIV-related conditions and other

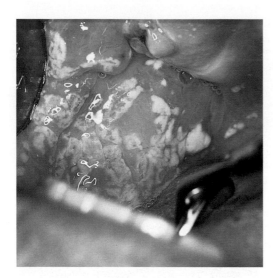

Fig. 4.4 Pseudomembranous candidosis (thrush).

immunosuppressive states has led to the routine use of the term 'acute' being abandoned. The pseudomembrane consists of a network of candidal hyphae containing desquamated cells, microorganisms, fibrin, inflammatory cells, and debris. This pseudomembrane lies on the surface of the tissue and candidal hyphae penetrate superficially into the epithelium to provide anchorage.

CLINICAL FEATURES

Clinically, this appears as a thick, white coating or series of patches on the affected tissue (Fig. 4.4). The pseudomembrane can be wiped away and, since the more superficial layers of the epithelium may be included, a red and bleeding base is left behind. This may be considered a reasonable preliminary clinical test to distinguish thrush from other white lesions of the mucosa and confirmation may also be obtained by taking a direct smear from the lesion. This may be fixed by gentle heat and immediately stained, using the periodic acid–Schiff (PAS) reagent. The hyphae are readily identified under the microscope. A swab should be taken and sent to the microbiological laboratory for culture and sensitivity.

Any of the mucosal surfaces of the mouth may be affected by thrush, as may the posterior pharyngeal wall. In this last instance, the condition must be taken particularly seriously, since extension into the oesophagus and trachea is possible and may prove fatal. This is likely to occur only in the severely debilitated patient, although the pre-existing condition may not have been previously recognized. In a few patients laryngeal candidosis of a less active form may be associated with oral lesions. This has been noted in patients taking antibiotics and in those taking oral steroid preparations. In general, the laryngeal discomfort and hoarseness resolve with treatment of the oral lesions.

MANAGEMENT

The treatment for pseudomembranous candidosis is summarized in Table 4.7. It is evident, however, that treatment of symptoms alone is insufficient and that steps must be taken to determine

any predisposing cause. In some patients the essential underlying factor is understood and under reasonable control, but in others, in particular those patients with AIDS, the debilitating nature of the condition may be expressed in virtually continuous candidosis of the mouth. In these circumstances it is necessary to maintain long-term antifungal treatment. A particular difficulty arises in the case of patients with leukaemia or other neoplastic diseases under treatment with cytotoxic and other drugs. In these cases not only the underlying disease process, but also the therapy, tend to predispose towards candidosis.

Erythematous candidosis

This can be 'acute' or 'chronic' depending on the duration of the oral lesions. Acute erythematous candidosis was formerly known as 'acute atrophic candidosis' or 'antibiotic sore mouth' and usually occurred as a result of medical treatment involving antibiotics or steroid preparations. A significant number of patients (adults and children) are now using steroid inhalers for pulmonary disease and these can predipose to the development of either erythematous or pseudomembranous candidosis (Chapter 14).

CLINICAL FEATURES

Acute erythematous candidosis resembles 'thrush' without the overlying pseudomembrane. Clinically, the mucosa involved is red and painful. This is, in fact, the only variant of oral candidosis in which pain and discomfort is marked. As would be expected from this description, the epithelium is thin and atrophic with candidal hyphae embedded superficially in the epithelium. The condition may follow or be concurrent with thrush, or may occur as the only manifestation of the infection. As has been pointed out above, this form of candidosis is common in patients with the suppressed immune function of AIDS as well as patients undergoing prolonged antibiotic or steroid therapy. It is not always possible for patients on steroids to discontinue treatment and the continuous lowering of the resistance of the tissues to infection makes treatment by the usual means relatively ineffective.

MANAGEMENT

Topical antifungal therapy (Table 4.7) is usually effective. Erythematous candidosis as a result of antibiotic therapy usually resolves after cessation of the course, although this may take some time. In a patient known to be susceptible to this condition and for whom it is necessary to prescribe further antibiotic treatment, it would be wise to add oral antifungal treatment to the regime. In the authors' experience, a minority of these patients appear to develop a chronic glossodynia (burning tongue) that persists despite the lingual mucosa appearing normal and after elimination of candidal infection (see Chapter 17). Patients who regularly require a steroid inhaler should be instructed to rinse their mouth with water after use. Use of a spacer device for the inhaler may be necessary (Chapter 14, Fig. 14.2).

Hyperplastic candidosis

Chronic hyperplastic candidosis is also known as 'candidal leukoplakia' and is associated with chronic infection of the oral mucosa with candidal species, usually *C. albicans*. This chronic form of candidosis is considered to be a premalignant lesion and is more likely to occur in patients who smoke. Currently, there is a great deal of controversy concerning the role of *Candida* species in the development of epithelial neoplasia. The premalignant nature of candidal leukoplakia is discussed fully in Chapter 10.

CLINICAL FEATURES

Chronic hyperplastic candidosis classically presents as a fixed white patch at the commissures of the mouth. Other areas of the mouth, particularly the palate, may be affected but the tongue is less commonly involved. Clinically, the lesion(s) appear as raised, irregular white plaques, which may be 'speckled' or nodular in appearance. There is frequently evidence of oral candidosis elsewhere, particularly on the palate of patients with full dentures and/or angular cheilitis.

MANAGEMENT

Definitive diagnosis depends on histopathological examination of a biopsy, which is essential to confirm the presence of *Candida* species and to ascertain the degree of epithelial atypia—if any. Management involves the eradication of predisposing factors, such as smoking and institution of appropriate antifungal therapy—either topical or systemic. An initial course of fluconazole for 2–3 weeks can be combined with topical therapy (see Table 4.7), which may be required on a longer-term basis. Attention must be given to denture hygiene and other factors predisposing to oral candidosis, either local or systemic. Haematological investigations should be undertaken to check for haematinic deficiencies such as iron deficiency, and a blood glucose test is advisable to exclude diabetes. Excision of persistent lesions or those with a significant degree of dysplasia is preferably carried out with a laser. Long-term follow-up is essential.

Candida-associated, denture-induced stomatitis

This is by far the most common form of oral candidosis and is also referred to as chronic erythematous candidosis (or, more colloquially in the past, as 'denture sore mouth'—a misnomer because the condition is nearly always painless). This form of denture stomatitis represents the end-result of secondary candidal infection of tissues, traumatized by a dental appliance. This need not be ill-fitting, although most of the dentures involved are old. The appliance is commonly but not exclusively a denture—an orthodontic plate may produce a similar result.

CLINICAL FEATURES

The clinical picture is of marked redness of the palatal mucosa covered by the appliance (the equivalent mandibular denture-bearing area does not appear to become involved) often with a sharply defined edge (Fig. 4.5). If a relief area is present on the denture, there may be a corresponding area of spongy 'granular looking' tissue, but otherwise the affected mucosa is smooth. Newton introduced a classification for this condition: type 1, characterized by pin-point hyperaemia of the palatal mucosa; type 2 (the most common type), in which there is diffuse erythema

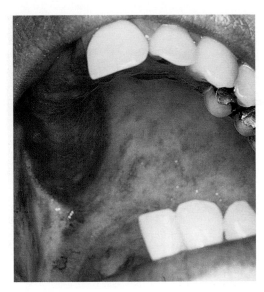

Fig. 4.5 Candida-associated, denture-induced stomatitis (chronic erythematous candidosis) affecting the area of mucosa covered by a partial denture.

limited to the area of the denture; type 3, in which there is a hyperplastic nodular reaction of the palatal mucosa (Table 4.8). There is rarely any complaint of soreness by the patient in spite of the intense erythematous appearance of the tissues. *Candida*-associated denture stomatitis, because of its restricted distribution to the denture-bearing area, is sometimes mistaken for an allergic reaction to acrylic resin, a condition that is relatively rare.

MANAGEMENT

By taking swabs or carrying out direct inoculation from the fitting surface of the denture involved it is practically always possible to isolate a heavy growth of *Candida*. Swabs from the mucosal surface may also provide a prolific growth. Biopsy is rarely indicated but may be done in persistent or atypical cases to confirm the diagnosis. Histopathology often shows few candidal hyphae within the epithelium.

Since there are two contributing factors to this condition (tissue trauma and infection), treatment must be directed at both in order to obtain rapid resolution of symptoms. Denture hygiene is an important part of the treatment together with the elimination of trauma by the adoption of suitable prosthetic techniques, the use of tissue conditioners being particularly valuable as an initial treatment. The use of an antifungal cream or miconazole

Table 4.8 Newton's classification of *Candida*-associated denture stomatitis

Type	Description
1	Pin-point hyperaemia
2*	Diffuse erythema, limited to the fitting surfaces of denture
3	Nodular appearance of palatal mucosa

* Type most commonly seen.

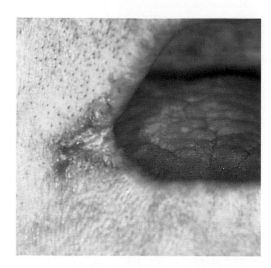

Fig. 4.6 Angular cheilitis with candidal involvement.

gel on the fitting surface of the appliance may prove a useful adjuvant to treatment and helps to speed the resolution of the abnormal tissues (Table 4.7). Careful and regular cleaning of all surfaces of the denture is also of great importance. A lacquer containing miconazole is now available and painted on to the fitting surface of the upper denture.

Candida-associated angular cheilitis

Angular cheilitis presents as erythema and cracking at the angles of the mouth and is commonly a *Candida*-associated lesion (Fig. 4.6). The pathogenesis, clinical presentation, and management of angular cheilitis are fully described in Chapter 6. The treatment of *Candida*-associated angular cheilitis is summarized in Tables 6.4 and 6.5.

Median rhomboid glossitis

Median rhomboid glossitis is classified as a '*Candida*-associated' lesion and characteristically presents as an area of depapillation on the midline of the dorsum of the tongue, immediately in front of the circumvallate papillae. The lesion is classically 'rhomboid-shaped'—hence the name. Its suface may be red, white, or yellow in appearance. This lesion is further discussed in Chapter 6.

Secondary oral candidoses: chronic mucocutaneous candidosis syndromes

Apart from the more common forms of oral candidosis, there is a spectrum of conditions in which candidosis of the oral cavity, the skin, and other structures such as the fingernails may occur, with or without association with other generalized disease processes. This group of conditions is generally known as chronic mucocutaneous candidosis (CMC). The oral lesions in CMC may be initially thrush-like, but eventually resemble lesions of chronic hyperplastic candidosis. The skin lesions may include widespread and disfiguring lesions of the face and scalp. Granulomatous lesions of the lips may also occur, similar to those that affect the skin. A variant (familial chronic mucocutaneous candidosis) is

Table 4.9 Chronic mucocutaneous candidosis (CMC) syndromes

Type	Features
Familial CMC	First decade—persistent candidosis: mouth, nails, skin. Iron deficiency.
Diffuse CMC (*Candida* granuloma)	First 5 years—chronic candidosis: mouth, nails, skin, pharynx. Susceptible to bacterial infections
Candidosis–endocrinopathy syndrome	Hypothyroidism, hypoadrenocorticism, and mild chronic hyperplastic candidosis involving the mouth
Candidosis–thymoma syndrome	Haematological disorders. Pseudomembranous or hyperplastic candidosis: mouth, skin, nails.

* Taken from Bagg, T. *et al.* (1999). *Essentials of microbiology for dental students.* Oxford University Press, Oxford.

genetically determined and is transmitted as an autosomal recessive condition. In the candidosis–endocrinopathy syndrome white candidal plaques in the mouth and candidal infections of the nails are associated with disorders of the parathyroids or adrenals. A classification of chronic mucocutaneous candidosis syndromes is shown in Table 4.9.

MANAGEMENT

Chronic mucocutaneous candidosis is difficult to treat and in many cases reduction, but not eradication, of *Candida* species is attainable. Predisposing factors for oral candidosis should, however, be eliminated (see above) wherever possible. Treatment is with long-term systemic antifungal therapy such as fluconazole and may need to be prescribed at doses higher than the normal therapeutic range. Regular monitoring of liver function is essential.

Viral infections

A number of viral infections may occur in and around the mouth and many of these present as vesciular lesions of the oral mucosa. The vesicles show a marked tendency to break down with the production of ulcers.

Diagnostic tests for viral infections have already been discussed in Chapter 2. The initial diagnosis of viral infection is, however, usually on the basis of clinical presentation. Tissue culture systems take at least 24 hours to confirm the presence of a virus and serological tests take 10–14 days. Table 4.10 shows the principal viruses that affect the oral and perioral region. Of these, three are human herpes virsuses (Table 4.11). There are currently eight human herpes viruses (Table 4.11) and all are enveloped, icosahedral viral particles, with a double-stranded DNA genome.

The human herpes viruses possess the property of latency (that is, they can remain dormant and become reactivated later). The clinical disease caused by the virus may differ depending on whether the infection is primary or secondary (that is, a reactivation).

Table 4.10 Principal viruses that affect the oral and perioral region

Herpes simplex virus
Varicella zoster virus
Epstein–Barr virus
Group A Coxsackieviruses
Paramyxoviruses
Human papilloma viruses

Table 4.11 Human herpes viruses

Herpes simplex virus (type 1)
Herpes simplex virus (type 2)
Varicella-zoster virus (type 3)
Epstein-Barr virus (type 4)
Cytomegalovirus (type 5)
Human herpes viruses 6, 7, and 8*

* Associated with Kaposi's sarcoma.

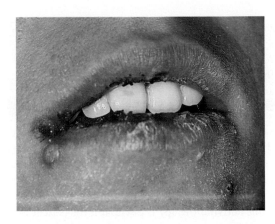

Fig. 4.7 Patient suffering from primary herpetic gingivostomatitis with involvement of the lips and perioral skin.

Herpes simplex virus infections

Primary herpetic gingivostomatitis

The herpes simplex virus (HSV) is a DNA virus of which two main groups are known in man, together with a number of slightly modified transitional types. Herpes simplex, type 1, affects the oral mucosa, pharynx, and skin whereas Herpes simplex, type 2, predominantly involves the genitalia. The lesions produced by these two types of the virus appear to be identical, but there are suggestions that the long-term consequences of infection may be different since the type 2 virus has been implicated in the production of cervical carcinoma. The type 1 virus is implicated in the majority of oral and facial lesions.

Primary herpetic gingivostomatitis is the most common viral infection affecting the mouth and it affects patients in two main age groups—young children and young adults. In early childhood the infection may be subclinical. The incubation period is about 5 days.

CLINICAL PRESENTATION

The patient with primary herpetic gingivostomatitis may give a history of recent exposure to a patient with a herpetic lesion. The initial symptoms are of malaise with tiredness, generalized muscle aches, and, sometimes, a sore throat. At this early stage the submandibular lymph nodes are often enlarged and tender. This prodromal phase may be expected to last for a day or two and is followed by the appearance of oral and, sometimes, circumoral lesions (Fig. 4.7). Groups of vesicles form on the oral mucosa and rapidly break down to produce shallow ulcers.

Although the vesicles may be relatively small, the breakdown of confluent groups may result in the formation of large areas of ulceration. The distribution of the lesions is variable—any of the oral mucosal surfaces may be involved. Apart from the ulcerated areas, the whole of the oral mucosa may be bright-red and sore. In young children, particularly, there may be a marked gingivitis that closely resembles that of acute leukaemia. It is evident that such an appearance should indicate screening for haematological changes. Apart from the intraoral lesions, there may be lesions of the lips and circumoral skin, which, because of the relative stability of the skin compared to the oral mucosa, may retain a much more obviously vesicular appearance. In a few cases, the primary infection may become widespread and disseminated throughout the body, so that encephalitis, meningitis, and other life-endangering conditions may follow. Such potentially fatal cases have been mainly reported in patients who are immunocompromised.

In the vast majority of untreated cases there is a slow recovery from the symptoms over a period of some 10–14 days. Most cases of primary herpetic gingivostomatitis are diagnosed on clinical grounds. HSV can be grown in tissue culture systems but this takes at least 24 hours. Serology can also be used to detect either an increase in the IgE antibody titre between the acute and convalescent phase, or specific IgM antibodies.

MANAGEMENT

Specific therapy for viral infections is generally unsatisfactory and management is, therefore, symptomatic with general supportive measures, such as rest, fluids, and antipyretics/analgesics. For oral infections, the use of an antiseptic (for example, chlorhexidine gluconate) or tetracycline mouthwash may reduce secondary infection and an analgesic mouthwash (for example, benzydamine) will reduce discomfort, particularly whilst the patient is eating. Systemic analgesics and antiypretics may also be required. In most immunocompetent patients, HSV infections are self-limiting and last 10–14 days.

Management of most viral infections affecting the mouth is symptomatic—general supportive measures include:

- rest
- fluids
- antipyretics/analgesics (systemic)
- antiseptic/analgesic mouthwashes

Aciclovir is active against herpes virses but does not eradicate them. It can be used for the systemic and topical treatment of herpes simplex infections affecting the skin and mucous membranes. Prophylactic use of aciclovir for prevention and recurrence of HSV infections is justified in the immunocompromised.

Systemic antiviral therapy is essential if the patient is immunocompromised, as this group is more susceptible to general dissemination of the HSV virus. In these cases, the clinical presentation of the infection may be atypical. An acute herpetic stomatitis represents the primary infection and, although subsequent immunity may not be complete, it is only very rarely that a second acute attack follows, unless the patient is immunocomprised. Recurrent intraoral herpes infections are therefore rare in the immunocompetent patient but crops of vesicles restricted to part of the oral mucosa, particularly the palate, have been described.

If the signs and symptoms of primary herpetic gingivostomatitis fail to improve after 2 weeks, then the patient should be referred for a specialist opinion to exclude blood dyscrasias and other underlying systemic conditions.

Secondary (recurrent) herpes simplex infections

Following resolution of the primary herpetic infection, there is an approximately 30–40 per cent likelihood that recurrent lesions will follow, regardless of the intensity of the primary attack. The usual site of the recurrent lesion is on or near the lips and the lesion is known as 'herpes labialis' or a 'cold sore'. Less commonly, the skin and mucosa of the nose and nasal passages are involved, as may be, occasionally, almost any site on the face. In an individual patient, however, the areas involved tend to remain the same in successive episodes. The recurrences may be provoked by a wide range of stimulae, including sunlight, mechanical trauma, and, particularly, mild febrile conditions such as the common cold. Emotional factors also play a part in precipitating recurrences in many patients. HSV particles can be detected in the saliva of approximately 30 per cent of patients who develop cold sores.

CLINICAL PRESENTATION

In the prodromal stages of a recurrence the patient may feel a mild degree of tiredness and malaise. This is quickly followed by a period of irritation and itching over the area of the lip involved in recurrence and, within a few hours, vesicles appear surrounded by a mildly erythematous area (at this stage the patient is highly infectious). In a short time the vesicles burst and a scab is formed. From this point the process is one of slow healing over a period of some 10 days, but secondary infection may occasionally delay the healing process and lead to the production of small pustules in

the area. Healing is without scarring and the affected area returns, after a short period of erythema, to an apparently normal stage until the onset of the next recurrence. This may be after a period of a few weeks or even days in some individuals, but generally the intervals between recurrences are on the order of months, this evidently depending to a large extent on the degree of exposure of the patient to the particular stimulus involved.

MANAGEMENT

There is no therapeutic measure available that provides reasonably consistent results and that entirely prevents further recurrences. Aciclovir cream, used as early as possible and at least five times a day in the early stages, may prevent progression of the lesion. This is now perhaps the most effective and acceptable form of treatment for recurrent herpes, although there is no real suggestion that a permanent cure may be obtained. A similar antiviral drug, penciclovir, can be used topically for cold sores, (herpes labialis). The 'prodrug' of penciclovir is famciclovir, which is a systemic antiviral agent recommended for HZV infections and genital herpes.

Topical therapy for 'cold sores' (herpes labialis) should be applied in the prodromal phase of the lesion. Aciclovir and penciclovir creams are available for topical application.

Varicella zoster virus infections

Varicella zoster virus (VZV) is a DNA virus morphologically similar to the HSV and apparently responsible for two completely dissimilar diseases in humans, namely, chickenpox and herpes zoster. There is, however, little evidence that contact with one of these diseases is responsible for the initiation of the other. It seems more likely that the zoster eruption represents the reactivation of the virus in a previously infected patient with only partial immunity, a situation parallel to that in recurrent herpes simplex. The zoster virus is also thought to remain latent in the relevant sensory ganglion and to pass down the nerve to the skin or mucous membrane on reactivation.

Chickenpox

Primary infection with VZV manifests as chickenpox, which is a common disease of childhood. It has an incubation period of 14–21 days, during which patients are infectious. The infection is spread by direct contact or droplet infection and is established first in the upper respiratory tract.

CLINICAL PRESENTATION

Just before the rash, oral lesions may appear on the hard palate, pillar of fauces, and uvula and appear as small ulcers, with a red halo. The rash initially manifests as pink, maculopapular lesions that develop into itchy vesicles on the back, chest, face, and scalp. Other clinical manifestations include malaise, fever, and lymphadenopathy. Adults can be quite severely affected. Rare complications of chickenpox include pneumonia and encephalitis. Treatment is symptomatic but it is important for the patient to avoid contact with any immunocompromised individuals.

Shingles

Most patients with herpes zoster are middle-aged or older (70 per cent over the age of 50), but it can occur in much younger patients and a few neonatal cases have been described. Predisposing factors that have been suggested include a wide range of debilitating diseases and immunosupression, either of iatrogenic or naturally occurring origin.

CLINICAL PRESENTATION

The characteristic superficial lesion of herpes zoster is a vesicular eruption in an area of distribution of a sensory nerve. The band-like distribution of shingles on the trunk is well known, having given the name to the virus (*zoster*, girdle). When the eruption affects the trigeminal nerve, the facial skin and oral mucosa in the sensory area may be affected. The trigeminal nerve is involved in about 15 per cent of cases. Of the three divisions of the trigeminal nerve the ophthalmic is the most frequently involved, but the other two divisions are also not uncommonly affected. Occasionally, when the disorder affects one division of the trigeminal nerve, the adjacent division becomes involved as well. Cervical nerves may also be affected. The initial symptoms are of pain and tenderness in the affected area—a discomfort much more severe than that experienced in HSV infection. The prodromal pain of shingles is severe and is occasionally misdiagnosed as toothache. The prodromal phase may last for 2 or 3 days and is succeeded by the appearance of vesicles in a rash, which may be either sparse or so dense as to be almost confluent. Frequently, the vesicles appear over a period of days rather than together, and these may become secondarily infected. When the ophthalmic division of the trigeminal nerve is involved there may be corneal ulceration, which requires most careful management to avoid permanent scar formation. Within the mouth, the vesicles behave much as those of herpes simplex infections, rapidly breaking down to form ulcers. The unilateral distribution of the oral lesions, and confinement to the area of a single branch of the trigeminal nerve, may give a clue as to the nature of the infection but this cannot be relied upon. If untreated, the vesicles and oral ulceration fade over a variable period from 2 to 4 weeks, or even longer. The skin vesicles may form firm crusts and, particularly if these are disturbed, marked scarring may occur. Following the fading of the rash the major complication of the condition—postherpetic neuralgia—may appear. In this condition anaesthesia, paraesthesia, and trigeminal neuralgia-like pains may affect the area and may persist for a period of years, occasionally reappearing after a prolonged absence. This is a highly refractory condition that may fail to

Table 4.12 Ramsay Hunt syndrome

Involvement of facial nerve with VZV
Facial nerve palsy (lower motor neurone)
Vesicles in external auditory meatus
Vesicles on palate
Other symptoms, e.g. dizziness, loss of taste

respond to any form of medical treatment (see Chapter 15). In a very few patients the facial nerve may become involved during an episode of zoster reactivation, probably via the geniculate ganglion. Facial weakness, loss of taste sensation, and symptoms such as dizziness resulting from labyrinthine disturbance may occur. This is the Ramsay Hunt syndrome (Table 4.12). Vesicular lesions in this condition are most often seen on the palate and around the external auditory meatus. In most cases, this is a self-limiting condition that resolves with restoration of function, but in some patients there may be permanent facial weakness.

MANAGEMENT

Treatment of shingles is with high doses of systemic aciclovir or famciclovir. This is particularly important when the ophthalmic division of the trigeminal nerve is affected. There is some evidence that early use of systemic antiviral therapy may reduce the postinfective complication of postherpetic neuralgia (Chapter 15). In the case of the oral lesions, topical treatment as for herpes simplex stomatitis (tetracycline mouthwash) is used, with the same rationale and with similar, if slower, results. Perhaps one of the most important functions of the clinician faced with a case of herpes zoster is to be aware of the possibility of corneal involvement and to place the patient under appropriate care if any symptoms, however mild, appear.

> Shingles (particularly if affecting the trigeminal nerve) should be treated as soon as possible by systemic antiviral therapy; such as aciclovir or famciclovir.

Epstein–Barr virus infection

The Epstein–Barr virus (EBV) plays a part in the pathogenesis of a number of conditions affecting the orofacial region, including infectious mononucleosis (glandular fever). The EBV is considered to be an oncogenic virus and associated with the formation of malignant lymphomas (Burkitt's lymphoma) in Africa and linked to nasopharyngeal carcinoma, particularly in southern China. The association of EBV with oral hairy leukoplakia in immunocompromised patients, particularly those with HIV infection, is discussed in the section on AIDS.

Infectious mononucleosis

This is a relatively common infection, usually manifesting symptoms in early adulthood. Children may suffer a subclinical infection. The diagnosis is confirmed by laboratory tests, which should include a blood film and differential white cell count. During the acute phases of the infection, patients produce 'atypical' mononuclear cells (Dauncy cells) and there will be a lymphocytosis. In the past, the Paul–Bunell test was used to detect the heterophile antibody in patient's serum, which agglutinates sheep erythrocytes. In most laboratories this test has been replaced by a slide agglutination test called the 'monospot'.

CLINICAL PRESENTATION

The patient with glandular fever feels ill and has a fever and enlargement of the lymph nodes that may extend over the whole of the body. The severity of these symptoms is very widely variable, ranging from a minor attack that may pass almost unnoticed to a condition requiring hospitalization.

In the early stages of this infection a sore throat and oral ulceration may be very troublesome. The ulceration is quite non-specific, but may be widespread. As in similar circumstances symptomatic treatment of the oral ulcers with antibiotic mouthwashes is the only helpful procedure. Petechiae may be visible at the junction of the hard and soft palate. Management of this condition is symptomatic but recovery can be quite protracted in severe cases.

Coxsackievirus infections

This group of viruses is divided into Coxsackie group A and group B viruses. Group A viruses are principally responsible for two infections that affect the oropharyngeal region: 'hand, foot, and mouth disease' and herpangina. These are relatively uncommon but tend to occur as mini-epidemics because they are highly contagious. The putative viruses, clinical presentation, and treatment of these infections are summarized in Table 4.13. Treatment for both these infections is symptomatic.

Hand, foot, and mouth disease

Hand, foot, and-mouth disease (not the same as 'foot and mouth disease') is caused by a Coxsackie A virus, usually type 16 but less commonly types 5 and 10. A number of minor epidemics of this condition have occurred and been described in detail, one involving students and staff at a dental hospital. The oral lesions in this outbreak consisted of small ulcers, resembling minor aphthous ulcers, relatively few in number and distributed over the oral mucosa. However, oral lesions, observed by one of the authors, also in dental hospital personnel, and confirmed by a full range of investigations, have, in fact, consisted of bullae that later ruptured to produce transiently painful erosions of the mucosa. The lesions of the hands and feet consist of a red macular rash, each macule apparently surrounding a deep-seated vesicle. The constitutional symptoms experienced are of a mild nature, a slight

Table 4.13 Clinical features of Coxsackievirus infections

Hand, foot, and mouth disease—Coxsackie A16 (others: A5, A10)
Intraoral vesicles/ulcers
Macular rash with vesiculation on
palmar surface of hands
plantar surace of feet
Malaise
Duration: 7 days
Mini-epidemics
Herpangina—Coxsackie A (most types)
Sore throat and malaise
Vesicles/ulcers on palate and pharynx
Duration: 3–5 days

malaise with minimal pain and discomfort. The symptoms resolve in about a week.

Herpangina

Herpangina is predominantly caused by Coxsackie A viruses. It is a mild infection, seen predominantly (but not entirely) in children, that tends to occur in minor epidemics. The patient complains of a moderate degree of malaise and of a sore throat, while occasionally there is also a minor degree of muscle weakness and pain. Small vesicular lesions appear in the posterior part of the mouth, in particular, on the soft palate. These lesions are not particularly characteristic of the condition, but resemble other virus-induced lesions and are recognizable only by their typical distribution. This is a self-limiting condition. The lesions fade after some 3–5 days and complications are extremely rare.

Paramyxovirus infections

Paramyxoviruses include the mumps virus and the morbillivirus that causes measles. These infections are included in this chapter because they both have orofacial manifestations.

Mumps

Mumps is characterized by bilateral swelling of the parotid glands, although unilateral glandular swelling can occur. Involvement of the submandibular gland is less common. The salivary gland ducts usually appear red and inflamed and patients occasionally report a dry mouth. Trismus may be present and the glands are extremely painful and tender to touch. Complications of mumps include pancreatitis, encephalitis, orchitis, oophoritis, and deafness. The elderly are at greater risk of developing complications. Management is symptomatic with general supportive measures (see also Chapter 8).

Mumps

- Incubation period: 14–21 days
- Transmission: respiratory secretions and saliva
- Salivary gland enlargement, usually bilateral parotid involvement
- Trismus
- Diagnosis: usually on clinical presentation

Measles

Measles usually presents as a systemic, febrile illness with an initial nasal discharge, (catarrhal stage). Koplik's spots are bluish-white, pinpoint spots, with dark-red aveolae, that appear on the buccal mucosae and disappear after 3–4 days. A maculopapular skin rash then appears but resolves after a few days—disappearance of the rash heralds recovery. In a few cases there are potentially serious complications resulting from infection with measles, including encephalitis and pneumonia. Management is symptomatic with general supportive measures. Antibiotics may be required for complications such as secondary otitis or pneumonia.

Human papillomavirus infections

There are over 100 different human papillomaviruses (HPV) and they can cause warty lesions on the skin and mucous membranes. The common wart (verruca vulgaris) is commonly seen on the skin and oral mucosa, where it is indistinguishable from a squamous cell papilloma (Chapter 9). The clinical presentation is of a 'cauliflower-like' lesion. Intraoral lesions or those affecting the lips are often the result of autoinoculation by chewing warts on the hands. Heck's disease is a rare oral manifestation of HPV infection in the mouth and is discussed in Chapter 9. Venereal warts (condyloma acuminatum) may occur in the mouth, as a result of orogenital sexual contact and appear as soft, pink papillary lesions, particularly on the palate and tongue. Cancer of the cervix has been associated with HPV infection.

Human immunodeficiency virus and AIDS

The human immunodeficiency virus (HIV) is a retrovirus responsible for the acquired immune deficiency syndrome (AIDS). The first human retrovirus, human T-cell lymphotrophic virus type I, was isolated in1980 from a patient with T-cell leukaemia. The clinical manifestations of HIV infection were first recognized in 1981. The country of origin of the virus is unknown, although there is fairly strong presumptive evidence that the initial centre of activity was in central Africa. HIV infection is, however, a rapidly expanding worldwide problem, although, quite clearly, prognostication in these circumstances is a very difficult process and there can be no degree of certainty about the many projections of future patient numbers that have been made. Transmission of the virus is currently thought to be predominantly via blood and blood products and semen. Perinatal and postnatal transmission occur in about 20 per cent of infants born to infected mothers.

The pathogenesis of disease caused by HIV infection is complex and outside the scope of this book. The most significant effect of the virus is in the infection and consequent inactivation of CD4-expressing cells, that is, the helper and delayed-type hypersensitivity T cells. Infection with the virus is a slow process, but eventually the host's immune system is functionally disabled.

A classification of the stages of HIV infection has been proposed and is shown in Table 4.14.

The management of patients with HIV infection is complex but involves antiretroviral therapy and the treatment of opportunistic infections (for example, candidosis, herpes virus infections, and *Pneumocystis carinii*) and malignancies associated with AIDS. Azidothymidine (AZT) was the first antiretroviral drug to be licenced for treating HIV and is a protease inhibitor. The prognosis for patients has improved with the introduction of multiple drug therapies. Triple therapy consists of a combination of drugs, including a protease inhibitor (for example, AZT), nucleoside reverse transcriptase inhibitors, and non-nucleoside reverse transcriptase inhibitors. The cost of these drug regimens is high and considered to be unaffordable by Third World countries. Their long-term effectiveness has yet to be proven.

Table 4.14 Classification of the stages of HIV infection*

Group	Description
I	Seroconversion illness
II	Asymptomatic
III	Persistent generalized lymphadenopathy
IVA	Constitutional disease
IVB	Neurological disease
IVC	Secondary infectious disease
IVD	Secondary cancers
IVE	Other conditions

* As proposed by the Center for Disease Control, USA.

Oral manifestations of HIV infection

The oral manifestations of HIV infection are considered to be of great significance and have been classified as two groups: group 1, lesions commonly associated with HIV infection; and group 2, lesions less commonly associated with HIV infection (Table 4.15). The most significant consideration concerns the changes that may appear in the oral cavity of a patient with HIV infection that has not, as yet, been diagnosed. The likely oral changes are dependent on the increasing reduction in immune surveillance, presenting either as infections or as neoplasms. The most likely infection is candidosis.

Table 4.15 Oral manifestations of HIV infection

Diseases strongly associated with HIV infection
Candidosis
    Erythematous
    Pseudomembranous
Hairy leukoplakia
Periodontal disease
    Linear gingival erythema
    Necrotizing ulcerative gingivitis
    Necrotizing ulcerative periodontitis
Kaposi's sarcoma
Lymphoma
Lesions less commonly associated with HIV infection
Mycobacterial infections
Melanotic pigmentation
Necrotizing (ulcerative) stomatitis
Cystic salivary gland disease
Thrombocytopenic purpura
Non-specific ulceration
Viral infections including *Herpes simplex*, *Herpes zoster*, and human papilloma virus infection

ORAL CANDIDOSIS IN HIV INFECTION

As has been pointed out previously in this chapter, oral candidal infection should always be considered as an indicator of generalized ill health and, in the case of the early AIDS patient, it may be the earliest presenting sign. Other viral, fungal, and bacterial oral infections are much less likely, but do occur. The otherwise unexplained onset of an infection, particularly when associated with other persistent signs and symptoms, such as generalized lymph node enlargement, malaise, intermittent fevers, and weight loss, should arouse suspicions. Oral candidosis has already been described in this chapter and angular cheilitis is further discussed in Chapter 6. Erythematous candidosis commonly occurs in HIV-infected individuals and affects the hard and soft palate, tongue, and buccal mucosae. Pseudomembranous candidosis is frequently chronic and angular cheilitis may also be present.

HAIRY LEUKOPLAKIA AND HIV INFECTION

'Hairy leukoplakia' has been described in a large number of patients who are HIV-infected. It occurs on the lateral margins of the tongue and has a folded, corrugated, or 'hairy' appearance and generally is asymptomatic. Although *Candida* may be associated with the lesion, it does not seem to be a 'candidal leukoplakia' or chronic hyperplastic candidosis, as described earlier in this chapter. The lesion appears to be associated with the Epstein–Barr virus (herpes, type 4), as demonstrated both by histochemical and immunological studies. It is suggested that hairy leukoplakia is a powerful clinical indicator of immunosuppression in HIV-infected patients and that it is a predictor of the eventual onset of AIDS. This does not seem to be a lesion with significant premalignant potential. No cases of malignant transformation in hairy leukoplakia have as yet been described.

PERIODONTAL DISEASE IN HIV INFECTION

Three periodontal manifestations of HIV have been described: a linear gingival erythema that appears as a red band on the marginal gingiva and is not particularly associated with poor oral hygiene; a necrotizing ulcerative gingivitis, associated with pain and spontaneous bleeding; and a necrotizing ulcerative periodontitis that is destructive and rapidly progressive.

KAPOSI'S SARCOMA

The neoplasm that is most likely to occur in the AIDS patient is Kaposi's sarcoma (Fig. 4.8). The mouth and, in particular, the mucosa of the hard palate is a common site for this lesion, which is, in fact, a form of diffuse lymphoma rather than a discrete neoplasm. The lesion is described as a pigmented, nonpainful, slightly nodular lesion of the mucosa with a characteristic histological appearance. Before the recognition of AIDS this was considered to be a rare lesion, confined to elderly patients of several restricted racial groups (Bantu, Jewish, and Italian) or to patients on immunosuppressive therapy. Its appearance in patients of other kinds is now said to be virtually pathognomonic of active AIDS. Homosexual men are considered to be more at risk from Kaposi's sarcoma than other groups with HIV infection. The herpes virus 8 (HHV-8) is now considered to have a role in the aetiology of this sarcoma.

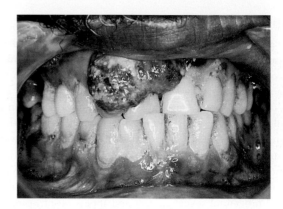

Fig. 4.8 Kaposi's sarcoma of the gingivae.

LYMPHOMA

Non-Hodgkin's lymphoma is commonly associated with HIV infection and may present as a swelling or ulcerative lesion in the mouth.

Group 2 lesions include a wide range of opportunistic infections (Table 4.12) including HPV-associated lesions that may affect the oral cavity. Swelling of the salivary glands, xerostomia (Chapter 8), and melanotic pigmentation has also been associated with HIV infection.

Discussion of problem cases

Case 4.1 Discussion

Q1   What advice would you give this lady?

The patient can be advised to use a topical antiviral preparation, such as aciclovir or penciclovir cream. This should be applied five times daily starting in the prodromal stage of the lesion, that is, when she first feels a 'tingling' or 'pricking' sensation of the lips. In resistant cases, or when the lesions recur at regular intervals, then it would be justified to prescribe a prophylactic course of systemic aciclovir (for dose, see manufacturer's data sheet). Exposure to sun appears to precipitate this lady's lesions and she should use a sunblock lip preparation with a high sun protection factor (SPF). It is advisable to remind the patient that cold sores are highly infectious and she should be careful not to share towels, cups, or cutlery with other family members. Orogenital transmission is also a risk during sexual activity.

Q2   Does the lesion on her lip pose a hazard to members of the dental team?

Herpetic whitlows were considered to be an occupational hazard for dental health-care workers, prior to the use of protective gloves, and resulted from contact with a patient presenting with a herpetic lesion on their lips. Patients who bite their nails may autoinoculate their HSV and develop a herpetic whitlow, which is extemely painful and difficult to treat.

Case 4.2 Discussion

Q1   How would you manage this patient?

You should inform the patient about his candidal infection and explain that it is important to check for an underlying cause or precipating factor. Detailed questioning about his medical history and general health is essential, with particular emphasis on recent antibiotic or steroid therapy (including steroid inhalers for asthma). There may be a family history of diabetes and the patient should be asked specific questions, relating to symptoms of diabetes. At this stage, the patient can be asked if he knows any reason why he might be susceptible to infections. He may then volunteer that he is in a risk group for HIV infection. It is not always appropriate in the dental surgery to ask patients about their lifestyle or sexuality, but the patient may wish to divulge this information. Patients should be able to discuss their medical history in privacy and it must always be considered confidential, by all dental staff.

The patient should be prescribed topical or systemic antifungals (for example, fluconazole), while awaiting the results of microbiological sampling, and a topical analgesic mouthwash to reduce oral discomfort. He should be advised to maintain his fluid intake and eat soft foods. Further investigations, including a full range of blood tests, and follow-up need to be carried out at a specialist oral medicine (or oral surgery) unit. The patient may request HIV testing but this should only be done after professional counselling—this is usually available in a department of genitourinary medicine.

Projects

1. Widespread and often inappropriate use of antibiotics has resulted in the emergence of bacteria that are resistant to therapy. It is well recognized that resistance to antibiotics is transferred from one bacterium to another. Find out about the different methods of genetic exchange in bacteria.

2. What laboratory tests are currently used for the diagnosis of HIV infection? Why is professional counselling recommended for patients prior to HIV testing?

5

Oral ulceration

Traumatic ulceration
- Aetiology
- Clinical features
- Management

Recurrent aphthous stomatitis (RAS)
- Clinical features
- Aetiology of RAS
- Histopathology and immunopathogenesis of RAS
- Systemic conditions and 'RAS-like' lesions
- Management of RAS

Behçet's disease

during the healing phase of ulceration. All traumatic ulcers should be reviewed. If they persist then a biopsy should be carried out to exclude squamous cell carcinoma.

> If a putative traumatic ulcer persists for more than 10–14 days after elimination of the aetiological factor, then the patient should be referred for a specialist opinion and possible biopsy to exclude the possibility of an oral carcinoma.

Factitious (self-inflicted) oral ulceration can also occur (see Chapter 17) and may be difficult to diagnose and manage. Psychiatric advice is required in some cases.

Recurrent aphthous stomatitis

Recurrent aphthous stomatitis (RAS) is the most common oral mucosal disease affecting humans and has been reported as affecting 20–25 per cent of the general population at any time. A higher prevalence has been reported in North American students, particularly at examination times, and in upper socio-economic groups. Interestingly, RAS is infrequently found in Bedouin Arabs.

Clinical features

The clinical features of RAS consist of recurrent bouts of one or several, shallow, ovoid, painful ulcers, occurring at intervals of a few days or up to 2–3 months. Three clinical presentations of RAS are recognized: minor recurrent aphthous stomatitis (MiRAS), major recurrent aphthous stomatitis (MjRAS); and herpetiform ulceration (HU). The clinical presentation of these types of RAS are shown in Table 5.2. Patients may sometimes present with a mixed pattern of RAS but this is relatively uncommon.

Minor recurrent aphthous stomatitis (MiRAS)

This is the most common form of RAS and approximately 80 per cent of patients have lesions of this type. It is reported that 56 per cent of the patients are females and that the peak age of onset of the ulcers is in the second decade (10–19 years). However, many patients experience their first ulcers at an age well outside these limits. Indeed, it is by no means uncommon to find this form of ulceration in much younger children.

In its most characteristic form MiRAS presents the picture of a number of small ulcers (one to five) appearing on the buccal mucosa, the labial mucosa, the floor of the mouth, or the tongue. Moreover, the ulcers are usually concentrated in the anterior part of the mouth. The pharynx and tonsillar fauces are rarely implicated in this form of ulceration. The prodromal stage of ulceration is variable, but there is usually a sensation described as 'burning' or 'pricking' for a short period before the ulcers appear. Following this phase, ulceration occurs directly by loss of the epithelium. The ulcers are usually less than 1 cm in diameter and, in most instances, their size is approximately 4 or 5 mm in diam-

Table 5.2 Clinical features of RAS

Feature	Type of RAS		
	Minor (MiRAS)	Major (MjRAS)	Herpetiform (HU)
Peak age of onset (decade)	Second	First and second	Third
Number of ulcers/bout	1–5	1–3	5–20 (up to 100)
Size of ulcers (mm)	< 10	> 10	1–2
Duration	7–14 days	2 weeks– 3 months	7–14 days
Heal with scarring	No	Yes	No*
Site	Non-keratinized mucosa especially labial/buccal mucosa. Dorsum and lateral borders of tongue	Keratinized plus non-keratinized mucosa, particularly soft palate	Non-keratinized mucosa, but particularly floor of mouth and ventral surface of tongue

* Unless a number of ulcers coalesce.

eter. However, the classification of 'minor' RAS does not depend on the dimensions of the lesions alone, but on a number of clinical features. It is quite possible to have large minor ulcers and small major ones. The appearance of the ulcer base is grey-yellow, often with a red and slightly raised margin, and, unless influenced by the site (as in the depth of the buccal sulcus where they appear elongated), they are usually oval in shape (Fig. 5.1). The ulcers are painful, particularly if the tongue is involved, and may make eating or speaking difficult. If the lips are implicated, there may be a minor degree of oedema in the surrounding area but this is not common. Lymph node enlargement is seen only as a response to secondary infection in severely affected patients. The course of these ulcers varies from a few days to a little over 2 weeks, but usually their duration is of the order of 10 days. After this period the ulcerated areas re-epithelialize and heal over in an interval of some days, but resolution may or may not be simultaneous in all the ulcers of a group. Minor aphthae heal without scar formation. Thus, if scars should form, it is probable that the condition is not MiRAS, but the major type. Following healing of the ulcers, there is a variable ulcer-free interval—3–4 weeks is most common—but many patients are able to predict with some degree of accuracy the periodicity of the condition. In a few patients, however, the recurrence of the ulcers appears to be entirely random and, in some cases, there may not be an ulcer-free period between attacks, with new aphthae developing before existing ones have healed.

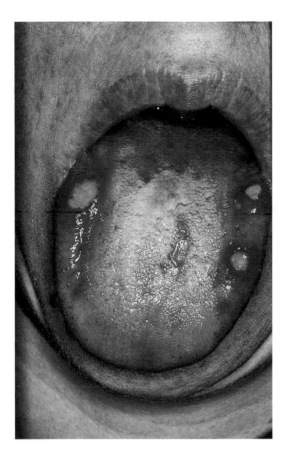

Fig. 5.1 Aphthous stomatitis (minor type) on tongue.

Major recurrent aphthous stomatitis (MjRAS)

Major RAS varies from the minor form in a number of important clinical features. The ulcers are generally larger than those of MiRAS (Fig. 5.2) and they are of greater duration, up to a period of months in some cases. As a result of the long periods of time involved, there is probably a marked tendency to the production of a heaped-up margin which, when a single ulcer is seen in isolation, may lead to the suspicion that the lesion is malignant. On eventual healing, the ulcers may leave a substantial scar and

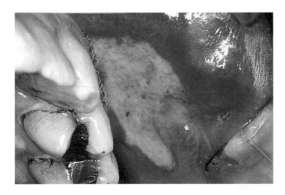

Fig. 5.2 Aphthous stomatitis (major type), on labial mucosa, of 6 weeks duration.

this, together with the tissue destruction that may occur during the active phase of ulceration, may lead to gross distortion of the involved tissues (Fig. 5.3). MjRAS may produce lesions throughout the entire oral cavity, including the soft palate and tonsillar areas, and ulceration often extends to the oropharynx (Fig. 5.4). The involvement of the posterior oral tissues is so characteristic of MjRAS as to be diagnostic, even though the ulcers may initially be small.

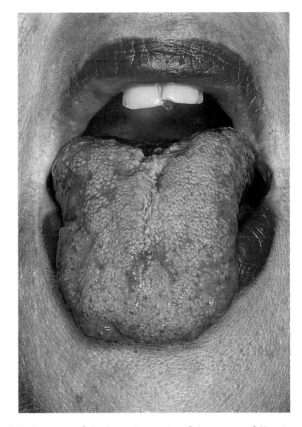

Fig. 5.3 Scarring of the lateral margin of the tongue following recurrent major aphthous stomatitis.

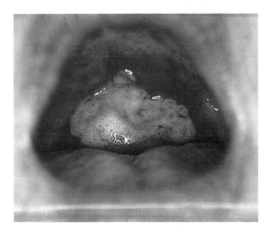

Fig. 5.4 Aphthous stomatitis (major) on the soft palate.

ulceration, it follows that the drugs exert their maximum effect at this time. With the establishment of the ulceration and the fall in sensitized lymphocyte concentration, the specific blocking effect of the steroid becomes less important, and only the anti-inflammatory action of the drug operates. For this reason it is important that the patient should understand that, whatever preparation is used, it is of maximum value at the time that the earliest prodromal signs of ulceration are noticed.

> If using a topical steroid for RAS, aim to use a preparation that is less likely to give side-effects because of systemic absorption.

The drugs most commonly adopted for local oral application in RAS are hydrocortisone hemisuccinate (as pellets of 2.5 mg) and triamcinolone acetonide (in an adhesive paste containing 0.1 per cent of the steroid). There is little risk of adrenal suppression provided that the recommended dose (four times daily) is adhered to. Little is known about the long-term effect of small dosages of topical steroid therapy in children but prescribing of these should be approached with caution, in this group of patients.

> Hydrocortisone succinate (2.5 mg) tablets (Corlan®) are dissolved four times daily in vicinity of aphthous ulcer. Start in the prodromal phase of RAS.

> Triamcinolone (Adcortyl®) in orabase paste should be applied on a moist finger to dried ulcers, four times daily. Many patients find this preparation difficult to use but it appears to be retained better, if applied at night.

In MiRAS unresponsive to these preprations and in MjRAS it may be necessary to use a more potent steroid preparation, such as a betnesol (or triamcinolone) rinse or steroid spray (see Chapter 3).

SYSTEMIC THERAPY FOR RAS

In severe cases of RAS, particularly MjRAS, it may be necessary to use some form of systemic therapy. However, all drugs have side-effects and risks that must be weighed against their benefits. Apart from prednisolone, a number of systemic drug therapies have been advocated for the treatment of MjRAS (Table 5.8) and, in some cases, Behçet's disease (see next section). Thalidomide has been used successfully for severe RAS that has failed to respond to other treatment modalities. It has also proved useful in HIV-associated oral ulceration. Thalidomide is a TNFα inhibitor that has anti-inflammatory effects. Its use is limited because of its teratogenic effects. Thalidomide must not be used for women of child-bearing age. Peripheral neuropathy is a side-effect of therapy and regular nerve conduction tests (electromyography, EMG) must be carried out. Patients should receive counselling, prior to starting drug treatment. Colchicine affects the function of polymorphs by inhibiting their migration to sites of inflammation. The use of cimetidine (H_2-receptor blocker), carbenoxolone sodium, and many other treatment modalities have also been tried for RAS (Table 5.8) with little success.

> Thalidomide can be used for severe RAS and Behçet's syndrome but patients must receive counselling. Thalidomide must not be used for women of child-bearing age. Peripheral neuropathy is a recognized side-effect of therapy and patients must have nerve conduction studies on a regular basis.

Behçet's disease

Behçet's (pronounced 'Betchet's') syndrome was first recognized in Turkey and was originally thought to be a disease of Mediterranean origin. However, a large number of cases have since been reported in Japan and other countries. Women are more commonly affected than men. Behçet's syndrome is a rare disease characterized by a classical triad of RAS (any of the three clinical variants), genital ulceration, and inflammatory eye lesions. Other manifestations include skin, joint, neurological, vascular, and intestinal disorders. Up to 90 per cent of affected patients have RAS. Genital ulcers are similar to those of the oral mucosa and healing may take place with scar formation and lead to residual tissue loss and deformity similar to that in the oral cavity. The ocular involvement initially takes the form of anterior uveitis, a superficial inflammatory lesion of the anterior part of the eye, which may become more severe in later episodes and, perhaps, progress to involve other structures of the eye. This may lead to permanent damage by scar formation or, even, to blindness.

The sequence of involvement of the oral and genital mucosa is variable, and the two may not be involved simultaneously. Indeed, there may be a considerable interval between the involvements. Ocular involvement, however, is usually late, occurring sometimes after many years of intermittent oral and genital ulceration. In the generalized form of the disease, skin lesions of various kinds may appear, the most characteristic being papules that proceed to pustule formation. It is interesting to note that in some patients with skin lesions there is a marked skin reaction to trauma. The tendency of sterile blisters to develop at venepuncture sites is known as 'pathergy', and it may be useful as a diagnostic indicator. Pathergy is less commonly reported in UK patients with Behçet's disease.

The neurological disease that may occur in these patients is the result of the appearance of centres of inflammation and necrosis within the central nervous system. The symptoms are variable, depending upon the location of the lesions, but in the early stages they may resemble those of multiple sclerosis. There is a vasculitis, perhaps complicated by thrombotic episodes, that may be either localized and minor or involve major vessels. The effect on the joints is that of a non-specific arthropathy. It has been suggested that major and minor criteria should be used to arrive at a diagnosis of Behçet's disease. The major criteria are oral ulceration, genital ulceration, eye lesions, and skin lesions. The minor criteria include lesions of the nervous system, vascular system, joints, gastrointestinal tract, and pulmonary system. However, there is no agreement

Table 5.9 Criteria for the diagnosis of Behçet's disease

RAS plus any two of:
Recurrent genital ulceration
Eye lesions (anterior uveitis, posterior uveitis, retinal vasculitis)
Skin lesions (erythema nodusum, papulopustular lesions)
Positive pathergy test (read by physician 24–48 h)

as to the number or types of lesion necessary to arrive at the diagnosis. An international working party has redefined the criteria for the diagnosis of Behçet's as the presence of RAS plus any two of: recurrent genital ulceration, eye lesions, skin lesions or a positive pathergy test (Table 5.9). It is the authors' viewpoint that, as this is a progressive condition, often beginning as RAS without any other system involvement, it is impossible at any given time to differentiate with any degree of accuracy between uncomplicated RAS and RAS that might eventually proceed to orogenital ulceration or Behçet's disease.

Management

The management of Behçet's syndrome usually requires a multidisciplinary approach. However, the local management of oral aphthae in Behçet's syndrome is exactly that for all other forms of RAS and is similarly limited in effect. Systemic therapy is therefore required in most cases and drugs used include: systemic steroids, azathioprine, cyclophosphamide, colchicine, ciclosporin, and, more recently, anti-TNFα therapy and mycophenolate. Thalidomide appears to be successful in some cases with mucocutaneous involvement but its use is restricted because of its teratogenicity and side-effects (see above).

Discussion of problem cases

Case 5.1 Discussion

Q1   How would you manage this gentleman and what therapeutic options are available?

The history and clinical examination of the ulcers in this case are consistent with major RAS. It is important specifically to enquire about genital ulceration and other symptoms, which might be suggestive of Behçets disease. The short history of ulceration is, however, suggestive of a recent precipitating cause or factor, which should be sought. It is important to establish whether the patient stopped smoking after his myocardial infarction and then developed RAS, as smoking cessation can precipitate RAS in some individuals. Stress may also have been a contributory factor. The possibility of HIV infection must also be considered, but is unlikely in this case. Oral ulceration has been reported in patients on nicorandil, a potassium-channel activator that is used for unstable angina, and it is important to rule this out as a cause of this patient's oral ulceration. (This must not be stopped before liaising with the cardiologists.) Blood tests should be arranged to check for raised inflammatory markers, haematinic deficiencies,

and anti-endomysial autoantibodies. A full biochemical and immunological profile is also advisable.

In view of the severity of the RAS and this patient's poor quality of life, some form of systemic therapy needs to be considered and the options include systemic steroids, azathioprine, ciclosporin, thalidomide, and colchicine. In the case of a young patient with a history of coronary artery disease, long-term prednisolone is contraindicated although a short, reducing course of prednisolone may give short-term relief of ulceration. RAS does, however, eventually recur after stopping the steroid. Topical analgesics may be required and an antifungal should also be considered, particularly if there is a high oral carriage rate of *Candida albicans*.

Colchicine has been reported as successful therapy for RAS and azathioprine may be worth considering, either alone or as a steroid-sparing agent. Another treatment option for this male patient is thalidomide, although this is associated with a number of significant side-effects and the patient will need counselling and close monitoring.

Q2   How would you manage this dental emergency?

There are a number of factors to be considered when arranging extraction of this man's tooth, including his medical and drug history (previous myocardial infarction, aspirin) and anxiety about dental treatment. He is probably best treated under local anaesthesia, with sedation if required. The aspirin may predispose to postextraction haemorrhage but this is unlikely to be significant and there is no indication to stop the medication. It is important to check for haemostasis after the extraction and, if necessary, suture and/or pack the socket. If the patient develops angina then he should use his glyceryl trinitrate spray sublingually. If there are more severe cardiac complications, then the patient must be treated accordingly (see Chapter 19 on 'Medical emergencies').

Case 5.2 Discussion

Q1   How would you manage the patient in your practice?

Although the patient appears fit and well, she should be questioned about any gut, eye, or skin problems and asked if she has suffered from genital ulceration. Her doctor can arrange for blood tests but it is important to diplomatically point out that these should include estimation of ferritin, folate, and B$_{12}$ levels, as a full blood count and film are insufficient. (It is important to establish a good working relationship with general medical practitioners in your area.)

If this patient's clinical examination is consistent with a diagnosis of MiRAS and there is no inclination of systemic disease, then there are a number of treatment options available that the dentist can prescribe. Analgesic rinses can be helpful, particularly before meals, and an antiseptic rinse will reduce secondary infection and aid plaque control, particularly if toothbrushing is painful. Hydrocortisone pellets can be used topically in the prodromal phase of ulceration and may speed up resolution of the ulcers.

Triamcinolone paste is difficult to apply but may be useful, if applied last thing at night. Any obvious cause of mechanical trauma due to broken teeth or dental appliances should be eliminated, in case these are precipitating the aphthous ulcers. More potent topical steroids, in the form of rinses or inhalers (see Table 5.8) may be required. In most cases, these simple measures can reduce the discomfort and duration of RAS. It does, however, need to be pointed out to this patient that there is not, at the present time, any satisfactory 'cure' for this condition and the risks of systemic therapy probably outweigh the benefits in her particular case.

Project

1. Find out which systemic drugs have been reported as causing oral ulceration, including RAS.

6

Diseases of the lips and tongue and disturbances of taste and halitosis

Diseases of the lips
- Swelling of the lips
- Angular cheilitis (angular stomatitis, cheilosis, perlèche)
- Lip fissures
- Allergic cheilitis
- Actinic cheilitis (solar keratosis)
- Exfoliative cheilitis
- Perioral dermatitis
- 'Lick eczema'
- Cheilocandidosis

Diseases of the tongue
- Developmental abnormalities and morphological variations
- Tongue fissures
- Coated tongue
- Hairy tongue
- Atrophy of the lingual epithelium
- Traumatic irritation of the tongue
- Enlargement of the foliate papillae
- Geographic tongue ('erythema migrans', benign migratory glossitis)
- Median rhomboid glossitis

Disturbances of taste and halitosis
- Disturbances of taste
- Halitosis

Inadequate dentures with
reduced vertical dimension

Skin creasing with saliva leakage and
maceration at corners of mouth

Systemic disease
or deficiency

Trauma

Host defences
compromised

Candida spp (mouth)

S. aureus (nose/mouth)

Angular cheilitis

Fig. 6.1 Factors involved in the pathogenesis of angular cheilitis. (Adapted with permission from Fig. 26.13 in Bagg, J., *et al.* (1999). *Essentials of microbiology for dental students*. Oxford University Press, Oxford.)

Angular cheilitis is a multifactorial condition with a number of local and systemic predisposing factors (Fig. 6.1).

> Angular cheilitis is a multifactorial condition with a number of local and systemic predisposing factors.

In most cases, deep folds at the angles of the mouth become traumatized as a result of continual wetting by saliva. These angular folds are the result either of anatomical configurations or, in many cases, unsatisfactory dentures, particularly those with a decreased vertical dimension. Secondary infection by *C. albicans* (Fig. 6.2), *S. aureus* (or both), and other bacteria, including B-haemolytic streptococci, follows. In some cases angular cheilitis is the result of an underlying systemic condition or deficiency that results in the host's defences, being compromised (Table 6.2). A systematic diagnostic approach must be used in these patients (Table 6.3) and management is dictated by the results of investigations (Table 6.4). Antimicrobial therapy for angular cheilitis is summarized in Table 6.5. Antifungal therapy has been fully discussed in Chapter 4.

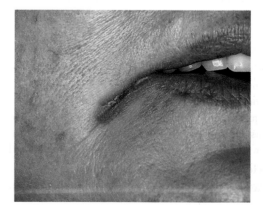

Fig. 6.2 Angular cheilitis with *Candida* present.

A few other conditions may result in a more specific form of angular cheilitis. For instance, facial eczema may present at the angles of the mouth and mimic a simple angular cheilitis. In this situation the diagnosis largely depends on the history of the

Table 6.2 Angular cheilitis as a marker of systemic disease

Anaemia
Iron, B$_{12}$, or folate deficiency
OFG (including Crohn's disease)
HIV infection
Diabetes mellitus
Sjögren's syndrome (and other causes of salivary gland hypofunction)

Table 6.3 The investigation of patients presenting with angular cheilitis

History: *key questions*
Generalized ill health?
Known systemic disease?
Xerogenic medication?
Antibiotic or steroid medication?
Social history, including tobacco use?
Ill-fitting dentures?
Dentures worn at night?
Therapeutic radiation?
Cytotoxic drugs?
Examination: *check for*
Signs of anaemia
Lymphadenopathy
Salivary gland swelling
Intraoral candidosis
Denture-induced erythematous candidosis
Commissural leukoplakia (chronic hyperplastic candidosis)
Oral dryness
Manifestations of OFG
Ill-fitting dentures/reduced vertical dimension
Special investigations
Microbiology
Sampling—technique (smear, swab, and oral rinse, if available).
Sampling—site (angles, palate, fitting-surface of denture, anterior nares)
Blood tests
Indicated if suspicion of underlying systemic factor or local therapeutic measures fail to resolve angular cheilitis
Full blood count
Serum B$_{12}$, ferritin, serum and red cell folate (or whole blood folate)
Blood glucose
Other tests
As indicated by clinical findings

Table 6.4 The management of patients with angular cheilitis

Elimination of predisposing local factors
Check dentures and denture hygiene
Instruct patient to leave out dentures at night
Referral for treatment of underlying deficiencies or systemic disease
Provision of appropriate antimicrobial therapy (topical or systemic)—as indicated by microbiology (see Table 6.5)

Table 6.5 Antimicrobial therapy for angular cheilitis*

Candida *isolated*
Intraoral†: nystatin pastilles or amphotericin lozenges (eliminate oral reservoir of infection)
Angles: nystatin ointment
S. aureus *isolated*
Angles: fusidic acid cream
Anterior nares: mupirocin cream or fusidic acid cream.
Mixed infections
Miconazole gel or cream‡

* Systemic fluconazole may be required to treat angular cheilitis resistant to topical therapy or for immunocompromised patients.

† Chlorhexidine solution has antibacterial and anticandidal activity and can be used as a rinse. Chlorhexidine may partially inhibit the action of nystatin.

‡ Miconazole can also be used if infecting micro-organisms are unknown—it has anti-staphylococcal activity. Miconazole is not the drug of choice for *Candida* infections because of variable sensitivity and possible development of azole resistance.

patient. It is unlikely that a patient would initially present with eczema affecting the angles of the mouth only. The rapid response to local steroid applications (such as 1 per cent hydrocortisone cream) helps to confirm the diagnosis. In Crohn's disease angular cheilitis is a significant diagnostic indicator when associated with other markers of the disease (Chapter 12). This is a parallel to the anal fissures seen in this condition and, similarly, responds readily to local steroid therapy.

Lip fissures

Vertical cracks in the lips are less commonly seen than angular cheilitis and the most common site is in the midline of the lower lip. Such fissures are often remarkably resistant to conservative treatment and surgical excision has been occasionally advocated for the more resistant lesions. The majority of these fissures are infected by *Staphylococcus aureus* and the most satisfactory form of treatment consists of the elimination of the secondary infection (by the use of suitable antibiotic creams) followed by the use of steroid creams. With such a regime most of these cracks can be persuaded to heal, at least temporarily. A short course of a systemic antibiotic may be required in some persistent cases—the drug of choice is indicated by culture and sensitivity of the putative bacteria. Should the predominant organism involved not be a *Staphylococcus*, but *Candida*, then the treatment should be modified suitably. The basic principle, however, of the elimination of secondary infection followed by the use of topical steroid is the one most likely to be successful. Lip cracks of this nature show a marked tendency to reoccur and a permanent cure is unlikely. Lip fissures are commonly seen in patients with Down's syndrome, together with angular cheilitis—possibly as a result of mouth breathing. Lip fissuring is also a feature of OFG (Chapter 12).

> Chronic lip fissures are often resistant to conservative treatment and may require surgical management.

Allergic cheilitis

Irritation and scaling of the lips may result from a contact allergy to a wide variety of substances, in particular, to the constituents of lipsticks. However, other topical preparations used on the lips, such as lip ointments or moisturizers, toothpastes, and, occasionally, foods, may cause an allergic cheilitis. In general, the irritation is confined to the vermilion of the lip, but may extend beyond it in an eczema-like irritation of the perioral skin. This form of contact sensitivity is often difficult to diagnose and requires detailed history taking. For instance, a lipstick allergy may be caused by the minimal amounts transferred in kissing and so may remain quite unsuspected. In some instances the irritation may follow the action of sunlight on the lips. This may not be a primary actinic reaction, but may be secondary to a photosensitizing effect of substances, such as those in lipsticks, which might in other subjects cause direct contact cheilitis. This is rather different from the actinic cheilitis that may occur in some patients who work in full sunlight for many years (see below). In the case of a simple contact cheilitis, treatment consists of tracing the sensitizing substance and eliminating it. Patch-testing may be necessary to confirm the putative allergen. Temporary relief may be given by use of topical steroids, but these should not be continued on a long-term basis.

Actinic cheilitis (solar keratosis)

In a number of predominantly male patients, long exposure to sunlight, often the result of outdoor work in a sunny climate, is followed by the onset of a cheilitis in which epithelial atypia may occur with progression to carcinoma in some cases. This is almost always most marked in the lower lip—the so-called 'lip at risk'. Crusting and induration of the vermilion margin occurs, the induration being due, in part, to a fibrotic reaction of the connective tissues (Fig. 6.3). Biopsy is necessary for a full assessment—the clinical appearance alone is an insufficient guide to the presence of worrying changes in the epithelium. If, on biopsy, significant dysplasia is found, then excision of the vermilion area by a lip shave operation or laser treatment should be considered. Chemical exfoliants can also be used.

> Prolonged exposure to sunlight, either occupational or recreational, can result in the development of an actinic cheilitis.

Exfoliative cheilitis

Exfoliative cheilitis is an uncommon condition affecting only the vermilion borders of the lips and characterized by the pro-

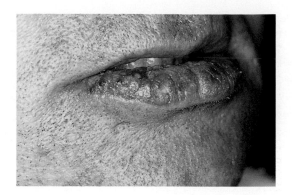

Fig. 6.3 Solar keratosis of the lower lip.

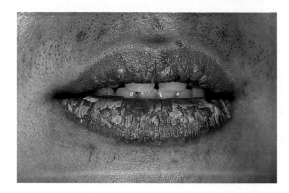

Fig. 6.4 Exfoliative cheilitis.

duction of excessive amounts of keratin. This forms brown scales that may be spontaneously shed or may be removed by the patient (Fig. 6.4). It has been suggested that this condition is exclusively seen in female patients, but several cases have recently been reported in males. The histology of the lesion is of a simple hyperparakeratosis and it is not considered to be a premalignant lesion. There is no apparent systemic background to this condition but some patients report an association with stress, the degree of keratin formation apparently increasing at times of increased anxiety. All systemic investigations in these patients prove negative and all forms of treatment have as yet proved unhelpful. Local and systemic steroids, cautery, cryosurgery, and many other forms of treatment have been attempted without success. In those with an apparent anxiety-related condition, mild tranquillization has been reported as helpful, although the mechanism for this is far from clear. Antidepressant medication has also been prescribed for a few of these cases, with some degree of success. The authors' experience with this condition is that affected individuals often appear to have a personality disorder. The extent to which there is a fictitious element involved is difficult to quantify. Most patients tend to peel off the exfoliating skin, but this could be a normal response under the circumstances. Eventually, this condition appears to resolve spontaneously but, while present, it is sufficient to cause the patient considerable distress.

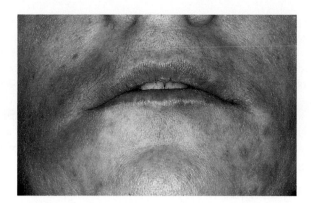

Fig. 6.5 Perioral dermatitis in a young female patient.

Perioral dermatitis

This relatively uncommon condition is often a considerable diagnostic problem and the patients are from time to time seen in the oral medicine clinic for investigation. The patients are almost always young adult females and complain of an erythematous rash on the facial skin around the mouth (Fig. 6.5). In some cases, but not all, there are papules present. In some patients there is a history of the use of steroid creams on the face, but this is not by any means invariable. Perioral dermatitis can also be due to a contact allergy (see allergic cheilitis).

The diagnosis is essentially clinical—there are no systemic changes detectable. Many of those patients with papules present respond to a long-term low-dose regime of tetracyclines, much as in acne. Paradoxically, some patients respond well to low-potency steroid creams, such as 1 per cent hydrocortisone. As in all cases where the facial skin is involved, caution must be exercised in the use of more potent steroid preparations because of the possibility of atrophic changes. In view of the wide range of presentation and reaction to therapy, it is possible that perioral dermatitis represents a reaction pattern rather than a single entity, and that more than one basic aetiological process may be involved.

'Lick eczema'

This is a further perioral condition that often causes diagnostic confusion. The patients are young—often children—and complain of a sharply delineated zone of irritable, scaly skin around the mouth. This condition, as its name implies, is simply the result of a licking habit that the patient may strongly deny, even when actually performing the licking action during the examination! The treatment is to stop the habit. If this is done, the lesion rapidly fades. Such a well-ingrained habit (of which the patient may be entirely unconscious) may, however, be difficult to eradicate. A removable appliance with a rough or sharp edge to interfere with the tongue action is often successful.

Cheilocandidosis

There have been several reported cases in which the lips become the site for a heavy candidal infection. These lesions are reported as occurring bilaterally, predominantly on the lower lip, and appear as ulcerated granular areas from which *C. albicans* can be freely cultured. This is reported to occur in generally healthy patients, but there are strong suggestions of prior local abnormality that might lead to a secondary candidal infection, for example, solar irritation in some Australian patients. In some cases the cheilitis has been associated with chronic intraoral candidosis. These lesions have been considered by several authors to represent candidal infection affecting intrinsically unstable epithelium and it is suggested that, as in chronic hyperplastic candidosis (candidal leukoplakia), early treatment by antifungals might lead to resolution, whereas delay might lead to increasing epithelial dysplasia.

Diseases of the tongue

The tongue may be involved in a wide range of oral mucosal diseases. Apart from this involvement in generalized oral conditions, several lesions are quite specific to the tongue. Many of these depend on alterations in the specialized epithelial covering of the tongue and, in particular, in the filiform papillae. These structures appear to be particularly susceptible to changes brought about by systemic abnormalities. For instance, in anaemias (in which the oral mucosa as a whole may undergo some change), the predominant oral abnormality may be of the tongue. When a lesion of any kind is present on the tongue, it may be brought rapidly to the notice of the patient because of the mobility of the organ and its rich supply of sensory nerve endings. This, however, is by no means invariably the case and there are many examples of lesions (for example, the widespread ulceration of major erosive lichen planus) in which the patient complains of far less pain than might be expected. Of greater significance is the fact that neoplasms of the tongue may grow to a considerable size before secondary infection leads to symptoms of pain (an early carcinoma of the tongue may be quite painless).

Developmental abnormalities and morphological variations

Significant developmental abnormalities of the tongue are rare. Ankyloglossia (tongue tie) is usually congenital and may be associated with microglossia. Contrary to popular opinion, there is no evidence that ankyloglossia interferes with speech, although patients may find that the restricted mobility interferes with the mechanical cleansing action of the tongue. Macroglossia can occur in a number of systemic conditions, such as congenital hypothyroidism, Down's syndrome, acromegaly, and amyloidosis.

Tongue fissures

The normal gross structure of the tongue includes fissures, which may show variation in number, depth, and arrangement. There is considerable doubt as to the extent to which the pattern of fissures may change during disease processes, although it does

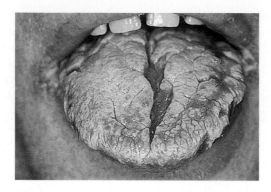

Fig. 6.6 Deep fissures of the tongue in a patient with chronic mucocutaneous candidosis.

seem that in a few conditions, for example, chronic mucocutaneous candidosis, the fissures appear so exaggerated and of such abnormal form that they must be considered as part of the pathological change (Fig. 6.6). In general, however, there is little evidence of changes in fissure pattern due to less exaggerated pathologies. There is no doubt, however, that fissures of normal form and distribution may play a part in the modification, or even the initiation, of pathological processes, since conditions of anaerobic stasis are present in the depths of these structures and present opportunities for selective bacterial growth. This being so, it is common to find superficial infections and similar conditions concentrated at and alongside the fissures. Similarly, in a situation that may lead to a sore and irritated tongue, the fissures may be the first and the most severely affected part. The use of a chlorhexidine mouthwash may be helpful for patients with a symptomatic fissured tongue.

The so-called 'scrotal tongue' is a normal morphological variant with multiple fissures on the dorsum of the tongue. The appearance of an irregular border of the tongue (often said to resemble a 'pie-crust edge') is known as a 'crenated tongue' and can be one of the features of bruxism in some patients.

Coated tongue

The tongues of all normal individuals have a coating consisting of a layer of mucus, desquamated epithelial cells, organisms, and debris. In the healthy individual the tongue is mobile, there is a rapid flow of saliva, and this coating is kept to a minimum. With the slightest disturbance to the health of the individual, however, the balance is upset and the coating may quickly become very much thicker. A lack of mobility of the tongue, which may be caused by the most minor painful lesions, a disturbance in saliva flow, an excess of tobacco or of alcohol, a gastric or respiratory upset, or a febrile condition, may result in a build-up of the tongue coating sufficient to produce a white or coloured plaque. The colour of such a coating depends on a variety of factors, such as tobacco usage and dietary habits, and is of very little diagnostic significance. Such a coating may, however, be unpleasant to

the patient and its removal may be quite difficult since very often it is firmly adherent to the tongue. Patients frequently become overly aware and self-conscious about their coated tongue and need reassurance. In a few patients their coated tongue becomes an obsession. Vigorous brushing of the tongue is often advocated and tongue scrapers are now commercially available. Use of these is sometimes found to be most unpleasant by the patient. Effervescent mouthwashes, such as those containing ascorbic acid, may be helpful, particularly if combined with brushing of the tongue.

Hairy tongue

In hairy tongue the lesion does not consist simply of a coating on the surface of the tongue but represents an elongation of the filiform papillae, often to many times their original length. With this elongation the papillae often take on a dark colour, black or brown being common (Fig. 6.7). The mechanism for the formation of these coloured hairy tongues is quite unknown, there apparently being many initiating factors. For instance, hairy tongue frequently follows a course of antibiotic therapy and may resolve quite rapidly on completion of treatment. Other hairy tongues apparently appear completely spontaneously and no cause is ever found for them. Equally doubtful is the source of the pigment involved. It is usual to relate this to pigment-producing organisms entrapped within the papillae but, in fact, no such organisms have ever been demonstrated. In the past, the presence of hairy tongue was often ascribed to candidal infection but, again, it has never been shown that there is any true association between candidosis and the production of the elongated papillae.

Treatment of hairy tongue is remarkably difficult. Those cases associated with antibiotic therapy frequently, but not invariably, resolve when the medication is finished. The use of effervescent and mucus-solvent mouthwashes may be helpful in reducing secondary irritation and thereby producing suitable conditions for the resolution of the abnormality but, again, the results are variable. The authors have used chemical cauterization, with trichloracetic acid, to treat hairy tongue, but only small areas can be managed at a time, because of discomfort afterwards. Long-term

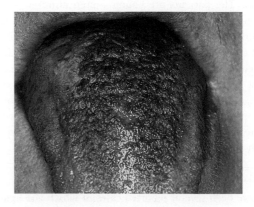

Fig. 6.7 Black hairy tongue.

results of this chemical counterization were disappointing. 'Sucking a dry peach stone' has been advocated for the management of hairy tongue but this approach does seem to be potentially hazardous! Some patients with this condition use tongue scrapers or brush their tongue vigorously but these measures are rarely effective.

Atrophy of the lingual epithelium

At the opposite extreme from the proliferation of the filiform papillae seen in hairy tongue are the atrophic changes in the papillae found in a number of generalized diseases but, in particular, in haematological and nutritional abnormalities. Atrophic change in the oral epithelium as a whole may be the consequence of a wide range of abnormalities (for instance, iron deficiency, megaloblastic anaemias, and nutritional deficiencies of various kinds). These atrophic changes are sometimes, but not invariably, found predominantly in the filiform papillae, and the surface of the tongue may become red, shiny, and painful. It is now accepted that a wide spectrum of generalized abnormalities may be responsible for the production of similar epithelial changes. Conversely, a wide range of oral signs and symptoms may occur in different patients with similar conditions. It is certainly true, however, that all patients with painful, depapillated, or reddened tongues should undergo blood tests including estimations of serum, ferritin, B_{12}, folate, and glucose to eliminate the possibility of an underlying haematinic deficiency or undiagnosed diabetes.

A sore tongue may be found in association with many generalized conditions, particularly the anaemias and salivary gland hypofunction. For instance, in rheumatoid arthritis, where there may be an anaemia of chronic disease, it is not unusual to find a sore tongue. Similarly, in Sjögren's syndrome, in which the salivary flow is reduced, the tongue may become dry, reddened, or painful (Chapter 8). There are, however, some patients in whom no cause can be found for the atrophic changes. In older patients the atrophy may be regarded as an age change, but it is not clear to what extent this may represent subclinical systemic changes. In some conditions in which depapillation of the tongue has taken place, the original morphology of the lingual epithelium may not return on healing. For instance, in major erosive lichen planus a large area of the tongue may be ulcerated. On healing, the epithelium is often virtually devoid of filiform papillae appearing as a flat, featureless tissue.

In addition to those patients in whom a recognizable pathological condition exists, there is a group, largely of older female patients, who complain of tenderness and soreness of the tongue, and who show no obvious signs to account for these symptoms. All tests may show negative results and it is tempting to classify such symptoms as being psychogenic in origin. There is no doubt that in some patients this may be so, but the possibility of habit-induced irritation must always be considered in such cases. Glossodynia and burning mouth syndrome (BMS) are considered fully in Chapter 17.

Traumatic irritation of the tongue

The mobility of the tongue makes it particularly susceptible to trauma, which may be acute (as that following the fracture of a carious tooth) or chronic (as that caused, for example, by the adoption of a habitual activity such as rubbing the tongue over the edges of the anterior teeth or a denture). The lesions produced vary greatly, from mildly erythematous patches often seen on the tip of the tongue to frank ulceration. These traumatic ulcers are often extremely painful and, although they may be evidently related to the sharp edge in question, they may show some degree of induration due to localized inflammatory changes together with whiteness of the surrounding epithelium—changes that arouse immediate suspicion of malignancy. It has been amply demonstrated, however, that superficial ulcers of the tongue, surrounded by a white margin, are virtually always benign and of traumatic origin. The easiest way to allay these suspicions is to remove the offending tooth or appliance, or to deal with it in some other suitable way in order to eliminate the trauma completely. Traumatic ulcers resolve very rapidly and virtually all trace may be expected to have disappeared within a week of removing the irritant. If this resolution has not occurred in the expected time, then the lesion must be viewed with suspicion and a biopsy taken. In the tongue, as in other areas, there is little evidence of a relationship between physical trauma and malignancy, but the possibility must obviously be considered.

More difficult to diagnose are the more chronic forms of lingual irritation resulting from habits of various kinds (for example, tongue biting). These often result in no obvious oral lesion, but frequently cause the patient a great deal of concern. In these cases it may be difficult to decide whether any systemic factor is involved in the production of the symptoms described by the patient and it may be necessary to carry out a full series of haematological investigations before coming to the conclusion that a habit is the only factor involved. In particular, there are a number of patients in whom the irritation of the tip of the tongue and, often also the lower labial mucosa, follows the most minor change in morphology of the anterior dentition, for example, by the replacement of a crown or the insertion of a replacement partial denture. Frequently, there is no discernible abnormality in the restoration to account for this. Nonetheless, it is evident from the mild erythema of both the tip of the tongue and the mucosa of the lower lip that trauma is occurring. It is often difficult to help such patients in the absence of any discernible fault in the restoration.

Enlargement of the foliate papillae

The foliate papillae appear as bilateral, pink nodules on the side of the tongue, at the junction of the anterior two-thirds and posterior third. They can become enlarged and inflamed (foliate papillitis) and cause soreness to the patient. The appearance of these may cause concern to patients, who should be adequately reassured.

Geographic tongue ('erythema migrans', benign migratory glossitis)

Depapillation of the tongue is also a marked feature of the condition usually described as geographic tongue or 'erythema migrans'. The pattern of depapillation is quite characteristic with the affected areas occurring as red patches surrounded by white borders. The patches are distributed over the surface of the tongue in a 'map-like' fashion (hence the name 'geographic tongue') and tend to vary position, apparently moving about the surface of the tongue, hence the name erythema migrans (or benign migratory glossitis) (Fig. 6.8). The appearance of the lesions may be the patient's only complaint but some patients complain of tenderness of the tongue, particularly when eating highly flavoured food. This condition often proves extremely worrying to the patient in view of its often quite spectacular appearance. The age range of the patients involved is very wide. Although geographic tongue is generally considered to be a condition affecting adults, the authors have seen patients from the age of 3 years upwards. The association of geographic tongue with psoriasis has been reported in a number of studies. A further suggested association is between geographic tongue and deep fissuring. Again, there is no clear evidence that this is other than a random association of two relatively common conditions. Erythema migrans can occur elsewhere on the oral mucosa and has been reported affecting the palate and labial mucosa.

The aetiology of erythema migrans is unknown. It is rarely associated with any underlying systemic disorder although, should there be a haematinic deficiency such as anaemia, there may be an increase in the tenderness of the tongue. Diagnosis is in general simple, being based on the characteristic appearance and behaviour of lesions, although it may sometimes be necessary to see the patient on several occasions to confirm the migratory nature of the condition. If the tongue is symptomatic, then appropriate blood tests should be carried out to eliminate any underlying haematinic deficiency. In some patients the lesions may be somewhat less defined and with a marked white border, although, in most cases, at least a small area of white demarcation may be seen. In other patients the lesions may occur in a more static manner or in a single site and this may cause confusion with a traumatic lesion. There are, however, few cases of geographic tongue that cannot eventually be diagnosed on a clinical basis alone. Biopsy is rarely necessary to confirm diagnosis, but should be considered if there is a possibility of sinister pathology. No successful treatment is known for a painful geographic tongue, but an analgesic mouthwash may provide symptomatic relief. Most patients learn to avoid foodstuffs that irritate their tongue. Some authorities have suggested the use of zinc supplements for geographic tongue but the evidence for this being efficacious is mainly anecdotal.

Median rhomboid glossitis

The tongue may be involved in candidal infection (Chapter 4). This is particularly so in the chronic infections consequent to immunological defects (such as chronic mucocutaneous candidosis) or in debilitating chronic diseases. In such cases the tongue may not only be covered by plaques of candidal pseudomembrane, but may also become deeply fissured and apparently fibrosed. It should be stressed that candidosis of the tongue, as in the oral cavity in general, may well signal underlying systemic disease, such as diabetes or iron deficiency. Lesions of superficial midline glossitis are usually seen in apparently healthy patients. These are, by definition, in the midline of the tongue in sites varying from immediately in front of the vallate papillae (where the condition is known as 'median rhomboid glossitis' because of the characteristic shape of the lesion in that site) towards the anterior dorsal surface of the tongue. Median rhomboid glossitis has for long been considered to be a developmental abnormality in some way connected with the site of the embryonic tuberculum impar. It has now been recognized that these lesions are often associated with the presence of *Candida*.

Median rhomboid glossitis appears as an area of depapillation on the dorsum of the tongue and may have a red, white, or yellow appearance (Fig. 6.9). Long-term therapy with topical antifungal agents, for example, nystatin pastilles, may be effective in reducing the size of the lesion, and recent success has been reported with systemic antifungal agents (for example, fluconazole). Not all lesions disappear fully with this treatment. Any doubt as to the nature of the condition should be resolved by biopsy and histopathological examination. In general, however, the characteristic appearance, site, and texture of the lesion is such as to enable a confident initial diagnosis to be made on clinical

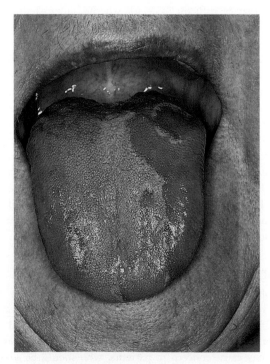

Fig. 6.8 Geographic tongue (erythema migrans).

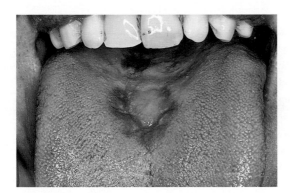

Fig. 6.9 Median glossitis.

grounds. Patients presenting with this lesion should undergo blood tests to exclude an underlying haematinic deficiency or diabetes. Median rhomboid glossitis may also be seen in patients infected with HIV.

Disturbances of taste and halitosis

Disturbances of taste

'Hypogeusia' is a reduced taste sensation and 'ageusia' is a complete loss of taste. An unpleasant or altered taste sensation is known as 'dysgeusia. Patients complaining of disturbance of taste sensation are among the most difficult to manage. There is often nothing other than the patient's own description to characterize the condition and objective tests are often not helpful. Physiological tests to determine the patient's ability to differentiate the basic taste sensations of sweet, sour, bitter, and salt may be done, but these in themselves may give little information, since the sense of taste as a whole depends on a mixture of associations of taste and scent.

Disturbances of taste

Dysgeusia—unpleasant or altered taste sensation
Ageusia—complete loss of taste
Hypogeusia—reduced taste sensation

True neurological disturbance of the sense of taste is extremely rare, but may occur in some generalized abnormalities of the central nervous system. A somewhat more common (although still rare) neurological disturbance is that due to surgical trauma to the chorda tympani following operations on the middle ear. If the nerve is disturbed, either during operation or by postoperative oedema, an area of taste disturbance may develop on the side of the tongue corresponding to the terminal distribution of the chorda tympani with the lingual nerve. In a few patients with Bell's palsy (Chapter 15) there is a similar loss of taste sensation due to involvement of the chorda tympani on the affected side.

Medication can affect taste, and drugs commonly implicated include the antirheumatic (for example, allopurinol and phenylbutazone) and antimetabolite (for example, methotrexate) drugs. Penicillamine and captopril (an angiotensin-converting enzyme (ACE) inhibitor) have been reported as causing taste disorders. Metronidazole can also cause an unpleasant taste. Any drugs causing xerostomia can also indirectly affect taste perception.

The most common cause of a disturbance of taste sensation or of a foul taste in the mouth is the presence of a pyogenic infection, most usually the result of periodontal disease, infection in the nose or sinuses, or a discharge from a lesion such as an infected dental cyst. An infective focus may be very difficult to detect, particularly when present in a relatively inaccessible area such as a salivary gland. The clinical examination of such a patient should always include a careful search for pus-contaminated saliva from any of the major salivary glands as well as radiographic assessment for the presence of possible intrabony infected lesions, sinusitis, and similar possible infective foci. Clearly, such patients are suffering not from a true disturbance of taste sensation, but from the chronic imposition of unpleasantly tasting material into the oral cavity.

Table 6.6 lists some conditions that may give rise to alterations or loss of taste. Anosmia (absence of smell) can either be transient due to upper respiratory tract infections or permanent as a result of tearing of the olfactory nerve following maxillofacial or head injuries and will result in some diminution of taste. The underlying cause for the alteration in taste may be elicited from the patient's history and examination of the oral cavity, but it is advisable to check for zinc deficiency.

Patients with evidence of cranial nerve deficits or reporting neurological symptoms should be sent for specialist evaluation

Table 6.6 Conditions associated with alterations in taste

Dental conditions	*Systemic disease*
Periodontal diseases	Uraemia
Carious lesions	Neurological disorders (e.g. Bell's
Discharging dental sinus	palsy, brain tumours, damage to
Restorations with marginal	chorda tympani)
deficiencies	Anaemia
Dry socket	
	Deficiencies
Associated structures	e.g. zinc
Salivary glands	
• Salivary gland hypofuction	*Drugs*
• Sialadenitis	ACE inhibitors, lithium salts, gold,
Sinuses	carbimazole, metronidazole,
• Sinusitis	penicillamine, xerogenic drugs
Lungs	
• Respiratory disease	*Smoking*
Stomach	
• Gastro-oesophageal	*Psychogenic*
reflux disorder	Oral dysaesthesia
	Psychosis (delusions, hypochondriasis)

and appropriate imaging. When all such examinations have been performed, there remains a group of patients in whom no abnormality of any kind is detected, but who continue to complain of an unpleasant taste. These patients are often obsessional, but it is very difficult to determine whether this is the cause or the consequence of their complaint (see Chapter 17). Alterations in taste can be one of the symptoms of oral dysaesthesia. Some of the most difficult patients to treat among those with disturbances of taste sensation are those who are wearing relatively recently acquired dentures. Few taste buds are covered by the denture and the olfactory nerve endings are in no way affected but, nonetheless, some such patients complain of an abnormality or even complete loss of taste sensation. The explanations for this are not convincing, but it would seem that variations in texture between the uncovered palate and the denture may play a part.

The dentist's responsibility in such cases as those described above is to eliminate, by detailed examination, any of the local causes. The patient may then need to be referred appropriately to eliminate non-orodental causes. If this examination is negative and if all concerned are sure that there is no nasal or similar aetiology, then there is little point in attempting treatment. Mouthwashes may occasionally help but, in general, the patient who is obsessionally concerned with a persistent taste is completely resistant to local treatment.

Halitosis

A closely related problem is that of halitosis—bad breath. This may occur in the healthy, or in those with significant oral or generalized disease. It is often a transient problem, but, if not, warrants investigation. The causes of halitosis may be divided into local (Table 6.7), systemic (Table 6.8), and drug-induced (Table 6.9) causes. Patients who smoke or eat a great deal of garlic and highly spiced foods will have a characteristic odour on their breath. Local causes of halitosis include poor oral hygiene, chronic periodontal or dental disease, and ear, nose, and throat (ENT) problems, such as sinusitis or chronic tonsillitis (Table 6.7). Systemic disease, as in renal or hepatic failure, respiratory disease, and uncontrolled diabetes leading to ketosis, is a rare cause of halitosis but should be considered (Table 6.8). Some drugs are reported as causing halitosis (Table 6.9). The most common drug-induced form of halitosis is probably that due to the lack of oral hygiene resulting from iatrogenic dry mouth (discussed in Chapter 8).

The problem of delusional halitosis is further discussed in Chapter 17.

Discussion of problem cases

Case 6.1 Discussion

Q1 How would you manage this case?

The history is suggestive of erythema migrans (geographic tongue). Examination of the tongue will confirm the diagnosis and exclude other pathological conditions.

Table 6.7 Local causes of halitosis

Mouth
Poor oral hygiene
Food packing and stagnation
Chronic periodontal disease
Acute necrotizing ulcerative gingivitis
Dry socket
Pericoronitis
Chronic dental sepsis
Infections
Malignant tumours
Haemorrhage
Nose and pharynx
Pharyngitis
Tonsillitis
Sinusitis (postnasal drip)
Malignant tumours
Foreign bodies

Table 6.8 Systemic diseases causing halitosis

Lower respiratory tract infections
Diabetic ketoacidosis
Kidney failure
Liver failure
Febrile illness (dehydration)

Table 6.9 Drugs that may produce halitosis

Paraldehyde
Isosorbide dinitrate
Disulfiram
Alcohol
Cytotoxic drugs (indirectly)
Xerogenic drugs (indirectly)

The recent history of increasing soreness suggests a possible underlying factor, such as anaemia, due to iron deficiency—particularly in view of her reported tiredness. This girl should be asked further questions about her general health, including any gastrointestinal symptoms and drug history. Signs of iron deficiency anaemia include pallor of the mucous membranes, angular cheilitis, aphthous stomatitis, glossitis, oral candidosis, and koilonychia.

Blood tests should be undertaken including a full blood count (FBC), serum B_{12}, red cell and serum folate, and serum ferritin estimations. It may also be worthwhile to carry out a serum zinc assay. Iron deficiency anaemia in a female student with no obvious gastrointestinal disease is most likely to be due to excess menstrual loss and/or poor diet. The 'geographic tongue' can be treated symptomatically with an analgesic rinse (for example, benzydamine) and avoidance of 'irritating' foods. Any haematinic deficiency should be investigated and appropriately managed.

Case 6.2 Discussion

Q1   What advice would you give to this girl's mother?

Q2   What other factors must be considered when providing dental treatment for a patient with Down's syndrome?

Enlargement of the tongue (macroglossia) is a well recognized feature of Down's syndrome. The tongue may become ulcerated as a result of occlusal trauma. An enlarged tongue and constant dribbling may predispose to the development of angular cheilitis in Down's syndrome, particularly if there is mouth breathing. Microbiological sampling should be carried out and an appropriate antimicrobial agent applied. *Staphylococcus aureus* is commonly isolated from lip fissures, which may respond to topical fucidin with the addition of a low-potency steroid preparation. Nasal carriage of *S. aureus* needs to be addressed, if reinfection is to be avoided. Persistent lip fissures often require surgical excision, although cryosurgery has also been advocated. When considering elective surgical intervention in a patient with Down's syndrome, a risk assessment should be undertaken in relation to anaesthesia and susceptibility to infective endocarditis (see below).

There are a number of factors that need to be considered when providing dental treatment for patients with Down's syndrome. Congenital cardiac anomalies are present in about 40 per cent of infants with Down's syndrome but most can be successfully corrected by surgery. Antibiotic prophylaxis may, therefore, be needed for dental procedures likely to create a bacteraemia. Other potential problems for the dentist include increased susceptibility to infection and periodontal disease. There may be reduced cooperation and understanding of the need for oral hygiene, but the majority of patients with Down's syndrome can be successfully treated in routine dental practice. The carriage rate of hepatitis B is reportedly higher in patients who are institutionalized.

Case 6.3 Discussion

Q1   How would you manage this case?

Q2   What is the differential diagnosis of the lip condition?

The most likely diagnosis of this patient's chronic lip condition is actinic cheilitis due to sunlight damage, as a result of his outdoor occupation. Solar UVB radiation is most damaging and responsible for premalignant and ageing damage. It is important to check the face, scalp, and other exposed skin for actinic keratoses, particularly in fair-haired individuals. Other conditions to be considered in the differential diagnosis are lichen planus and lupus erythematosus. An allergic cheilitis is also possible but less likely unless it is superimposed on an already sun-damaged lip. Biopsy is essential and management depends on the histopathology and degree of epithelial dysplasia.

Actinic cheilitis is considered to be a premalignant condition and can transform into squamous cell carcinoma, which can be quite aggressive compared to others at this site. In cases where there is significant dysplasia but no frank carcinoma, one form of treatment is a vermilionectomy, in which the vermilion border is completely excised and the labial mucosa advanced to join the skin. Laser ablation can also produce good cosmetic results with fewer postoperative complications. Chemical exfoliation with 5-fluorouracil can be used but sometimes causes quite significant discomfort and inflammation until healing takes place. All patients with actinic cheilitis or evidence of sun-damage elsewhere on the skin must be given advice about sun avoidance (if possible) and the use of sunscreens (lip salves or creams) with a high sun protection factor. Older men in particular can be encouraged to wear a hat outdoors, especially if they have thinning hair or are bald. Patients diagnosed with actinic cheilitis should be followed up on a regular basis.

Project

1. There is a wide range of mouthwashes commercially available for the management of halitosis (bad breath). What are the constituents of these preparations? Is there any evidence that they are effective in treating halitosis?

7

Swellings of the face and neck

Facial swellings
- Differential diagnosis

Swellings in the neck

Cervical lymphadenopathy
- Differential diagnosis
- Examination of the lymph nodes
- Inflammatory causes
- Neoplastic causes of lymph node enlargement

Swellings of the face and neck

Problem case

Case 7.1

A 65-year-old man attends your surgery for the provision of new dentures. The patient has smoked (30 cigarettes per day) since he was a teenager. When questioning this gentleman about his medical history you notice that he has a 'croaky' voice. He reports a 2-month history of increasing hoarseness. On examination you can palpate a hard, fixed, nontender jugulo-omohyoid lymph node.

Q1 What other questions would you ask this gentleman?

Q2 How would you manage this case?

Facial swelling

Differential diagnosis

Although dental infections are by far the most common cause of swellings about the face seen by the dental surgeon, there are many other possibilities that must be considered in a differential diagnosis. These include facial swellings due to allergy or angioedema (often misdiagnosed as a purely dental problem) and the swellings in oral Crohn's disease (orofacial granulomatosis), which are equally susceptible to a mistaken initial diagnosis. Similarly, facial swelling due to infections of non-odontogenic origin—such as that, for instance, in acute sialadenitis—is commonly assumed to be of dental origin. Masseteric hypertrophy can give rise to some diagnostic problems in patients presenting with facial swelling and is discussed in Chapter 16 ('Temporomandibular disorders').

There are a large number of conditions, both localized and generalized, that can cause facial swelling (Table 7.1). Some of these conditions are considered elsewhere in this book. Readers are, however, advised to consult textbooks of pathology, medicine, and surgery for details of other conditions.

Swellings in the neck

Cervical swellings generally present either at the side or the middle of the neck and their differential diagnosis is outlined in Table 7.2. Cervical lymphadenopathy will be discussed in more detail.

Table 7.1 A 'surgical sieve' for the differential diagnosis of facial swelling

Congenital (e.g. lymphangioma, haemangioma)
Infectious
Orodental infections
Salivary gland infections (Chapter 8)
Cutaneous infections
Neoplastic
Sarcomas
Carcinoma (Chapter 10)
Traumatic
Post-injury
Postoperative
Surgical emphysema
Immunological
Allergic
Hereditary (Chapter 14)
Endocrine and metabolic (Chapters 13 and 18)
Cushing's syndrome
Acromegaly
Myxoedema
Nephrotic syndrome
Others, e.g.;
Orofacial granulomatosis (Chapter 12)
Idiopathic or drug-induced angioedema (Chapter 14)
Corticosteroid therapy (Chapter 3)
Masseteric hypertrophy (Chapter 16)

Cervical lymphadenopathy

Differential diagnosis

Normal lymph nodes are not palpable. Enlargement of a node or a change in texture, so that it may be palpated through the skin, indicates that it is either the primary site of a pathological process (for example, lymphoma) or secondarily involved (for example, in an infective or neoplastic process elsewhere in the body). Differentiation between these two situations is important. The

Table 7.2 The differential diagnosis of swellings in the neck

Side of neck

Cervical lymphadenopathy

Salivary gland enlargement (Chapter 8)

Actinomycosis

Carotid body tumours

Branchial cyst

Pharyngeal pouch

Cystic hygroma

Middle of the neck

Thyroid enlargement (multinodular goitre—neoplasia, ectopic)

Thyroglossal cyst

Dermoid cyst

'Plunging' ranula

Ludwig's angina

Table 7.3 Cervical lymphadenopathy: important infective and neoplastic causes

Infective causes

Lymphadenitis

   Orodental

   Antral

   Tonsillar

   Aural

   Nasopharyngeal

   Scalp

   Facial

Tuberculosis

Brucellosis

Infectious mononucleosis (glandular fever)

HIV infection

Toxoplasmosis (cat scratch fever)

Syphilis

Neoplastic causes

Lymphoma

Leukaemia

Secondary neoplasia

vast majority of cervical lymph node enlargements are due to either infection or neoplasia (Table 7.3). However, lymph nodes can be enlarged in some connective tissue disorders (for example, sarcoidosis) and (rarely) as a side-effect of drug therapy (for example, phenytoin).

Examination of lymph nodes

Lymph nodes may be examined by palpation, ultrasound-guided fine needle aspiration (USG-FNA) and appropriate imaging techniques. Histopathological examination of an excised node is only indicated in specific situations, such as occult primary head and neck tumours and lymphoma.

When examining the lymph nodes of the head and neck (Fig. 7.1), each of the main groups must be palpated in turn, using a systematic approach. From a position behind the patient, the pre-auricular, parotid, facial, submandibular, submental, deep, cervical (upper, mid, and lower), supraclavicular, posterior triangle, and occipital groups of nodes are palpated in turn on each side. When examining the cervical nodes it is helpful to relax the surrounding tissue by bending the patient's head forward and laterally towards the side examined. If a palpable node is found, its texture is noted and it is moved between two fingers to discover any attachment to skin or underlying tissue.

In addition to a detailed extra- and intraoral examination, the examiner should check the skin of the scalp, face, and neck. Plain radiographs of the hard tissues may be required to identify any odontogenic inflammation related to the patient's dentition. Secondary neoplasms in bone usually present as an ill-defined radiolucency. If there are no foci of infection or evidence of mucosal lesions responsible for the cervical lymphadenopathy, then the patient should be referred to a maxillofacial (or ENT) surgeon for further examination of the ear, nose, and throat. Flexible nasoendoscopy or rigid oesophagolaryngoscopy may be required, together with specialized imaging techniques such as MRI and ultrasonography (see Chapter 2).

Inflammatory causes

Acute infections

Lymphadenitis arising from an acute infection such as a periapical abscess or a pericoronitis is usually unilateral. The appearance of the nodes is rapid, and they are soft and are painful when touched. There may be oedema of the soft tissue surrounding the nodes giving the visual impression of greater enlargement than is, in fact, the case. The facial lymph node, lying just anterior to the anterior border of masseter at the level of the occlusal plane, is commonly involved in children.

Chronic lymphadenitis

In chronic infections the affected nodes are firm but may not be tender. In tuberculosis the involved nodes become attached to the skin and this produces the so-called 'collar stud abscess'. In long-standing cases of chronic infection, calcification of a node may present as a solitary hard, nonfixed swelling. More widespread smaller calcifications in the cervical nodes are more common. They are usually discovered incidentally during radiography, are asymptomatic, and cannot be palpated. Widespread lymph node enlargement may be the first clinical sign of infection with the HIV virus—the submandibular nodes are often prominently affected (Chapter 4).

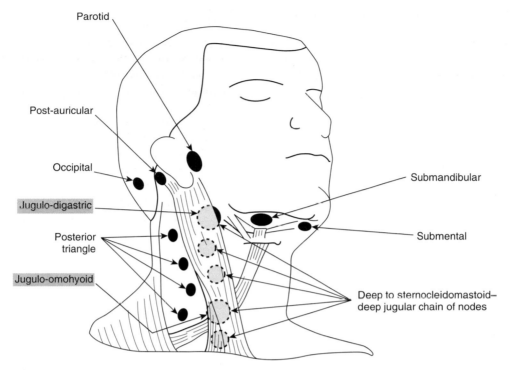

Fig. 7.1 Principal groups of lymph nodes in the head and neck.

Neoplastic causes of lymph node enlargement

Lymphoma

The lymph nodes of the neck are often involved early in lymphomas, both of the Hodgkin's and non-Hodgkin's types. Affected nodes are initially discrete, rubbery in consistency, and painless. Diagnosis is by histopathological examination. Burkitt's lymphoma more commonly arises as a central lesion of the jaws, although the cervical lymph nodes may be affected first in a few patients.

Leukaemia

The orofacial manifestations of leukaemia are fully discussed in Chapter 13. Patients with an underlying diagnosis of leukaemia rarely present with a neck mass. It is, however, important to appreciate that dental infections and non-odontogenic infections commonly occur in leukaemic patients and give rise to either facial swelling and/or cervical lymphadenopathy.

Secondary neoplasia

Spread to lymph nodes of the neck may occur at any stage in the growth of a malignant neoplasm of the oral cavity, pharynx, antrum, or adjacent structures. The nodes are initially painless, hard, and usually unilateral. The presence of painless enlarged lymph nodes tends to be more suggestive of a pathological process other than infection. 'Troisier's sign' is the presence of a left supraclavicular node in the presence of gastric cancer—so-called because as a physician it was the first sign that caused him to suspect his own gastric carcinoma.

Discussion of problem case

Case 7.1 Discussion

Q1   What other questions would you ask this gentleman?

Persistent hoarseness is highly suggestive of malignant disease of the larynx and must be excluded, as a matter of urgency. The hard, fixed jugulo-omohyoid lymph node is a particularly worrying feature and suggestive of metastatic spread. The patient should be specifically asked about other symptoms, such as difficulty swallowing (dysphagia) or breathing (dyspnoea), dry cough, earache, haemoptysis (coughing up blood), and weight loss.

Q1   How would you manage this case?

It is important to examine the mouth and oropharynx for obvious mucosal lesions. The patient should be immediately referred for further investigation by an ENT or head and neck surgeon. A direct referral can be faxed to the hospital unit concerned or arranged by the patient's doctor, who should also be telephoned. It is essential to check that your referral has been received as administrative errors are always possible.

Squamous cell carcinoma of the larynx is multifactorial but consumption of tobacco and alcohol are recognized as risk factors. In the European Union, carcinoma of the larynx is in the top 10 most common malignancies for males. Other causes of persistent hoarseness include chronic laryngitis due to inflammatory conditions or vocal fatigue (overuse), vocal cord paralysis, and, less commonly, syphilis, tuberculosis, hypothyroidism, myaesthenia gravis, and functional dysphasia. Benign tumours rarely cause hoarseness.

Project

1. Magnetic resonance imaging (MRI) and ultasonography are techniques that can be used to investigate soft-tissue swellings in the head and neck. What are the indications, comparative advantages, and disadvantages of these two techniques?

8

Salivary glands and saliva

Saliva and the salivary glands
- Saliva
- The salivary glands

Assessment of the salivary glands
- Examination
- Measurement of salivary flow
- Salivary gland imaging
- Sialochemistry
- Biopsy

Salivary gland disease
- Sialadenitis
- Sialosis
- Necrotizing sialometaplasia
- Sarcoidosis
- HIV-associated salivary gland disease
- Salivary gland tumours

Disturbances of salivary flow
- Xerostomia
- Sjögren's syndrome
- Excessive saliva

Salivary glands and saliva

Problem cases

Case 8.1

A 48-year-old male attends for a 6-month review appointment at your practice. On updating his medical history you learn that he is about to start a course of external beam radiotherapy for tonsillar carcinoma.

Q1 What advice would you give to this patient concerning his future oral health?

Case 8.2

A 55-yearold female presents to your practice for routine review. She reports xerostomia. On examination you notice that she has a dry oral mucosa. New carious lesions, on the proximal surfaces of previously sound lower incisors, have developed since her last visit.

Q1 What questions would you ask this lady?

Q2 What advice would you give?

Q3 What is the most frequent cause of xerostomia?

Case 8.3

A 45-year-old male patient presents to your practice and complains that over the past month he has been experiencing pain and swelling under his tongue and lower jaw—on the left side. The pain and swelling is worse just before eating and improves considerably after a meal.

Q1 What further questions would you ask this patient?

Q2 Clinically how would you examine this patient?

Q3 How would you manage him?

Q4 Is this patient likely to complain of a dry mouth?

Saliva and the salivary glands

A number of conditions affecting the salivary glands are managed surgically. These include cysts and neoplasms arising in the glands and also conditions arising as a result of the presence of calculi or other obstructions in the glands or ducts. However, with the elimination of these two groups of important salivary gland diseases there remains a number of conditions that should be considered within the scope of oral medicine. This chapter will consider sialadenitis, sialosis, necrotizing sialometaplasia, and disturbances in salivary flow rate. The clinician should be cognizant with the functions of saliva and the anatomy of the salivary glands. This information is helpful in understanding the nature of the investigations required to study salivary gland disease, their ensuing sequelae, and the therapies available.

Saliva

Saliva is a glandular secretion that is essential for the maintenance of healthy orodental tissues. Saliva is a complex fluid and many of the functions of saliva have a protective role, some of which are shown in Table 8.1. The physical properties of saliva vary according to the different types of salivary glands, with parotid secretions having a serous (watery) consistency. The submandibular and sublingual glands secrete a more viscous saliva due to their higher glycoprotein content. A severe reduction in salivary flow rate can have devastating consequences on oral health and, subsequently, on the psychological and social well-being of the sufferer.

Table 8.1 Functions of saliva

Function	Description
Lubricant	Coats and protects the mucosa against mechanical, thermal, and chemical irritation
Cleanses the teeth	Clears food from the oral cavity and oral mucosa
Ion reservoir	Facilitates remineralization of the teeth
Buffer	Neutralizes plaque pH after eating
Antimicrobial	Secretory immunoglobulins, enzymes, and other salivary proteins help regulate the oral flora
Pellicle formation	A protective layer of salivary protein that forms over enamel acts as a diffusion barrier
Digestion	Salivary amylase initiates the digestion of starch
Facilitates taste	Saliva is a solvent and therefore allows the interaction of foodstuff with taste buds
Water balance	Dehydration causes a reduction in salivary flow rate with an associated oral dryness; this should stimulate a need to increase fluid intake

- Saliva is important for the maintenance of oral health.
- A diminution of salivary flow can have a detrimental impact on the quality of life of a patient.

The composition of saliva is affected by a number of factors, including the type of salivary gland. The majority of amylase is produced by the parotid glands but the blood group substances are secreted mainly by the minor mucous glands. The unstimulated flow rate is more important than the stimulated flow rate for oral comfort. However, the stimulated flow rate is important to facilitate chewing and swallowing during mastication. The submandibular gland contributes approximately 65 per cent of the resting whole salivary flow rate. Only 15–20 per cent is derived from the parotid, with the sublingual and minor glands both delivering 7–8 per cent. In contrast, the parotid provides 45–50 per cent of the stimulated whole salivary flow rate. Salivary flow rates exhibit diurnal variation with an average unstimulated flow rate throughout the day of approximately 0.3 ml/minute—in sleep this may fall to 0.1 ml/minute. Many textbooks mention that approximately 1500 ml of saliva is produced each day. More recently, however, it has been suggested that this figure is an overestimation of total daily salivary flow rate, and a daily flow rate of 500–600 ml/day may be a more realistic estimate. The breakdown of salivary flow over a 24-hour period is shown in Table 8.2.

The salivary glands

The parotid glands are the largest salivary glands. They are wedge-shaped and situated in front of the ear and behind the ramus of the mandible. The apex of the wedge is the deepest part of the gland. The peripheral branches of the facial nerve (CN VII) are intimately associated with the parotid gland. This relationship is inadvertently demonstrated when an inferior dental nerve anaesthetic block is administered incorrectly, and causes a temporary drooping of the upper eye lid.

Parotid saliva is transferred along the parotid duct into the oral cavity. The thick-walled parotid duct (Stenson's duct) emerges at the anterior border of the parotid gland and runs over the surface of the masseter before hooking medially over the anterior muscle border. The orifice of the duct is covered by a small flap of mucosa called the parotid papilla and this is situated opposite the maxillary second permanent molar.

The two submandibular glands are approximately half the size of the parotids. The superficial part of the submandibular gland

Table 8.2 Salivary flow over a 24-hour period

Sleep
40 ml saliva will be produced over 7 hours
Awake
300 ml of unstimulated saliva over 16 hours
200 ml of stimulated saliva during meals—over 54 minutes

is wedged between the body of the mandible and the mylohyoid muscle, with the smaller deep part hooking around the posterior border of the muscle to lie on the floor of the mouth—above the mylohyoid. The submandibular (Wharton's) duct runs forward, along the floor of the mouth to open into the subligual papilla, just lateral to the lingual frenum. The secretions are a mixture of serous and mucous fluids.

The sublingual glands are the smallest of the three pairs of salivary glands and are located just below the floor of the mouth beneath the sublingual folds of mucous membrane. There are numerous sublingual ducts that open into the mouth along the sublingual folds. The secretions of these glands are predominantly mucous.

The minor salivary glands consist of numerous small mucosal glands situated on the tongue, palate, buccal and labial mucosa. They produce primarily a mucous secretion.

Assessment of the salivary glands

Examination

The parotid glands, lying partially concealed by the ascending ramus of the mandible, are not particularly easy to palpate. Tenderness and swelling are best detected by standing in front of the patient and by placing two or three fingers over the posterior border of the ascending ramus of the mandible. Backwards and inwards movement of the fingers with light pressure is almost always all that is needed to detect tenderness in the superficial part of the parotid. This manoeuvre is necessary to differentiate parotid tenderness from that of the temporomandibular joint or the masseter with which it is often confused. It must also be remembered that the painful signs resulting from temporomandibular joint/muscle dysfunction may extend to the upper pole of the parotid with which the joint is in close anatomical relationship. Swelling of a parotid gland may also be visualized by standing behind the patient who is seated in a reclined dental chair. When examining a parotid gland the duct papilla must also be examined intraorally for signs of inflammatory change. Parotid saliva can be visualized by lightly compressing the skin overlying the duct with the fingers. If the cheek is held retracted, the saliva expressed by this manoeuvre will be seen coursing downwards over the buccal mucosa from the duct papilla. It is helpful for the clinician to know that parotid saliva can expressed, but this method is not of value in quantitatively assessing the parotid flow rate of saliva.

The submandibular gland may be felt below the angle and body of the mandible, this simple palpation being reinforced by bimanual palpation with a finger in the floor of the mouth, gentle pressure being exerted between the examining hand (below the mandible) and the finger. As in the case of the parotid gland, the submandibular (Wharton's) duct should be observed for signs of inflammation and a subjective assessment made of the quality of the saliva. It is similarly difficult to specify the 'normal' palpation features of the submandibular gland. In some entirely normal individuals it is possible to palpate the gland, while in others it is not.

Measurement of salivary flow

Sialometry

Salivary flow rate is measured by sialometry and either resting (unstimulated/basal) or stimulated saliva may be collected. Whole saliva, representing contributions from all the salivary glands or secretions from individual major glands, can be measured. For example, a Carlson–Crittenden collector (a small cup placed over the orifice of the parotid gland duct) can be used to collect saliva from the parotid gland. The parotid or submandibular ducts can also be cannulated to measure flow rates. These techniques are relatively invasive and make measurement of unstimulated flow rates unreliable for individual glands. Stimulated whole saliva can be collected and measured by a variety of volumetric and gravimetric techniques. Sialometry should be measured under standardized conditions. Consideration must be given to the time of day, the type of stimulant used, and the pre-collection instructions, for example, asking the patient to refrain from smoking, drinking, and eating for a defined period. Despite the measurement of whole salivary flow rates being a relatively simple and non-invasive approach, it is not usually undertaken in general dental practice. Sialometry is probably most beneficial for the longitudinal assessment of flow rates for individual patients as there is considerable variation within the population.

A wide range of flow rates have been quoted for both basal and stimulated saliva in the general population, but it has been shown that changes in salivary flow are probably more important indicators of salivary function than a single flow rate measurement. Volunteers given atropine reported that a dry mouth developed when their resting flow fell to about 50 per cent of their normal flow rate. The normal rate of flow of unstimulated whole saliva is approximately 0.3 ml/minute and for stimulated whole saliva 1–2 ml/minute. Stimulated saliva is mainly secreted in response to masticatory and gustatory stimuli and the flow rate will rise significantly (4–6 ml/minute) when chewing a powerful sialogogue.

Salivary gland imaging

Plain radiography

Calculi can sometimes be seen on plain films, but it should be remembered that not all calculi are radio-opaque. When investigating a suspected salivary calculus, two views should be taken at 90°. For the parotid gland, a panoramic or oblique lateral view can be combined with rotated anterior–posterior or posterior–anterior view. For the submandibular gland, panoramic and lower occlusal views (true and oblique) are appropriate. In the interest of radiation dose reduction, it is advisable to take a sectional panoramic film where possible for these patients, limited just to the symptomatic side.

Sialography

Sialography is an imaging technique used to demonstrate the ductal system of the parotid or submandibular gland. A water-soluble radio-opaque contrast medium is injected into the duct orifice and 'post contrast' radiographs are then taken in two different planes. Following the removal of the cannula, a final 'drainage' film is usually taken to assess the clearance of the contrast medium. This gives some idea of the gland function and will often highlight an obstruction within the ductal system. Traditionally, sialography was carried out using an oil-based contrast medium, but this could cause problems if extravasated outside the ductal system and it could also damage the gland in patients with little or no salivary flow rate. Water-soluble, preferably non-ionic, contrast media are now used routinely in most centres.

> Sialography demonstrates a major salivary gland in three phases:
> * preoperatively
> * the filling phase
> * the emptying phase

Sialography is helpful in demonstrating structural abnormalities of the duct system. Strictures of the submandibular gland and duct dilatations are clearly seen. When there is atrophy of the salivary acini, an extravasation of contrast medium will be evident in the body of the gland (sialectasis). In Sjögren's syndrome there is sometimes a characteristic 'snowstorm' appearance (punctate sialectasis).

Sialography should not be undertaken in the presence of acute infection or when a calculus is known to be close to the duct opening. There is a risk that the contrast medium may displace the calculus further into the duct.

Suspected 'mass' lesions within the salivary glands should not be investigated with sialography as such lesions cannot be seen directly. Displacement of the ductal system, giving the 'ball in hand' appearance, may suggest the presence of such a lesion, but this pattern is not always seen and may result in lesions being missed. Patients with discrete masses within the salivary glands should be sent for ultrasound and possibly a magnetic resonance imaging (MRI) scan.

Scintigraphy (radioisotope imaging)

Salivary glands, in common with the thyroid, have the ability to concentrate certain radioisotopes. In salivary scintiscanning labelled technetium pertechnetate ($^{99}Tc^m$) is frequently used because it has a shorter half-life than iodine. An intravenous injection of the radioisotope is followed by scanning of the salivary glands at intervals of 30 seconds. Salivary gland function is then assessed with computer-assisted quantitative programmes. The rate of concentration of the isotope in the glands is plotted and, after 30 minutes, salivary secretory activity is stimulated by dropping citric acid solution on the tongue. The resulting activity of the glands is again followed by scanning at intervals of

30 seconds. Time–activity profiles of the glands are thereby produced and can build up a full picture of salivary secretory activity (Figs 8.1 and 8.2). This procedure measures gland uptake of the radioisotope and gives an indication of its clearance. The clin-ician can visualize and compare the activity of all the major salivary glands. Scintigraphy is therefore beneficial for comparing the function of a diseased gland (as in a localized chronic sialadenitis) with the remaining healthy glands or to detect a generalized loss of glandular function (as seen in Sjögren's syndrome). Scintigraphy provides no information about salivary gland anatomy.

> Scintigraphy is used to assess salivary gland function in salivary gland diseases such as Sjögren's syndrome.

Ultrasonography

Ultrasound may be used for superficial soft-tissue swellings and the initial investigation of suspected mass lesions. Ultrasound is particularly useful for differentiating between solid and cystic lesions but the sound waves are blocked by bone. Ultrasound may be used in cases of chronic infection where sialography is contraindicated and may identify the presence of sialectasis or of a calculus, though subtle changes are difficult to see.

Magnetic resonance imaging

MRI is used to investigate space-occupying lesions such as salivary gland tumours. However, only limited information is given on adjacent hard tissues. This technique provides good soft-tissue detail and localization of masses—the facial nerve is usually identifiable. Imaging techniques are discussed more fully in Chapter 2.

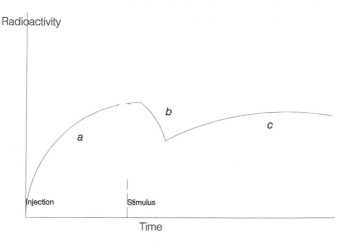

Fig. 8.1 Time–activity curve of normal salivary gland during scintiscanning—see text for details of the procedure. Part a of the curve represents the initial isotope uptake and part b the response to stimulus—the wash-out effect. Part c shows continuing slow uptake which reaches a maximum and then declines.

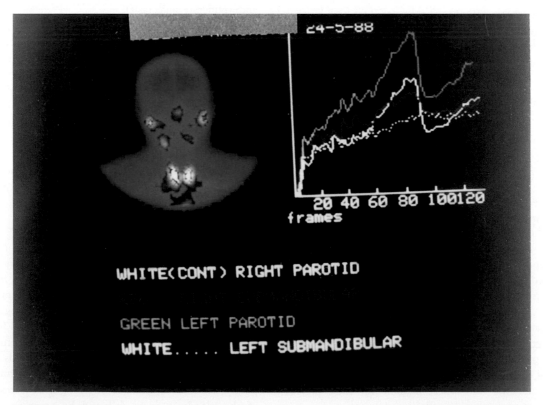

Fig. 8.2 The computer screen during a scintiscan of a patient with poor uptake and response to stimulus of the left submandibular gland.

Table 8.3 Clinical conditions in which saliva may play a diagnostic role

Monitoring	Condition
Blood groups	Useful in forensic medicine
Drug levels	Lithium, methadone, digoxin
Detection of drugs	Alcohol, amphetamines, benzodiazepines, opioids
Hormones	Cortisol, testosterone
Antibody detection	HIV infection, measles, mumps, rubella

Sialochemistry

The measurement of the biochemical constituents of saliva has been undertaken for many diseases of the salivary glands; however the results are frequently misleading or difficult to interpret. Sialochemistry is not routinely used for diagnostic purposes but it remains a potentially useful research tool. It can also be of value in measuring drug, antibody, and hormone levels. Table 8.3 identifies some conditions in which the use of saliva can contribute to the diagnosis.

Biopsy

Open biopsy of a major salivary gland can be hazardous and is best avoided. Parotid gland biopsy carries a risk of facial scarring, damage to the facial nerve, or the establishment of a salivary fistula. It is common practice to assess the histopathology of the salivary glands by an intraoral biopsy of the minor glands, notably the labial glands. Fine needle aspiration (see Chapter 2) of the major salivary glands may be undertaken.

Labial gland biopsy

This entails making a small incision inside the lower lip, through normal mucosa, under local anaesthesia and harvesting a number of small mucosal glands for histopathological analysis. This biopsy is particularly useful in establishing a diagnosis of Sjögren's syndrome, and the pathological changes mirror the focal lymphocytic sialadenitis that occurs in the major glands in this condition. The patient should always be warned of the possibility of localized lip parasthesia (or anaesthesia) following biopsy of the labial glands. This is a well recognized postoperative complication.

Salivary gland disease

Sialadenitis

Sialadenitis is the term used to describe inflammation of salivary glands, most commonly the result of viral or bacterial infection, but occasionally due to other causes (for example, allergic reactions, irradiation). Bacterial sialadenitis is usually a secondary consequence of either a localized or systemic cause of reduced salivary flow and is rarely the primary pathological process. Viral infections, however, frequently affect previously normal salivary glands. Generally speaking, sialadenitis is a clinical problem affecting the major salivary glands. However, it may also occur in minor salivary glands, either as a primary phenomenon (as in Sjögren's syndrome) or as a secondary feature of some other condition such as pipe-smoker's palate, in which the palatal salivary glands often become inflamed and enlarged (see Chapter 9).

Of the viral infections of the salivary glands by far the most common is mumps, which most commonly affects the parotid glands but also from time to time involves the other major glands. The mumps virus (an RNA paramyxovirus) is transmitted by direct contact or by droplet infection, and a clinical infection is heralded by a feeling of malaise and often by abdominal pain. The saliva of patients developing mumps is infectious for several days before parotitis develops and for approximately 2 weeks after the presentation of clinical symptoms. Following this, there is swelling of one or both parotid glands, sometimes associated with a swelling of the submandibular glands. In many cases, one of the parotid glands is by far the more severely affected. With the swelling of the gland there is pain and tenderness together with a general malaise and a fever. Patients often have trismus. The swelling of the salivary gland is at its maximum within 1 or 2 days of the onset of symptoms and is followed by a gradual resolution over 1 or 2 weeks. Mumps often occurs in minor epidemic form and is usually recognized on clinical symptoms alone. Rarely, confirmation may be obtained by antibody measurements. Treatment of mumps is entirely symptomatic, with the use of antipyretics, simple analgesics, ample fluid intake, and rest. Isolation is important since the disease is very contagious. Mumps is also discussed in Chapter 4.

A well-established complication of mumps is the onset of orchitis or oophoritis—occasionally sterility may ensue. These conditions are caused, not by direct viral infection, but by the production of autoantibodies directed against the tissues of the reproductive organs. After an attack of mumps, immunity is usually complete and, therefore, a recurrent swelling of the parotid region is not likely to be due to a recurrence of mumps. It should be remembered, however, that, rarely, salivary gland infections may be caused by other viruses, including cytomegalovirus and Coxsackieviruses. The widespread use of immunization against mumps will result in a fall in incidence.

> Sialadenitis can:
> - be chronic or acute
> - affect the minor or major salivary glands
> - have a systemic or local aetiology
> - have an infective or non-infective aetiology

A reduction in salivary gland flow rate, either from a localized or systemic cause, is a predisposing factor in acute sialadenitis. As has been pointed out, bacterial infection of the salivary glands is commonly secondary to an obstructive condition such as calculus formation or duct stricture; it is therefore a localized condition. This being so, it is evident that a single gland is normally affected. Most often this is a parotid gland. The reduced salivary flow predisposes the gland to an ascending infection from bacteria within the oral cavity. In this condition the gland is painful, tender, and swollen, and pain is radiated to the ear and the temporal area. Intraorally, the duct of the affected gland may be seen to be swollen and reddened, and the duct papilla enlarged. Purulent saliva may be milked from the duct by manual pressure. When pus can be expressed from the duct it should be sent for culture and sensitivity testing. In the absence of sensitivity tests, flucloxacillin is the antimicrobial of choice in the patient who is not sensitive to penicillin. There will often be an associated lymphadenopathy of the cervical nodes.

Sjögren's syndrome is a predisposing factor for bacterial infections, both acute and chronic. In patients in whom ill health has led to lowered resistance, ascending infection of any of the salivary glands may occur from the mouth via a salivary gland duct. This, once a common sequel to gastrointestinal surgery, especially in older patients, is now not so often seen due to improved perioperative care. In these cases the treatment is evidently nonsurgical, being dependent on antibiotic therapy, the maintenance of a correct fluid balance, and, if possible, the resolution of the predisposing condition.

Treatment of an acute parotitis tends to be somewhat protracted. Bacterial swabs should be taken and antibiotic sensitivities determined whenever possible. It is clear, however, that the use of antibiotics should be regarded only as first-line treatment. Any predisposing factor must be identified. It is possible that surgical treatment may be necessary, such as removal of a duct calculus or, occasionally, the excision of a severely damaged gland.

Chronic sialadenitis, either of the parotid or the submandibular glands, may follow the resolution of an acute infection or may occur without any evident primary acute phase. In these circumstances symptoms are relatively low-grade with tenderness and a minor degree of swelling of the affected gland, and occasionally with some degree of swelling and redness of the duct and the papilla. As in acute sialadenitis, purulent saliva may be expressed from the duct. Frequently in these cases, minor dilatations of the ductal system of the glands may be detected on sialography and, presumably, these provide foci of infection and stagnation. Such a recurrent chronic sialadenitis may occur following radiotherapy affecting the glands or may follow the minor damage due to the presence of a calculus. The principles of treatment are exactly the same as those of acute sialadenitis. In the patient with recurrent sialadenitis of a submandibular gland, excision of the gland might be required. Table 8.4 summarizes the main causes of sialadenitis.

Sialosis

Sialosis (sialadenosis) implies a painless, non-inflammatory, non-neoplastic swelling of the salivary glands. There are many precipitating factors for this condition, including the effect of antirheumatic drugs, drugs containing iodine, and adrenergic

Table 8.4 Causes of sialadenitis

Bacterial
Ascending sialadenitis
Recurrent parotitis of childhood
Viral
Mumps
HIV
Cytomegalovirus
Sjögren's syndrome
Irradiation

drugs. Similar experimental sialosis may be stimulated in animal models by the administration of isoprenaline. On the whole these drug-induced enlargements are reversible, although, in some cases, acute sialadenitis has been reported following withdrawal of the drug. Sialosis may also occur in hormonal abnormalities (diabetes mellitus, acromegaly) and in nutritional deficiency states, including anorexia nervosa and chronic alcoholism. The parotid glands are most frequently affected, and the swelling is commonly bilateral. The mechanism involved is not understood, but, histologically, there is hypertrophy of serous acini. Investigation of patients with possible sialosis should include the identification of predisposing causes. Thus, liver function tests and tests for blood glucose and growth hormone may be indicated. A detailed drug history should be recorded and the possibility of eating disorders considered (Chapter 17). Appropriate imaging should be undertaken. However, biopsy is rarely indicated.

Necrotizing sialometaplasia

This relatively uncommon, 'tumour-like' condition occurs more frequently in males, especially smokers, and is of unknown aetiology. It appears to be the result of a vasculitic phenomenon that occurs in minor salivary glands, usually in the palate. It is possible that ischaemia leads to infarction of salivary tissue. The consequence is relatively painless ulceration of rapid onset. The margins are often everted and may be indurated, resembling a carcinoma. Anaesthesia of the palatal mucosa has been reported as an early indicator of this form of ulceration. Histologically, the squamous metaplasia found in the salivary ducts, together with pseudo-epitheliomatous hyperplasia of the surrounding palatal epithelium, may give an incorrect impression of malignancy. This is a self-limiting condition that resolves in about 8 weeks time without anything other than symptomatic treatment. Lesions of necrotizing sialometaplasia are often excised for diagnostic purposes. As yet, there is no real information about the immediate cause of this condition or of its implications in relation to systemic factors.

Sarcoidosis

Sarcoidosis is a chronic granulomatous disorder that may rarely present as painless, persistent enlargement of the major salivary

Table 8.5 Causes of salivary gland swelling

Infective	Drug-associated
Bacterial	Alcohol
Ascending sialadenitis	Iodine compounds
Recurrent parotitis of childhood	Thiouracil
Viral	Sulfonamides
Mumps	Phenothiazines
HIV parotitis	Chlorhexidine
Inflammatory	*Endocrine*
Obstructive sialadenitis	Acromegaly
Sjögren's syndrome	Diabetes
Sarcoidosis	*Metabolic*
Sialosis	Alcoholic cirrhosis
Neoplasms	Malnutrition
Pleomorphic salivary adenoma	*Others*
Adenolymphoma	Sarcoidosis
Mucoepidermoid carcinoma	Necrotizing sialometaplasia
Acinic cell carcinoma	
Adenoid cystic carcinoma, etc.	

Table 8.6 Classification of salivary tumours*

Adenomas	Carcinomas
Pleomorphic adenoma	Mucoepidermoid carcinoma
Warthin's tumour (adenolymphoma)	Acinic cell carcinoma
Basal cell adenoma	Adenoid cystic carcinoma
Oncocytoma	Carcinoma arising in pleomorphic adenoma
Canalicular adenoma	Polymorphous low-grade adenocarcinoma
Ductal papillomas	Other carcinomas

* Source: Soames, J.V. and Southam, J.C. (1988). *Oral pathology*, 3rd edn. Oxford University Press, Oxford.

glands. There is often an associated reduction in salivary flow and there may be an accompanying 'Sjögren's-like' condition. Sarcoidosis is described more fully in Chapter 12.

HIV–associated salivary gland disease

Patients with HIV infection can develop salivary gland problems and xerostomia. The salivary gland swelling may be due to a 'Sjögren's-like' condition with lymphocytic infiltration and a dry mouth. However, there may be other pathology present in the salivary gland such as Kaposi's sarcoma or a lymphoma. It is also possible that salivary gland swelling may be a consequence of other viral infections such as cytomegalovirus or Epstein–Barr virus (Chapter 4). Chronic parotitis in children is highly suggestive of HIV infection.

Salivary gland tumours

Salivary gland tumours compromise about 3 per cent of all tumours. The majority occur in the parotid glands and only 10 per cent affect the minor salivary glands. There is a great variety of salivary gland tumours and in 1991 the WHO proposed a classification and nomenclature for these (see Table 8.6 for summary).

The clinical presentation, histopathological features, and management of these salivary gland tumours is outside the scope of this book, and readers are advised to consult other reference sources (see the project at the end of chapter).

Tumours affecting the minor salivary glands will be briefly discussed, as these present intraorally. Since the greatest concentration of these glands is in the area of the junction of the hard and soft palates, this is the region in which these neoplasms are most often seen. About 20 per cent of minor salivary gland tumours occur in the upper lip. The majority of these lesions are pleomorphic adenomas but more aggressive lesions such as adenocystic carcinomas may occur.

> Ten per cent of all salivary gland tumours affect the minor salivary glands. The majority of these are pleomorphic adenomas occurring in the palate.

Clinical features

The growth of pleomorphic adenomas is usually slow and painless and ulceration is unusual unless there has been some degree of trauma. The texture of such a tumour is usually firm and the overlying mucosa may appear virtually normal (Fig. 8.3).

The outstanding characteristic of these growths is their unpredictability, both in histological appearance and in clinical behaviour. More aggressive growth may occur in some tumours with ulceration of the underlying mucosa. These features must be considered as possible markers of a malignant lesion such as an adenocystic carcinoma, which may result in death, both by local tissue invasion and the production of distant metastases. The only clue as to the probable eventual behaviour of a salivary neoplasm is from the histological examination of tissue, and this must form the basis of the surgical treatment of the lesion.

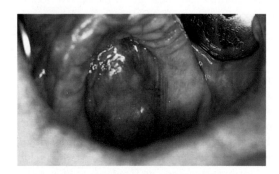

Fig. 8.3 A large pleomorphic adenoma of the palate.

Salivary gland tumours, because of their often slow and painless growth, are often very deceptive, and lack of complaint from the patient may produce a quite unwarranted sense of security. Any suspected salivary tumour should be referred at once for investigation and treatment without any attempt at minor surgical intervention, which might make later definitive treatment difficult. Most pleomorphic adenomas affecting the minor salivary glands are excised with a margin of surrounding normal tissue.

> Any suspected salivary gland tumour should be referred for investigation and treatment without any attempt at minor surgical intervention, which might make later definitive treatment difficult.

Disturbances of salivary flow

Xerostomia

Xerostomia is the subjective feeling of oral dryness, which may or may not be associated with hypofunction of the salivary glands. A lack of saliva may be due to either a loss of secretory tissue in the salivary glands, or a disturbance in the secretory innervation mechanism brought about by the action of xerogenic drugs or, much less commonly, by neurological disease. A significant proportion of patients complaining of xerostomia are found, after investigations, to have some systemic factor responsible for the reduction in salivary function. These systemic factors may be associated with a wide range of disease processes (such as renal and endocrine disturbances) but many of these patients suffer from Sjögren's syndrome; this will be discussed in more detail below. The causes of xerostomia are summarized in Table 8.7.

> Xerostomia is a symptom that should be investigated because it may be indicative of underlying systemic disease.

Therapeutic radiation to the head and neck region, for the treatment of malignancy, can also cause a marked diminution in salivary flow and severe oral dryness. Patients treated by whole-body radiation (for example, prior to bone marrow transplantation for leukaemia) and those given radioactive iodine (I^{131}) for thyroid cancer can also suffer from xerostomia. Early diminution of salivary flow due to radiation may be due to damage to the blood supply of the glands, but later effects are the result of destruction of the gland's secretory apparatus.

Neurological disease, either central or peripheral, may be responsible for a decrease in the secretomotor stimulation of the salivary gland and, hence, the dryness of the mouth. However, the most common cause for this is the action of drugs with the site of action being either central or in the autonomic pathway. Groups of drugs implicated as having this kind of action include antihistamines, antihypertensives, and sedatives. However, the more common ones to cause xerostomia are the psychotropic drugs and,

Table 8.7 Causes of xerostomia

Developmental
Aplasia or atresia
Salivary gland disease
Sjögren's syndrome (primary, secondary)
Sarcoidosis
HIV infection
Iatrogenic
Drug-induced
Therapeutic irradiation (e.g. external beam radiotherapy, total body irradiation
Graft-versus-host disease
Psychogenic
Oral dysaesthesia
Burning mouth syndrome
Anxiety/depression
Dehydration
Febrile illness
Diabetes mellitus
Diabetes insipidus
Renal failure
Diarrhoea
Alcohol
May cause salivary gland disease, liver disease, and dehydration
Local
Mouth-breathing

in particular, the antidepressants and tranquillizers. Over 400 drugs have been identified as having the potential to cause varying degrees of oral dryness, and the effects may be potentiated in patients taking multiple xerogenic drugs. Drug-related oral dryness should be a reversible side-effect, with resolution occurring following cessation of the drug.

Commonly used drugs that cause xerostomia

Antidepressants	Tranquillizers and hypnotics
Antihistamines	Antipsychotics
Decongestants	Diuretics
Antiparkinsonian agents	Appetite suppressants

Salivary hypofunction can also be due to an underlying cognitive disorder, such as depression or chronic anxiety. The ability of acute anxiety to cause a transient reduction in salivary flow is well known to students taking examinations and those engaged in public speaking. Patients with a sensory or cognitive disorder may also have a perception of oral dryness, but objective measurements of salivary flow may be normal and the mouth apparently moist. These individuals frequently complain of other symptoms, such as a bad taste and abnormal sensations in the mouth. Xerostomia is frequently reported by patients with burning mouth syndrome.

There are conflicting reports on the effect of age on salivary gland function, but there is some evidence that stimulated salivary flow rates are unimpaired with age in healthy, unmedicated individuals. Unstimulated whole salivary flow rates, however, have been shown to decrease with age in healthy non-medicated subjects. Age, in addition to drugs and disease, is important in reducing the secretion of resting whole saliva. Iatrogenic causes and systemic disease are risk factors for xerostomia that are more likely to be encountered in the middle-aged or elderly population.

Investigation of xerostomia

Symptoms of a dry mouth include thirst, difficulty in eating dry foods and swallowing, difficulty in speaking and wearing dentures, and the need to take frequent sips of water while eating. Patients may also complain of a burning sensation in the mouth and abnormal taste or halitosis—frequently they report cracked lips or soreness at the corners of the mouth. The questions listed in Table 8.8 are frequently helpful in identifying patients with oral dysfunction associated with a reduced salivary flow. Orofacial signs and symptoms associated with salivary gland hypofunction are given in Table 8.9.

Clinical signs associated with salivary gland hypofunction include dryness of the oral mucosa (which often appears like parchment), fissuring and lobulation of the tongue (Fig. 8.4), and evidence of oral candidosis, particularly in the form of

Table 8.8 Questionnaire to identify patients with salivary gland hypofunction

1. Does the amount of saliva in your mouth feel too little, too much or do you not notice it?
2. Does your mouth feel dry when you eat a meal?
3. Do you frequently sip liquids when you eat a meal?
4. Do you have difficulties swallowing any foods?

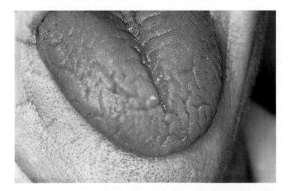

Fig. 8.4 A dry and somewhat lobulated tongue associated with xerostomia.

Table 8.9 Signs and symptoms suggestive of salivary gland hypofunction

Symptoms reported
Oral dryness
Burning, tingling sensation of tongue
The need for frequent drinks to be taken whilst eating or talking
Difficulty in chewing and swallowing dry foods
Altered taste (dysguesia) and smell
Recurrent salivary gland swellings/infections
Increase in rate of dental decay
Dry, sore, cracked lips and angles of mouth
Difficulty in talking (dysphonia)
Generalized mucosal soreness and ulceration of denture-bearing areas
Oral examination reveals
Swollen salivary glands
Absence of salivary film over oral mucosa
Dry, paper-thin 'parchment' appearance of oral mucosa or appearance of small amounts of frothy saliva in an otherwise dry mouth
Fissuring and lobulation of the tongue
Dry, cracked lips, angular cheilitis
Evidence of chronic oral candidosis
Development of new carious lesions, especially on incisal or cuspal surfaces

angular cheilitis. The saliva may appear stringy and thick and tends to accumulate as small beads on the mucosa. There may be difficulty in 'milking' saliva from the major ducts and there is often dental caries at sites not usually susceptible to decay. The salivary glands may also be swollen, either due to chronic infection or involvement in an autoimmune sialadenitis (Figs 8.5 and 8.6).

Salivary gland hypofunction increases a patient's susceptibility to: • caries   • candidosis, including angular cheilitis   • oral mucositis

Management of xerostomia and salivary hypofunction

Management depends on the underlying cause of the xerostomia and the degree of salivary gland impairment. Patients who have detectable salivary function can be encouraged to use some form of local stimulation, for example, chewing sugar-free gum or sugar-free pastilles. The antibacterial properties possessed by xylitol, which is often used as a sweetener in sugar-free gums, may have a significant additional anti-caries effect. Dentate patients must be discouraged from using sugar-containing or acidic sweets as these can exacerbate the tendency to demineralization of the teeth and cause dental caries. Systemic medication to stimulate salivary flow has been assessed in a number of clinical trials and, to date, pilocarpine seems to have been the most effective drug tested. However, such stimulating therapy is of little use if the xerostomia is due to near total loss of secretory units in the salivary glands. Pilocarpine also has disadvantages: it has a number of interactions with other drugs and may have adverse effects on the cardiovascular system. Minor side-effects such as sweating and the urge to urinate have been reported by patients taking systemic pilocarpine and are due to its cholinergic agonist activity.

Symptomatic relief of dry mouth

Intrinsic (increase gland activity)
- sugar-free gum,
- pilocarpine

Extrinsic
- saliva substitutes

The use of saliva substitutes may be of some help to patients complaining of a dry mouth and can be offered to provide symptomatic relief for patients who have insufficient salivary function to benefit from stimulation. A large number of different 'artificial salivas' are now commercially produced, and most are based on carboxymethylcellulose or mucins. If porcine mucin preparations are preferred by the clinician, care must be taken not to prescribe them to vegetarians and various religious groups. A number of preparations contain fluoride and this could be beneficial as a protective measure against caries. Clinical trials have indicated that artificial salivas can be useful for the management of xerostomia but patients frequently discontinue their use. Either they do not like the taste or consistency or find that frequent application is required, making use inconvenient and expensive. Many patients prefer to take frequent sips of water from a small container carried around with them. The use of sugar-free pastilles may sometimes be more helpful than sprays in a social setting. Cracking and drying of the lips can be controlled by a petroleum-based ointment such as Vaseline, and angular cheilitis is treated according to the micro-organisms cultured. Oral candidosis can usually be controlled with topical antifungal agents. Dentate patients require regular dental inspections, which may need to be at intervals of 3 months or less. Advice should be given about maintenance of oral hygiene, avoidance of sugary foods, and use of fluoride supplements. The use of astringent mouthwashes, especially those that contain alcohol, are best avoided. Fluoride-containing gels may be tolerated more successfully by patients with salivary gland hypofunction. They often last longer and this may render them more cost-effective. It is often difficult for patients to alter their diet which tends to be severely restricted to bland, soft foodstuffs. Many foods are too astringent and hard foods can traumatize the fragile oral mucosa. Nevertheless, individual dietary analysis is advisable for patients who have a high caries incidence.

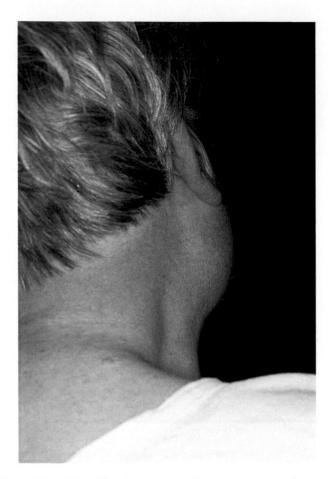

Fig. 8.5 Parotid swelling in a patient with autoimmune sialadenitis.

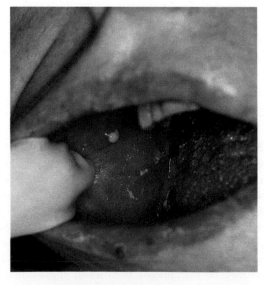

Fig. 8.6 Pus expressed from the parotid duct—the result of infection secondary to autoimmune sialadenitis as part of Sjögren's syndrome.

Chewing sugar-free gum:

- increases the flow of stimulated saliva to levels about 3 to 10 times resting values
- can help prevent caries: stimulated saliva has enhanced buffering capacity and a greater remineralizing potential than resting saliva
- will increase the resting salivary flow rate for up to 30 minutes beyond the period of chewing
- has an antimicrobial activity if it contains xylitol
- may be problematic in patients with hiatus hernia or gastric and intestinal ulcerations

Patients who complain of xerostomia, but have no clinical or objective evidence of a dry mouth, often have other oral symptoms suggestive of oral dysaesthesia and many complain of a burning sensation in the mouth. These patients can best be managed by counselling, including psychotherapy if appropriate. Psychotropic medication, particularly the use of tricyclic medication, is best avoided as it may exacerbate xerostomia. This subject is further discussed in Chapter 17.

Sjögren's syndrome

Sjögren's syndrome (SS) is an autoimmune disease of the exocrine glands that particularly involves the salivary and lacrimal glands. Traditionally, the symptoms of Sjögren's syndrome were thought to result from the destruction of salivary and lacrimal gland tissue. More recently, it has become clear that this is not the case and that many Sjögren's syndrome sufferers have substantial reserves of histologically normal acinar tissue that simply does not function properly. Re-evaluation of Sjögren's syndrome in this light gives a much more optimistic outlook for treatment development. Whereas there can be no possibility of recovery if the acinar cells have been destroyed, reversal of acinar cell hypofunction may be attainable if the cause of the hypofunction can be determined.

- Primary Sjögren's syndrome consists of dry eyes (xerophthalmia) and dry mouth and is not associated with a connective tissue disease
- Secondary Sjögren's syndrome consists of dry eyes and dry mouth and is associated with a connective tissue disease, most commonly rheumatoid arthritis
- Systemic lupus erythematosus, systemic sclerosis, primary biliary cirrhosis, and mixed connective tissue disease may also be associated with secondary Sjögren's syndrome

This process may occur as an isolated phenomenon, in which case it is termed primary Sjögren's syndrome (1°SS), or in conjunction with a connective tissue or collagen disease, in which case it is referred to as secondary Sjögren's syndrome (2°SS). The prevalence of this syndrome is unknown and it is thought that many cases remain undiagnosed. Recent data has suggested that the estimated prevalence of SS is between 1–3 per cent of the UK population. Middle-aged and elderly women are mainly affected and present with a complaint of dry mouth (xerostomia) and dry eyes (xerophthalmia), with or without evidence of a connective tissue disease. In patients with secondary SS, rheumatoid arthritis is the most commonly associated condition. Other associated diseases include systemic lupus erythematosus, primary biliary cirrhosis, and systemic sclerosis. In common with many autoimmune diseases SS shows a sexual dimorphism with a female to male ratio of approximately 9 to 1. Xerostomia is often severe in primary SS, but some studies suggest that it is less marked in secondary SS. A history of salivary gland swelling is common and is either due to infiltration of the gland by lymphoepithelial tissue or to recurrent infections (Figs 8.5 and 8.6). Swellings due to the replacement of salivary gland tissue do not tend to be painful. Salivary gland swellings of an infective nature are painful, and there is an associated local or systemic rise in temperature and pus may be expressed from the duct orifice (Fig. 8.6). Xerophthalmia (dry eyes) is the most common complaint but many sufferers also complain of 'itching' or 'grittiness' in the eyes or give a history of recurrent eye infections. This can give rise to keratoconjunctivitis sicca. Untreated, this can eventually lead to corneal damage and loss of sight. Patients with SS may also complain of a dry skin or vaginal dryness.

The early detection of Sjögren's syndrome can prevent serious ocular disease.

The assessment and management of patients with salivary gland enlargement continues to be a problem in the Sjögren's patients. Persistent glandular swelling in these individuals is a worrying feature as they have an increased risk of developing non-Hodgkin's lymphomas. These are often low-grade B-cell lymphomas and appear to be similar to lymphomas that develop in other mucosa-associated lymphoid tissue (MALT). Low-grade B-cell lymphomas of other MALT sites (MALTomas) include those of stomach. thyroid, and lung. Salivary gland imaging techniques, including CT and MR, can provide important diagnostic information but biopsy is indicated in some cases. Histopathology of enlarged salivary glands (particularly parotids) in SS usually reveals a benign lymphoepithelial lesion, but this is not always the case. Major gland biopsy is, however, not indicated for routine diagnostic evaluation of SS. Clinical signs, such as a rapid and progressive unilateral or asymmetrical gland enlargement or/and a change in the consistency of the gland from a soft swelling to a hard or nodular one, should prompt major gland biopsy. Open procedures give more useful information and better tissue sampling than a needle biopsy. There are few laboratory markers that will identify those patients at risk from malignant lymphoma, although a fall in serum immunoglobulins should prompt further investigations.

Diagnosis of Sjögren's syndrome

Patients should be questioned about the oral symptoms as outlined in the section above, but should also be asked about other symptoms (Table 8.10) and dryness elsewhere in the body. there is a generalized exocrine hypofunction. Measurement of salivary gland flow should be determined by sialometry, and glandular function is further assessed by scintiscanning with labelled pertechnetate. Sialography, using a water-based dye, may be indicated where there is a history or clinical signs indicating possible structural damage of the salivary glands. This may occur as a result of secondary chronic infection (Fig. 8.6). Persistent swelling of the glands can be investigated by sialography, but modern techniques, particularly MRI, give a much better picture of soft-tissue lesions and are essential if a tumour is suspected. Great emphasis has been placed on the diagnostic importance of a labial gland biopsy for patients with suspected Sjögren's syndrome. The number of lymphocytic foci within the glands is then measured and graded according to the scheme proposed by Chisholm and Mason. There is increasing evidence, however, that a number of patients may have a negative labial gland biopsy result while, on other criteria, being diagnosed as suffering from SS.

A problem in the definitive diagnosis of SS has been the variable criteria used in different centres and the fact that some of these have been unduly narrow, in the sense that they have high specificity but low sensitivity. In addition, many relied on lip biopsy for a definite diagnosis of SS and, as a consequence, the condition may have been underdiagnosed in the past. Some patients are not prepared to undergo labial gland biopsy, which they perceive as a relatively unpleasant procedure, albeit minor surgery. A biopsy positive confirmation of SS rarely alters the management of the patient and, as a consequence, many are prepared to accept a provisional diagnosis of SS. Currently, however, labial gland biopsy is the procedure with the greatest specificity and diagnostic value for the salivary component of SS.

An American–European SS consensus group has now revised the criteria for the classification of this syndrome, including the concept of biopsy-negative SS (providing that certain autoantibodies are present; see Figure 8.7). The criteria for the classification and diagnosis of SS may, however, undergo further modifications in future. Autoantibodies are usually present in SS, and a routine immune profile for rheumatoid and antinuclear factors, as well as anti-SS-A and anti-SS-B antibodies should be arranged, together with measurement of serum immunoglobulins. Salivary duct autoantibodies may also be present in SS, but their significance remains unclear; they are not included in the diagnostic criteria of SS. A full haematological and biochemical screen should also be undertaken to eliminate systemic diseases, such as diabetes. Patients with eye symptoms must be examined by an ophthalmologist. A preliminary estimate of xerophthalmia can be made by inserting a small strip of absorbent paper inside the lower eyelid (Schirmer test) to assess the volume of tears present (Fig. 8.8). Individuals who have clinical evidence or symptoms suggestive of a connective tissue disorder should be assessed by a rheumatologist. Oral symptoms are managed as for other cases of xerostomia, but many patients with Sjögren's syndrome have little or no salivary function and can only be given symptomatic relief in the form of salivary substitutes. Recurrent infections, particularly of the parotid glands, can be particularly troublesome and may result ultimately in surgical removal, with the attendant risks to the facial nerve. If there is any clinical suspicion of a tumour developing in any gland, then imaging and biopsy are mandatory. Calculus formation is often troublesome as a long-term result of chronic infection and stasis in the major salivary glands. A summary of the management of a patient with Sjögren's syndrome is given in Table 8.12.

There is, to date, no effective cure for Sjögren's syndrome, but symptoms can usually be controlled to some extent by the measures outlined above. Patients are often relieved at obtaining a definitive diagnosis and may benefit from membership of a Sjögren's syndrome support group.

Table 8.10 Extra-orofacial signs and symptoms associated with Sjögren's syndrome

Location of symptom	Description
Ocular	Persistent, troublesome dry eyes, recurrent sensation of sand or gravel in the eyes, need to use tear substitutes daily
Respiratory tract	Dryness of upper and lower respiratory tract, dysphonia, disturbances to sense of smell
Vaginal	Vaginal dryness, burning, history of recurrent fungal infections, painful intercourse
Skin	Dry skin, butterfly rash, vasculitis
Gastrointestinal tract	Dysphagia, constipation
General	Fatigue, weakness, depression
	Sleep disturbance, loss of sexual desire, depression

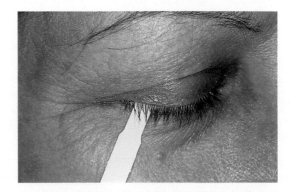

Fig. 8.7 The Schirmer test to assess the activity of the lacrimal glands.

Table 8.11 Revised international classification criteria for Sjögren's syndrome*

I   Ocular symptoms: a positive response to at least one of the following questions:

Have you had daily, persistent, troublesome dry eyes for more than 3 months?

Do you have a recurrent sensation of sand or gravel in the eyes?

Do you use tear substitutes more than 3 times a day?

II Oral symptoms: a positive response to at least one of the following questions:

Have you had a daily feeling of dry mouth for more than 3 months?

Have you had recurrently or persistently swollen salivary glands as an adult?

Do you frequently drink liquids to aid in swallowing dry food?

III Ocular signs, i.e. objective evidence of ocular involvement defined as a positive result for at least one of the following two tests:

Schirmer's I test, performed without anaesthesia (< 5 mm in 5 minutes)

Rose bengal score or other ocular dye score (> 4 according to van Bijsterveld's scoring system)

IV Histopathology: in minor salivary glands (obtained through normal-appearing mucosa)

Focal lymphocytic sialadenitis, evaluated by an expert histopathologist, with a focus score > 1, defined as a number of lymphocytic foci (which are adjacent to normal-appearing mucous acini and contain more than 50 lymphocytes) per 4 mm^2 of glandular tissue

V   Salivary gland involvement: objective evidence of salivary gland involvement defined by a positive result for at least one of the following diagnostic tests:

Unstimulated whole salivary flow (< 1.5 ml in 15 minutes)

Parotid sialography showing the presence of diffuse sialectasias (punctuate, cavitary, or destructive pattern) without evidence of obstruction in the major ducts

Salivary scintigraphy showing delayed uptake, reduced concentration, and/or delayed excretion of tracer

VI Autoantibodies: presence in the serum of the following autoantibodies:

Antibodies to Ro(SSA) or La(SSB) antigens, or both

For the diagnosis of primary SS:

In patients without any potentially associated disease, primary SS may be defined as follows:

• The presence of any 4 of the 6 items is indicative of primary SS, as long as either item IV (histopathology) or VI (serology) is positive

• The presence of any 3 of the 4 objective criteria items (that, is items III, IV, V < VI)

• The classification tree procedure represents a valid alternative method of classification, although it should be more properly used in clinical–epidemiological survey

For the diagnosis of secondary SS:

• In patients with a potentially associated disease (for instance, another well defined connective tissue disease), the presence of item I or item II plus any 2 from among items III, IV, and V may be considered as indicative of secondary SS

Exclusion criteria:

Past head and neck radiation treatment

Hepatitis C infection

Acquired immunodeficiency disease (AIDS)

Pre-existing lymphoma

Sarcoidosis

Graft versus host disease

Use of anticholinergic drugs (since a time shorter than 3-fold the half-life of the drug).

* Source: Vitali, C., Bombardieri, S., Jonsson, R., *et al*. *Ann Rheum Dis* (2002):61:554–558. Classification criteria for Sjögren's syndrome: a revised version of the European criteria proposed by the American–European Consensus Group.

Table 8.12 Sjögren's syndrome: assessment and clinical investigations

History
Dry mouth
Difficulty eating
Difficulty swallowing
Swelling of salivary glands
Dry skin
Vaginal dryness
Connective tissue disease
Examination
Mucosal dryness
No pooling of saliva on floor of the mouth
Dental status
Blood tests
Full blood count
ESR
Immunology
Inflammatory markers
Biochemical profile
Salivary gland imaging
Scintiscanning
Sialography
Biopsy
Labial gland biopsy.
Referral to
Ophthalmologist
Physician and/or rheumatologist

Typical results of investigations in Sjögren's syndrome

- Sialometry—low salivary flow rate
- Labial gland biopsy—lymphocytic infiltration
- Autoantibody screen—positive autoantibodies, in particular rheumatoid factor, antinuclear, SS-A, SS-B
- Salivary gland imaging—scintiscan will demonstrate reduced tracer uptake and secretion; sialography will show sialectasis
- Schirmer test—reduced lacrimal flow rate

Excessive saliva

An increased salivary flow rate is also known as sialorrhoea or ptyalism and, in contrast to xerostomia, it is an uncommon complaint. Hypersalivation may be transient or a chronic problem. There are several reasons why patients may complain of an increase in the production of saliva, but they are due to two main causes: hypersecretion and neuromuscular dysfunction. Excessive saliva is a frequent complaint of patients who are wearing an intraoral prosthesis for the first time. In fact, one of the commonly used methods of stimulating salivary flow for experimental purposes is to use an inert foreign body within the mouth. Most patients eventually become used to their new dentures or appliance and during this process the excess salivary flow usually disappears. In a few patients, however, this may prove an intractable problem. Infected or ulcerative lesions in the mouth may temporarily cause an increase in salivary flow, which adds to the discomfort of the initial condition. This can be a feature of primary herpetic gingivostomatitis. A similar effect is often seen in carcinoma of the mouth, in which the increased salivary flow may be accompanied by a reduced swallowing reflex and a constant dribbling of saliva. It can be difficult to distinguish between hypersalivation and drooling—the terms are not synonymous. In patients with hypersalivation saliva is normally cleared from the mouth by swallowing. Drooling occurs due to a failure to swallow saliva and is common in infants and also in those with poor neuromuscular coordination. Drooling is not necessarily caused by an overproduction of saliva, but it can occur because of it.

Very few drugs induce excessive salivation, a stark contrast to the number of drugs that reduce salivary flow rate. Anticholinesterases, which enhance neuromuscular transmission and are used in the treatment of myasthenia gravis, can cause hypersalivation. Interestingly, the antipsychotic drug clozapine has been implicated in causing a dry mouth and hypersalivation.

Excessive salivation may be due to:
- hypersecretion (for example, the provision of a new intraoral prosthesis, drugs)
- neuromuscular dysfunction (for example, cerebral palsy)
- oral dysaesthesia (patients with oral dysaesthesia are more likely to report xerostomia)

Systemic conditions, most notably neurological disturbances such as parkinsonism, cerebral palsy, and epilepsy, can cause patients to complain of excessive salivation. In these situations there may be no increase in the production of saliva but swallowing is uncoordinated and inefficient. Mercury poisoning and rabies are extremely rare diseases that have hypersalivation as a symptom.

Treatment for excessive salivation depends largely on the elimination of (or habituation to) the causative factor, whether it be a foreign body or an infective lesion. The use of drugs to suppress salivary flow is rarely indicated since virtually all drugs with a marked salivary suppressive effect also exert other, and often more significant, effects. Anticholinergic drug therapy is sometimes used in patients with cerebral palsy who drool excessively. One frequent oral side-effect of such medication is an increase in caries rate—often in a previously caries-free dentition. Alternatively, the major salivary gland ducts can be redirected to the oropharynx to treat drooling. In a few patients complaining of excessive salivation no increase in flow rate can be detected. In this situation there may be an underlying cognitive or psychiatric disturbance, and, indeed, some patients may display obsessional traits. The clinician can reassure the patient that there is no serious morbidity associated with this condition and sialometry may be helpful in demonstrating salivary flow rates within the normal range. In a minority of patients, behavioural therapy may be beneficial.

Discussion of problem cases

Case 8.1 Discussion

Q1   What advice would you give to this patient concerning his future oral health?

Therapeutic radiation can induce changes to mucosal, muscular, vascular, and osseous tissues. Alterations to salivary gland function are common as is a shift in oral microbial flora, resulting in a higher concentration of cariogenic bacteria. The irradiated patient has an increased risk of developing caries. Classically these occur at the cusp tips, incisal edges, and cervical thirds of the crown. The oncologist, radiotherapist, and dentist comprise a team of health-care professionals whose coordinated efforts are required for effective management of the radiotherapy patient. A pre-therapy dental evaluation is essential for the patient undergoing radiation therapy that may affect the oral cavity and/or salivary glands. The objective should be to establish good oral health for the patient prior to radiation treatments—failure to do so could result in complications.

Teeth that require extraction should be removed as soon as possible. It is advisable to liaise with the oncology unit to discuss the timing of extractions. Radiotherapy to the jaws can make a patient susceptible to osteoradionecrosis following oral surgery (including exodontia, especially when mandibular teeth require extraction). Teeth with a long-term questionable prognosis should be removed preferably before radiotherapy commences.

The patient should be warned that salivary flow may reduce dramatically following radiotherapy and the consequences of this on orodental health should be discussed with the patient. The patient should embark upon an intensive preventive programme—oral health education is of paramount importance. Nutritional guidance should be offered and the use of fluoride therapy considered. The clinician should realize that compliance with such a regimen may be a problem, especially if the patient did not maintain an oral self-care programme prior to radiotherapy. Therefore treatment plans should be realistic. Root canal treatment is not contraindicated in patients who are to undergo radiotherapy. Sialogogues can be beneficial including the use of systemic pilocarpine. The dose regimen and side-effects for this drug can be obtained from the *British National Formulary* or the manufacturer's data sheet.

Long-term patient follow-up is necessary on the part of both the dentist and hygienist. The patient may also experience non-specific oral mucositis following radiation and will be susceptible to oral candidosis. Post-irradiation sialadenitis is also a possible side-effect.

Case 8.2 Discussion

Q1   What questions would you ask this lady?

Questions should be asked to assess the severity of the dry mouth. the questions listed in Table 8.8 can help identify if a patient has oral dysfunction associated with salivary gland hypofunction. A full dental and medical history should be taken. It is also helpful to do a dietary analysis—the incidence of caries could increase as a result of more frequent intake of carbohydrate. Patients who develop a dry mouth may erroneously use mints or citrus-flavoured sweets to obtain symptomatic relief. A full medical history should be taken and specific questions that elicit the symptoms of Sjögren's syndrome should be used, for example, do you have dry eyes? do you have rheumatoid arthritis? A thorough drug history should be obtained. If you are in doubt as to the side-effects of any medication, a reference book such as the *British National Formulary* should be consulted. The local and regional UK Medicines Information service will also be helpful.

Q2   What advice would you give?

The treatment of this patient will depend upon the aetiology. If salivary gland hypofunction is suspected, then the patient should embark upon an intensive preventive regime (oral hygiene instruction, dietary advice, fluoride supplements, sialogogues, and possibly pilocarpine). The patient may merit referral to an oral medicine department if you suspect underlying systemic disease.

Q3   What is the most frequent cause of xerostomia?

The most frequent cause of xerostomia is the intake of drugs with anticholinergic activity.

Case 8.3 Discussion

The precipitating and relieving factors in the pain history are suggestive of an obstruction in a submandibular duct. The accumulation of saliva proximal to the blockage in the duct causes pain and swelling. The symptoms are worse just prior to a meal, when there is a rise in the production of saliva. The obstruction is most likely to be due to a salivary stone (calculus, sialolith). However, other causes could be a mucous plug, ductal stenosis, or a neoplasm.

Q1   What further questions would you ask this patient?

You would need to expand upon the pain history and establish if the pain is precipitated by any other gustatory or olfactory stimuli. It is unlikely that this pain has a spontaneous onset. Is the pain bilateral? Sialoliths are usually unilateral—affecting only one salivary gland.

Q2   How would you examine this patient?

You should palpate the submandibular gland and duct—both extra- and intraorally (bimanual palpation). The size of the salivary gland should be compared with that of the contralateral gland and the duct should be palpated for a stone or any irregularities of contour or consistency. A plain occlusal radiograph may be useful in identifying calculi. However, they are not all radio-opaque. Sialography may be required to identify the location of the obstruction. A scintiscan is a functional assessment of salivary gland activity and is of limited diagnostic value. Ultrasonography can be useful in identifying the site of any obstruction and the presence of calculi. It may also indicate the presence of an extra- or intraglandular tumour.

Q3 How would you manage him?

The management would depend upon the cause of the obstruction. The patient requires referral for salivary gland imaging and removal of the obstruction. A salivary duct calculus can sometime be successfully 'milked' along the duct and manipulated out of the orifice. A calculus lying in the submandibular duct that runs superficially along the floor of the mouth can be removed by incising the overlying mucosa—taking care not to damage the lingual nerve. The incision is often left unsutured to minimize possible duct obstruction due to scarring. Lithotripsy has been used for large salivary calculi. Submandibular salivary glands require surgical excision if they are severely damaged and associated with persistent symptoms.

Q4 Is this patient likely to complain of a dry mouth?

In a healthy patient, xerostomia is unlikely to accompany a condition that affects only one major salivary gland. It is usually a symptom of multiglandular disease.

Project

1. Find out about the clinical presentation, histopathological features, and management of tumours that may affect the salivary glands.

9

Inflammatory overgrowths, developmental and benign lesions, and pigmentation of the oral mucosa

Inflammatory overgrowths
- Epulides
- Fibroepithelial polyp
- Denture granuloma
- Focal epithelial hyperplasia (Heck's disease)

Developmental lesions
- Hamartomas
- Developmental white lesions

Benign neoplasms
- Squamous cell papilloma

Miscellaneous benign conditions
- Traumatic keratoses
- Nicotinic stomatitis (pipe-smokers' palate)
- Leukoedema

Pigmentation of the oral mucosa
- Amalgam tattoos
- Melanotic pigmentation
- Oral melanoma

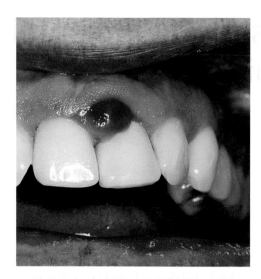

Fig. 9.1 A relatively early and immature fibrous epulis.

presence of multinucleated giant cells dispersed in a vascular stroma. With maturity the lesion may become less vascular and more fibrosed and may include some areas of bone formation. In its immature form, this epulis is characteristically red-purple in colour.

Epulides

Fibrous epulis
Vascular epulides
    Pyogenic granuloma
    Pregnancy epulis
Giant cell epulis (peripheral giant-cell granuloma)

Management

Treatment of all of these forms of epulis is by local excision. The origin of the lesion is often interdental and, in more advanced cases, the periodontal membrane may be quite deeply involved. If excision is not complete, there may be recurrence of the lesion and so, although radical surgical techniques are not called for, the initial removal should include all affected tissue. With repeated recurrence, it is sometimes necessary to remove the adjacent teeth in order to secure the elimination of the tissue of origin. In their tendency to recur, epulides may appear to be neoplasms, but the recurrence is due only to persistence of the conditions that caused the initial abnormal response. The timing for the excision of a pregnancy epulis is further discussed in Chapter 13.

Although the clinical diagnosis may be a confident one, it should always be confirmed by histological examination. Occasionally, a neoplasm may present in a form resembling a simple epulis and in a likely site for one. It should also be remembered that a central giant-cell granuloma may perforate

alveolar bone and appear as an epulis. Appropriate investigations (including blood tests for plasma calcium, phosphorus, and alkaline phosphatase) should be carried out on all patients presenting with a histologically confirmed giant-cell epulis to exclude hyperparathyroidism. Any symptoms or history that might imply undiagnosed hyperparathyroidism (such as renal calculi) should be taken into consideration (Chapter 18).

Fibroepithelial polyp

This lesion, similar in structure to the mature fibrous epulis, is essentially scar tissue produced as a response to trauma, such as repeated irritation of the buccal or labial mucosa, along the occlusal plane of the teeth, often caused by a bite. It is usually seen in adults and there is no sex differentiation. The lesion appears as either a sessile or a pedunculated swelling (Fig. 9.2) and is quite free of symptoms unless secondarily traumatized. The usual size of such a lesion when the patient presents for treatment is of the order of 1 cm in diameter, but occasional longstanding lesions are seen that are very much larger. The colour of the lesion is pink and the texture varies from soft to rubbery, depending on the maturity of the constituent fibrous tissue. Since this lesion is simply an exaggerated and chronically irritated mass of scar tissue, treatment need only be conservative, excision to the limit of the swelling or to the base of the pedicle being all that is required. Recurrence will occur only if trauma is repeated and is, in fact, uncommon. As with all other tissue overgrowths, absolute certainty of diagnosis can come only after histological examination, although a clinical diagnosis can often be made with a fair degree of confidence. An interesting clinical variant is one in which a fibroepithelial lesion (the so-called 'leaf fibroma') develops under the palate of an upper denture. In such cases the normal shape of the lesion is distorted and flattened into a thin disc that fits into a shallow depression in the palate. It retains a pedicle and may be displaced downwards on it like a hinged flap.

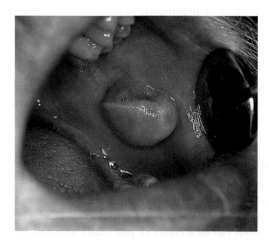

Fig. 9.2 A large fibroepithelial polyp of the buccal mucosa.

Denture granuloma

This is a lesion essentially similar to the fibroepithelial polyp, the irritating factor in this case being the flange of an overextended or ill-fitting denture. As in the case of the polyp, proliferative scar tissue is formed following chronic trauma. The typical fissured shape of the denture granuloma results from the indentation caused by the flange of the denture (Fig. 9.3). These lesions are rarely painful and, indeed, often cause astonishingly little trouble to the patient. This being so, occasional lesions are seen that are very large indeed, with multiple folds of proliferative tissue. The denture granuloma is a benign lesion and is treated by simple excision after removing the offending denture or drastically trimming it away from the affected area. The removal of the source of chronic irritation is in many cases sufficient to reduce considerably the size of the lesion within a relatively short time and even to make excision unnecessary.

Focal epithelial hyperplasia (Heck's disease)

This condition (otherwise known as Heck's disease) has been fully described and investigated only in recent years. The patients are predominantly children from Black African, Eskimo, and American Indian groups, although a very few cases have been reported in White Europeans. In this condition, multiple raised sessile lesions appear on the buccal and labial mucosa. The mucosa retains a relatively normal pink appearance and the texture of the lesions is soft. There is no ulceration (except in the case of secondary trauma) and the lesions are quite pain-free. Histologically, the epithelium, overlying a relatively normal corium, appears hyperplastic, with marked cellular irregularities. This condition is associated with specific types of the human papillomavirus, although there is thought also to be a genetic basis responsible for its high incidence in the groups mentioned above. No treatment is necessary. It is a self-limiting condition and regresses completely after a variable period.

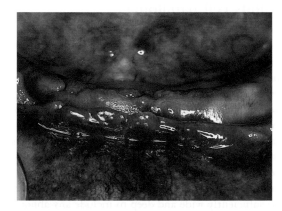

Fig. 9.3 A denture granuloma in the lower buccal sulcus.

Developmental lesions

Hamartomas

A hamartoma is a localized non-progressive tissue abnormality resulting from a defect in development. It is neither inflammatory nor neoplastic in nature but, since it may be confused with conditions of either type, it should be considered in relation to them. When present on skin or mucous membrane the term 'naevus' is often used even when the naevus cells (the melanocytes) are in no way involved. In such a lesion, a single element of the mucosa, epithelial, vascular, or lymphatic, is predominantly involved.

Angiomatous naevae

These are the result of developmental abnormalities in either the lymphatic or vascular components of the mucosa. Vascular naevae (haemangiomas) are relatively common lesions of the oral mucosa resembling the 'strawberry mark' of skin. Depending on the degree of dilatation of the abnormal blood vessels, the lesion may appear as a fine network of capillaries or as a more pronounced nodular structure, usually filled with slow-moving venous blood and, therefore, dark-blue in colour. The cavernous form may be mistaken clinically for a melanoma, but can be quickly differentiated by its tendency to blanch on pressure. This can be seen by pressing a glass slide down on to the surface. It should be emphasized that the vascular naevus is a static developmental abnormality that is asymptomatic and is best left undisturbed. A similar naevus involving the lymph vessels is the lymphangioma. It consists of a collection of dilated lymphatic vessels and spaces in a connective tissue stroma and is very similar to the vascular naevus in structure. Although it can appear on any part of the oral mucosa, it is seen much more commonly on the tongue than elsewhere. If the lesion is superficial it appears as a translucent white structure on the mucosa. If it is deeply situated the overlying surface of the tongue appears greyish and nodular. This is also an entirely innocuous lesion.

There may be problems of bleeding as a result of trauma to these lesions and action may be called for, although the bleeding rarely reaches dangerous proportions in these circumstances. Cryosurgery has been used to deal with this situation in the past, although not without some difficulties. There can be problems with postcryotherapy oedema of the tongue. The development of lasers has, however, provided an answer to this problem. If there is any doubt as to whether or not a lesion is a haemangioma, biopsy examination may be necessary, but angiomatous lesions often bleed copiously. No suspect vascular lesions should ever be subjected to any form of surgery except in hospital.

Developmental white lesions

A number of genetically determined white lesions of the oral mucosa exist, several of which are associated with lesions of other mucous membranes or of the skin. These are characterized by disturbances of keratinization and are often classified as 'genokeratoses' or 'genodermatoses' in the dermatological literature.

and the significance of this condition, one of the difficulties in this being that of definition. However, there can be no doubt that such a filmy coating appears on the buccal mucosa of a large number of completely asymptomatic patients when viewed in adequate lighting conditions.

Histologically, this lesion has been described as being parakeratotic, with large swollen cells in the superficial layers of the epithelium. This histological appearance is quite compatible with the observations that the grey surface film (consisting of the superficial oedematous cells) may easily be scraped away from the mucosa, leaving an apparently intact surface that again rapidly acquires the superficially grey appearance. Leukoedema is not associated with epithelial atypia and should not be regarded as a premalignant lesion.

Pigmentation of the oral mucosa

Pigmentation of the oral mucosa can occur as a result of environmental or occupational exposure to heavy metal salts, such as bismuth, lead, and mercury, some of which were used in the past as therapeutic agents for a number of diseases such as syphilis. Following absorption of the metals, they are deposited as metallic sulfides as a grey (or blue/black) line along the marginal gingivae.

Amalgam tattoos

Amalgam tattoos are a result of fragments of the material being embedded in the oral mucosa. These appear as isolated pigmented lesions (light-brown to dark-blue/black in colour). Amalgam tattoos may be radio-opaque, but this is not always the case (Fig. 9.5). They usually occur on the floor of the mouth or alveolar mucosa, near to existing or previous amalgam restorations. Marked amalgam tattoos may be seen on the attached gingivae, overlying teeth that have been apicetomized and apically sealed with amalgam.

Other foreign substances such as road grit can be implanted in the oral mucosa and occasional patients present with messages (often rude!) tattooed on their labial mucosae.

Melanotic pigmentation of oral mucosa

The significance of oral pigmentation in endocrine disturbances, and particularly in Addison's disease, is discussed in Chapter 13. An association between oral melanosis (particularly of the soft palate), smoking, and bronchogenic carcinoma has also been reported. Oral melanosis may occur in HIV infection (Chapter 4). A number of drugs may also stimulate increased pigmentation—including oral contraceptives, antimalarials, and major tranquillizers. There have been recent reports of minocycline causing pigmention of the skin and oral mucosa. Increased melanin production may also occasionally be seen in association with the oral lesions of lichen planus and with leukoplakias—this is reactive and of no clinical significance. However, in many patients, particularly those with heavily pigmented skins, oral pigmentation

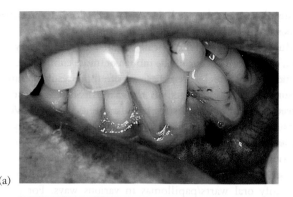

(a)

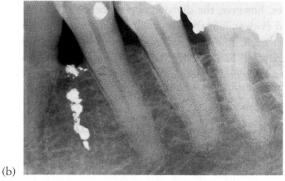

(b)

Fig. 9.5 (a) Amalgam tattoo. (b) Radiograph showing amalgam debris.

is quite normal. This may be patchy or diffuse, but the gingivae are almost always involved, even when the skin pigmentation is minimal.

The Peutz–Jegher syndrome is an autosomal dominant syndrome, comprising melanotic macules periorally and orally together with intestinal polyposis. Clinically, this syndrome manifests as multiple freckles occurring around the nose and eyes and on the lips and the oral mucosa. The intestinal polyps can be present throughout the gut and may give rise to symptoms, such as abdominal pain or cause intestinal obstruction. These polyps do not usually become malignant.

The Laugier–Hunziker syndrome (idiopathic lenticular mucocutaneous pigmentation) is a rare condition in which there is widespread melanin pigmentation affecting the oral and genital mucosa and longitudinal pigmentation of the nails.

The recognition of a localized and symptomless 'melanotic-like' lesion on the oral mucosa may cause considerable problems. Such a lesion may be entirely benign and static, but the initial stages of malignant melanoma may have a similar appearance to that of benign lesions. The first step must be to eliminate the possibility of an amalgam tattoo (see above).

Idiopathic melanotic macules are relatively common, benign lesions of the melanocytes, which appear as small brown or black patches on the oral mucosa or the lips. Oral melanocytic naevi are much less common and subdivided into 'junctional', 'compound', 'intramucosal', and 'blue' variants. Oral melanocytic naevi and melanotic macules should be excised to confirm the diagnosis

Table 9.1 Melanotic pigmentation of the oral mucosa: principal causes

Racial
Addison's disease
HIV disease
Reactive
Lichen planus and leukoplakia
Drug-related
Peutz–Jegher syndrome
Isolated melanotic lesions
Idiopathic melanotic macule
Melanotic naevus
Malignant melanoma

and, in particular, to exclude the possibility of a malignant melanoma. Table 9.1 summarizes the causes of melanotic pigmentation of the oral mucosa.

Oral melanoma

Intraoral melanomas are highly malignant oral tumours that usually occur as isolated dark brown or black patches on the oral mucosa. Amelanotic melanomas can manifest as red lesions. Oral melanomas are rare malignancies and tend to occur on the palate. In the early stages they may be symptomatic. The appearance is usually of a nodular or macular lesion that is firm to palpate. This ultimately ulcerates and causes discomfort or bleeds. Early diagnosis of any lesion suspected of being a malignant melanoma is essential as metastasis to the lymph nodes and other organs (lungs, liver, and bone) occurs early. The prognosis for oral melanoma is poor. Superficial spreading melanomas are rarely seen in the mouth and their appearance can be quite spectacular (Fig. 9.6).

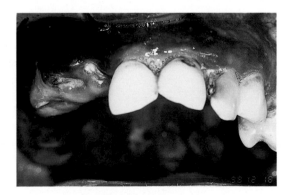

Fig. 9.6 Diffuse advanced oral melanoma.

Early diagnosis and treatment of oral malignant melanomas is essential, as they metastasize early to lymph nodes and other organs.

Discussion of problem cases

Case 9.1 Discussion

Q1   What is the differential diagnosis of this lesion and how would you manage this case?

An amalgam tattoo would be unusual at this site, although the authors have seen a few such cases. Malignant melanoma must be included in the differential diagnosis or possibly an early Kaposi's sarcoma. The most likely diagnosis of this isolated lesion is an idiopathic melanotic macule but excisional biopsy is indicated. The biopsy should be arranged as soon as possible, particularly in view of the patient's family history.

Case 9.2 Discussion

Q1   What is the most likely, clinical diagnosis of this lady's lesion?

This is likely to be a denture granuloma, caused by chronic trauma from the buccal flange of this lady's ill-fitting upper denture.

Q2   How is this lesion managed?

The flange of the denture should be trimmed back so that it is no longer traumatizing the mucosa and the patient should be discouraged from wearing her dentures at night. Surgical excision of the remaining hyperplastic tissue may be necessary but should not be carried out until the response to modifying the denture has been assessed. New dentures should be provided in the long term.

Q3   A more sinister oral lesion can occasionally present in a similar way. What is this and how can it be differentiated from the more common benign oral lesion?

Carcinoma of the maxillary antrum may infiltrate the maxillary bone and occasionally presents as a proliferative lesion in the buccal sulcus. The appearance of a tissue mass in this site, without any evidence of trauma from the denture, would immediately alert the clinician. Patients with antral carcinoma may also present with symptoms such as blocked nose, nasal discharge, pain, or paraesthesia over the cheek. Antral carcinoma can also present as a swelling in the palate, which tends to ulcerate. Radiography reveals opacity of the antrum, often with erosion of the antral walls. If there is any doubt whatsoever, immediate biopsy of the lesion must be carried out. Antral carcinoma has been described in particular risk groups, for example, workers in the wood or shoe industries and individuals who use snuff.

10

Precancerous lesions and conditions. Oral carcinoma and carcinogenesis

Precancerous lesions
- Leukoplakia
- Erythroleukoplakia
- Speckled leukoplakia
- Candidal leukoplakia (chronic hyperplastic candidosis)
- Malignant transformation of precancerous lesions
- Management of precancerous lesions

Precancerous conditions
- Oral submucous fibrosis (OSF)
- Sideropenic dysphagia
- Lichen planus
- Other precancerous conditions

Oral carcinoma and carcinogenesis
- Aetiological factors for oral squamous cell carcinoma
- Clinical features and diagnosis of oral carcinoma
- Staging systems for oral carcinoma
- The management of oral carcinoma
- Prevention of oral carcinoma
- Oral carcinoma as a genetic disease

10

Precancerous lesions and conditions. Oral carcinoma and carcinogenesis

Problem cases

Case 10.1

A 60-year-old edentulous gentleman presents to your dental surgery for the first time requesting a new set of dentures. His medical history is clear but he is a life-long smoker, averaging 20–30 cigarettes per day. His upper denture is badly stained with several teeth either fractured or missing.

During your oral examination you note an isolated ulcer on the left lateral border of the tongue, which is approximately 1 cm in diameter. Palpation of his neck reveals no obvious abnormality.

Q1   What questions would you ask this patient?

Q2   What features of the ulcer are important to note?

Q3   What is the most likely differential diagnosis in this particular case?

Q4   How would you manage this patient?

Introduction

There are a number of oral lesions that have a potential for malignant change. However, relatively few carcinomas develop within a recognizable precancerous lesion or in a patient with a precancerous condition.

A precancerous lesion is a morphologically altered tissue in which cancer is more likely to occur than in its apparently normal counterpart, that is, the lesion itself undergoes malignant transformation. Examples of precancerous oral lesions include leukoplakia and erthyroplakia.

> A precancerous lesion is a morphologically altered tissue in which cancer is more likely to occur than in its apparently normal counterpart.

An oral precancerous condition is a generalized state associated with a significantly increased risk of cancer developing somewhere in the mouth, that is, not necessarily in a pre-existing lesion. In precancerous conditions the linking factor appears to be epithelial atrophy such as that which occurs in oral submucous fibrosis and sideropenic dysphagia. Some authorities prefer the term 'potentially malignant' to precancerous because not all precancerous lesions undergo malignant transformation and a proportion regress or stay the same.

> A precancerous condition is a generalized state associated with a significantly increased risk of cancer developing.

Precancerous lesions

Leukoplakia

Definition of leukoplakia

Leukoplakia is currently defined as a predominantly white lesion of the oral mucosa that cannot be characterized as any other definable lesion—it is therefore a diagnosis of exclusion. Various attempts have been made by the World Health Organisation to define oral leukoplakia for use in epidemiological surveys and there have been a number of revised definitions. No doubt the current definition of leukoplakia will change as our understanding of its aetiology and progression increases.

> Leukoplakia is currently defined as a predominantly white lesion of the oral mucosa that cannot be characterized as any other definable lesion.

It is important to note that the term oral leukoplakia is a clinical term with no histological connotations. From a clinical point of view, it is useful to divide these lesions into homogeneous and non-homogeneous lesions. Non-homogeneous leukoplakias, including those with a 'speckled' appearance, have a worse prognosis with regard to malignant transformation than homogeneous lesions. Leukoplakias in particular sites, such as the floor of the mouth and the ventral surface of the tongue, are considered to be more at risk of malignant transformation than those elsewhere on the oral mucosa.

Incidence of leukoplakia

The incidence of oral leukoplakia is difficult to ascertain but reported prevalences throughout the world range from 0.2 to 4 per cent. However, there are marked variations in prevalence between different geographical areas (Western Europe and America) that probably reflect different ethnic and cultural groups and aetiological factors, such as smoking and chewing tobacco. Oral leukoplakia used to occur predominantly in males and affect older age groups but gender and age ratios are now changing.

Aetiological factors associated with oral leukoplakia

Two groups of leukoplakias may be recognized: idiopathic leukoplakias, in which no aetiological factors have been recognized, and leukoplakias in which an evident predisposing factor may be present. It is probable that the idiopathic group may include a certain number of lesions in which the aetiological factor remains unrecognized, but, even with this reservation, it would seem reasonable to accept the possibility of the existence of idiopathic lesions.

It is clearly established that there are a number of clinically significant aetiological factors that may contribute to the development of oral leukoplakia. The most important of these is the use of tobacco, either when smoked or chewed in one or other of the large number of tobacco-using habits that have been reported. The precise nature of the action of tobacco or of its smoke on the oral mucosa is not yet known, but there can be no doubt that a profound effect is often exerted. Apart from the tobacco itself, other substances involved in tobacco-chewing habits (such as betelnut and lime) may also be implicated in the production of leukoplakia. There have been many surveys concerned with the effect of tobacco habits on the oral mucosa and, in virtually all cases, it would appear that those individuals who use tobacco in any of its forms are much more likely to develop oral leukoplakia. It is also well established that the precise nature of the tobacco habit is of great significance in the determination of the exact form of the lesion produced and also of its eventual prognosis. In an investigation of the relationship between the incidence of leukoplakia and the sex, age, and tobacco habits of a Bombay (renamed 'Mumbai') population, it was shown quite clearly that the most important extrinsic factor by far was their smoking habit. Furthermore, the increased incidence of lesions in males was directly attributable to their increased use of tobacco compared to that of females. It is not difficult to extrapolate these findings to other series in which there has been a constant marked predominance of leukoplakia in male subjects. There is no doubt that those leukoplakias that are directly attributable to tobacco habits are, to a large degree, reversible, and it has been clearly demonstrated on many occasions that regression of a lesion may be induced by the cessation of the habit, although the regression may not be permanent.

> Individuals who use tobacco in any of its forms are much more likely to develop oral leukoplakia.

A second important aetiological factor in the production of oral leukoplakia is that of infection and, of the organisms involved. It appears that *Candida albicans* is by far the most important. It is well established (Chapter 4) that there may be a heavy infiltration of the pseudohyphal form of *Candida* into the epithelium of oral leukoplakias, and it has been shown that such lesions (candidal leukoplakias) are associated with an increased incidence of malignant transformation. The precise relationship between the candidal infection and the production of the leukoplakia is not known and, in particular, it has not yet been determined whether the infection is a primary or a secondary event. Histological studies would seem to provide evidence for either viewpoint, and it will probably be as the result of immunological studies that the final decision as to the exact aetiological factor in these cases is made. However, recent work has shown that, on an experimental basis, candidal infiltration into epithelium may of itself produce changes resembling those of leukoplakia, and there would also seem to be evidence that complex immune deficiencies may occur in some patients with leukoplakia, including a deficient immune response to *Candida albicans*.

There is also some evidence of an additive effect between the actions of tobacco and *Candida* in the formation of leukoplakias. It is currently suggested that heavy smokers are at increased risk, firstly, of developing candidal leukoplakia and, subsequently, of developing carcinoma within it. This is not a proven association but there is a considerable bulk of anecdotal information to support the concept. The role of viruses, such as the human papillomavirus (HPV), in the aetiology of oral leukoplakias remains uncertain. However, hairy leukoplakia, which occurs in HIV and other immunosuppressed patients, is associated with the Epstein–Barr virus (EBV).

Clinical features of leukoplakia

Leukoplakia appears as an intrinsic white area of the oral mucosa, sometimes homogeneous (Fig. 10.1), sometimes wrinkled, and sometimes with a verrucous (Fig. 10.2) or fissured surface. The white patch may vary from being transparent and filmy in appearance to being dense and thick. In some cases, the leukoplakia is a single, discrete, and well-circumscribed plaque area, whereas in other patients there may be widespread abnormality of the mucosa with a number of lesions distributed in varying sites. In a Danish population the highest incidence of leukoplakia has been found to be on the buccal mucosa and commissures, and then, in descending order of frequency, on the alveolar ridges, tongue, buccal sulci, floor of mouth, labial mucosa, and palate. However, in common with all other statistics regarding leukoplakia and associated lesions, it must be remembered that the figures refer to a specific population and that other populations in different areas and with different influencing factors (such as tobacco habits) may show diverse clinical features.

Histological features of oral leukoplakia

There is a wide range of histological changes that can occur in oral leukoplakias, and these range from hyperkeratosis without epithelial dysplasia, to squamous epithelial dysplasia and squamous cell carcinoma *in situ*. Keratinocytes show a number of cytological changes (cellular atypia) in epithelial dysplasia. The various histological changes are discussed in detail in standard textbooks of oral pathology. Not all the individual cellular atypia occurs in one lesion. It is conventional for oral pathologists to

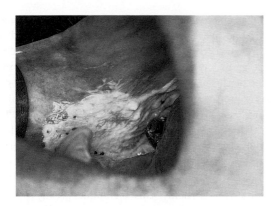

Fig. 10.1 Homogeneous leukoplakia of the floor of the mouth and labial mucosa.

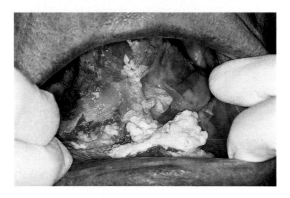

Fig. 10.2 Verrucous leukoplakia affecting floor of mouth, alveolar ridge, and ventral surface of tongue. (Histopathology showed moderate dysplasia.)

subjectively grade the degree of dysplasia as mild, moderate, or severe depending on the proportion of keratinocyte layers showing cellular atypia.

Erythroplakia

As implied by its name, erythroplakia is essentially a red lesion of the mucosa. An alternative term—erythroplasia—is taken from the name given to a somewhat similar lesion of the penis (erythroplasia of Queyrat), which has for some time been recognized as a premalignant lesion. The oral lesion is relatively uncommon and appears as a bright red patch that is well defined from the surrounding mucosa and has a velvet-like surface texture. There may be occasional white areas adjoining the lesion and, in some cases, patches of erythroplakia may be interspersed with leukoplakic lesions. It is most often seen on the buccal mucosa, although it may occur on other sites of the oral mucosa, such as the soft palate, ventral surface of the tongue, and floor of the mouth.

The most important feature of this lesion is the high incidence of cellular atypia shown on histological examination, and often this is associated with atrophy of the epithelium. A significant number of these lesions display epithelial atypia throughout all cellular layers—known as carcinoma *in situ*,

a diagnosis that warrants immediate surgical intervention. Paradoxically, it has been pointed out that some of these lesions display virtually no atypia and, indeed, may be of a simple inflammatory nature. It is quite evident that biopsy examination is essential in all these cases. As in the case of leukoplakia, it is by no means clear as to whether the *Candida* is a primary or a secondary feature of such lesions. However, it is generally felt (perhaps without any clear evidence) that the presence of *Candida* in the epithelium is likely to coincide with an increased tendency to malignant change. Whatever the aetiological factors involved, there seems little doubt that a high proportion of lesions clinically diagnosed as erythroplakia present sufficient epithelial abnormalities to be classified on histological examination as incipiently malignant. It would seem that erythroplakia warrants the description that has been applied to it of being the most serious of the oral precancerous lesions.

Speckled leukoplakia

This lesion can be considered as a variant of either leukoplakia or erythroplakia. It appears as a series of white nodular patches on an erythematous background and so, in appearance, is midway between these two conditions. Any area of the oral mucosa may be involved, but many lesions appear on the buccal mucosa near to the commissures (Fig. 10.3). Histologically, these lesions show a high incidence of atypia and, in many cases, the presence of candidal hyphae in the epithelium. The same doubts have been expressed about the exact role of *Candida* in these lesions as in the case of homogeneous leukoplakias, but there is no doubt that there are frequently two coincidental factors in all these lesions—the presence of *Candida* and the presence of epithelial atypia. Whether there is a causal effect remains to be determined. The lesions should always be considered as potentially malignant. Although accurate information is not as yet available, all available surveys suggest that speckled leukoplakias have a significantly higher rate of malignant transformation than homogeneous lesions.

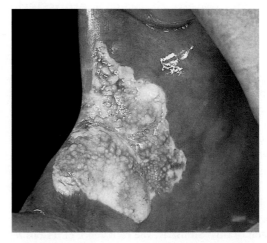

Fig. 10.3 Candidal speckled leukoplakia at the commissure—a characteristic site.

Candidal leukoplakia

Candidal leukoplakia is also known as chronic hyperplastic candidosis. The important role of *Candida* as an aetiological factor in the production of oral leukoplakia has already been discussed. It is not easy to ascribe a characteristic appearance to candidal leukoplakias and, indeed, a wide variety of lesions may be shown to include the organisms. However, it is generally accepted that candidal leukoplakias are frequently speckled and often have a somewhat irregular and nodular appearance. A high proportion of commissural lesions extending to the external angle of the lips are candidal leukoplakias (Fig. 10.3). Diagnosis of a candidal leukoplakia cannot be made by taking superficial swabs — the hyphae are within the lesion and very few may be on the surface. For a reliable diagnosis it is necessary to stain sections from a biopsy specimen with periodic acid Schiff (PAS) reagents. In this way the hyphae are readily seen within the superficial layers and stratum corneum of the epithelium. In view of the increased rate of malignant change in candidal leukoplakias, it is of evident importance that these lesions should be recognized and regarded with heightened suspicion.

Malignant transformation of precancerous lesions

Oral leukoplakia is a marker of an increased risk of cancer anywhere in the oral cavity, but to date there are no reliable clinical or histological features that can be used to predict whether the lesion will regress spontaneously, remain the same, or progress to cancer. It has been reported that malignant transformation occurs in between 4 and 8 per cent of oral leukoplakias and about 15 per cent will spontaneously regress. The site of involvement is important and in sublingual leukoplakias the rate of transformation is as high as 40 per cent. Erythroplakia has the greatest tendency to develop into a malignant lesion, with a transformation rate as high as 80 per cent and above.

The management of precancerous lesions

It is not within the remit of this book to deal in any detail with the surgical treatment of leukoplakias. It should be pointed out, however, that one of the problems in therapy lies in accurately defining the area at risk. It is evident that the oral mucosa as a whole must, to some extent, be exposed to the particular aetiological agent, whether the latter be intrinsic or extrinsic. Thus, it is often difficult to come to an arbitrary decision about the limits of surgical or laser excision necessary for optimum treatment. It is by no means uncommon for an apparently generous excision to prove inadequate or for entirely new fields of abnormality to appear. Indeed, it is clear that leukoplakia often represents more than a localized abnormality and that the whole of the mucosa may be involved, even though localized lesions may be the expression of this. Similarly, the recurrence of lesions repaired by mucosal grafts or allowed to epithelialize can be easily explained by the realization that such a manoeuvre is effective only in

removing specific epithelial cells that have become involved in a complex abnormality. If the pre-existing aetiological factors remain, then recurrent abnormality may be expected even though the aetiology may remain unrecognized. It may well be, in recurrent cases of this nature, that abnormal mesodermal–epithelial reactions are responsible for the initial lesion and are maintained by the presence of the influencing corium after surgery. There is increasing doubt regarding the recurrence of cryosurgically treated leukoplakias as carcinoma, even though it seems that some degree of undertreatment might be involved in such cases. Currently, excision of the lesions using a CO_2 laser is felt to be a safer alternative. Certainly, this technique greatly reduces the necessity for grafting of excised areas, there is little tissue distortion following re-epithelialization, and, in terms of postoperative discomfort, it is greatly preferable to cryotherapy.

Apart from surgical treatment it is possible to obtain a marked regression of a significant number of tobacco-induced leukoplakias by discontinuing the habit. Biopsy studies of such regression lesions have shown marked reductions in the incidence of atypia as well as in the extent of the lesions. This manoeuvre should be the first employed in the management of lesions in which a tobacco-mediated aetiology is suspected. Similarly, in those lesions with associated candidal infections, it is often possible to effect a marked improvement by the use of systemic antifungals. It is unlikely that a complete regression will be obtained in this way, but the reduction in the size of the lesion may make the eventual surgical management much simpler. The development of safer systemic antifungal agents, such as fluconazole, has facilitated their use in the routine management of candidal leukoplakia.

Leukoplakias with little or no dysplasia are often left untreated, particularly if patients are able to reduce or stop smoking or chewing tobacco. Lesions are monitored on a long-term basis, both clinically and histologically, as appropriate. This policy of 'watchful waiting' is clearly unsatisfactory and relies on the experience and subjective assessment of the clinician. The key to managing oral leukoplakia is likely to be the establishment of molecular assays that can redefine the assessment of the risk of malignant transformation and hopefully lead to successful methods of chemoprevention, such as the use of retinoids. Molecular markers are discussed in the next section of this chapter.

Precancerous conditions

Oral submucous fibrosis (OSF)

This is a disease that was first recognized in the 1950s, despite presumptive evidence that it must have been present long before that time. The vast majority of cases have been found in the Indian subcontinent, although similar examples have been reported in other Asiatic countries as well as an increasing number of patients in the UK.

Oral submucous fibrosis (OSF) is a condition in which fibrous tissue is laid down in the corium of the oral mucosa.

Simultaneous changes occur in the oral epithelium. In the early phase vesicles and small ulcers may be formed, but this stage is soon superseded by one of generalized epithelial atrophy. The effect of the fibrosis is a stiffening of the oral mucosa leading to difficulty in opening the mouth and to a binding down of the tongue. The appearance of the mucosa is of a blanched, 'marbled' nature, which seems to be quite characteristic of the condition. It is possible to palpate bands of fibrous tissue within the mucosa and it is reported that eventually the scar formation within the soft palate is sufficient to cause the near disappearance of the uvula.

The cause of OSF is not known with certainty, but recent work suggests that both a genetic susceptibility and a fibroblastic response to areca (betel) nut chewing may be involved.

Epidemiological studies indicate that this condition is induced by chewing areca nut and it is therefore particularly common in Asian communities. Studies indicate there is probably a genetic predisposition for OSF and the role of autoimmunity is also being investigated. The influence of nutritional factors, if any, remains unclear. Patients with OSF have an increased risk of developing oral carcinoma, which has been estimated to be as high as 10 per cent over 10 to 15 years. So far, there does not seem to be any satisfactory treatment for OSF although intralesional steroids have been used. Primary prevention by reducing the use of areca nut products would appear to be the best way forward to reduce the incidence of OSF.

A condition, know as 'betel-chewers' mucosa' has been described in which there is brownish-red discoloration of the oral mucosa (particularly the buccal mucosa) together with desquamation or peeling of the mucosa. The latter may be partly due to trauma from chewing. In addition, the mucosa often has a wrinkled appearance. This is not *per se* considered to be a precancerous lesion but may progress to oral submucous fibrosis and/or oral leukoplakia. Patients are often reluctant to stop chewing quid, although this is the key to successful management.

Sideropenic dysphagia

Sideropenic dysphagia is also known as the Paterson–Kelly (or Plummer–Vinson) syndrome and predominantly affects middle-aged females who have iron deficiency (see also Chapter 13). The oral and pharyngeal mucosa may appear atrophic and shiny red. Oral leukoplakias and multiple squamous cell carcinomas can develop in this condition but it is particularly associated with postcricoid carcinoma.

Lichen planus

The premalignant potential of oral lichen planus is discussed in Chapter 11 and the malignant transformation rate is cited as 0.4–3.3 per cent. Whether or not patients with atrophic or erosive forms of oral lichen planus are more susceptible to malignant change has yet to be proved by long-term prospective studies.

Other precancerous conditions

Discoid lupus erythematosus has been classified as a premalignant condition but only a few cases of malignant transformation of lip lesions have been reported. Tertiary syphilis is rarely reported these days because of early recognition and treatment. In the past, oral leukoplakias and squamous cell carcinomas developed in association with the atrophic glossitis of tertiary syphilis but the use of potentially carcinogenic agents such as arsenic to treat this condition may have predisposed to this transformation. Other rare conditions that have oral manifestations have been reported as precancerous and include xeroderma pigmentosum and epidermolysis bullosa. Overall, conditions in which there is epithelial atrophy appear to be associated with an increased risk of malignant transformation.

Oral carcinoma and carcinogenesis

Malignant tumours of the head and neck include squamous cell carcinoma (SCC) of the oral cavity, larynx, and pharynx, salivary/glandular cancers, malignant melanomas, lymphomas, and sarcomas. SCC is the most common neoplasm of the head and neck and accounts for more than 90 per cent of all oral malignancies. Worldwide, the annual incidence of SCC exceeds 300 000 with approximately 2000 new cases being registered per year in the UK. Each year nearly half that number die from oral SCC (OSCC). The high morbidity rate is due to a number of factors including late presentation, failure to respond to treatment regimens currently available, and a lack of suitable markers for early detection. The dental profession has a crucial role in the early detection of SCC, which, if treated early, has the best prognosis. Current approaches for controlling this cancer include improved prevention (risk factors such as tobacco are well recognized) and early detection of patients with suspicious oral lesions.

Aetiological factors for oral squamous cell carcinoma (OSCC)

The aetiological factors implicated in OSCC are tobacco use, alcohol consumption, sunlight (cancer of the lip), diet and nutritional status, chronic candidal infections, viral infections, and immune deficiency. Of these, tobacco use and alcohol are considered to be the most important. Consideration of all these factors is clearly outside the scope of this book but the role of tobacco, alcohol consumption, and diet will be briefly considered. The potential role of virus in oral carcinogenesis is discussed in a later section of this chapter.

The speculative relationship between *Candida* species and malignant transformation of oral leukoplakia has already been discussed in Chapter 4.

Tobacco use

Tobacco use, in any of its forms (cigarettes, cigars, pipe-smoking, tobacco-chewing, reverse smoking), is one of the most important aetiological factors in the development of OSCC. The relative risk of developing oral carcinoma from cigarette-smoking depends on a number of factors, including level of consumption and whether the cigarettes are high or low tar. However, a reasonable estimate is that an individual who smokes more than 20 cigarettes a day has a risk of developing oral carcinoma 10 times higher than that of a nonsmoker. Pipe- and cigar-smoking have been linked with cancer of the lip. In one region of India, where reverse cheroot smoking is practised amongst women, a greatly increased incidence of carcinoma of the palate in female patients has been reported. Reverse smoking is also common in other parts of the world. The increased incidence of oral cancer in India is likely to be due to the common practice of smoking bidis—a cheap type of cigarette (made from local tobacco rolled in a leaf)—and reverse smoking.

The chewing of betel quid is endemic throughout the Indian subcontinent, South-east Asia, and large parts of the western Pacific. Only three substances, nicotine, ethanol, and caffeine, are consumed more widely than betel. Quid consumption is higher in females and there is considerable regional variation in its constitutents. Quid has been defined as 'a substance or mixture of substances placed in the mouth or chewed and remaining in contact with the mucosa, usually containing one or both of the two basic ingredients, tobacco or areca nut, in raw or any manufactured or processed form'. Ingredients commonly used in the preparation of betel quid are listed in Table 10.1. Pan masala has all the ingredients of the betel quid, except the betel leaf, and is conveniently packaged in small sachets and tins (Fig 10.4).

A number of case control studies have reported an increased relative risk of developing cancers of the oral cavity due to the use of betel quid, with or without tobacco. Oral submucous fibrosis and oral leukoplakia, both considered to be premalignant, are associated with betel-chewing (see 'Precancerous lesions' and 'Precancerous conditions'). It is reported that this habit improves digestion and salivation, diminishes hunger pangs, and produces a feeling of euphoria, and some claim it has aphrodisiac powers. Children as young as 3 years of age participate in this practice. It is an essential element in social, cultural, and economic life in many parts of the world.

> Chewing of betel quid is associated with oral leukoplakia, oral submucous fibrosis, and squamous cell carcinoma.

Tobacco-chewing is traditionally practised by miners, as smoking is obviously dangerous underground. Miners who adopt this practice are, therefore, susceptible to developing oral leukoplakia, which may undergo malignant transformation.

It is important to appreciate that tobacco usage is not only an important risk factor for oral carcinoma but a common aetiological factor of oral leukoplakia (see above).

Alcohol consumption

Alcohol consumption as a risk factor for oral carcinoma is difficult to quantify, particularly as many patients who drink heavily also

Table 10.1 Ingredients commonly used in the preparation of betel quid

Betel leaf (also known as pan)
Areca nut (supari)—seed of areca catechu tree
Lime (calcium hydroxide)
Catechu (resinous extract from acacia tree)
Tobacco

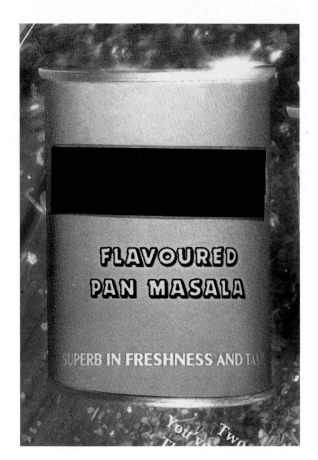

Fig. 10.4 Pan masala, on sale to the public.

have a high consumption of cigarettes. The general consensus, however, is that alcohol is an independent risk factor but the effect of alcohol and tobacco together is multiplicative, that is, greater than the added risk of alcohol or tobacco.

Diet and nutritional status

The role of diet and nutritional status in the prevention of oral cancer has been the subject of a number of studies and it is generally considered that deficiencies of vitamins A, C, and E may predispose to the development of oral carcinoma. Lack of dietary iron may lead to aerodigestive (including oral) carcinomas as is in the Plummer–Vinson syndrome. High consumption of fruit and fresh vegetables may lower the risk, and recent studies suggest that patients with head and neck cancers have a high fat and red meat intake.

Clinical features and diagnosis of oral squamous cell carcinoma

Not all oral carcinomas are preceded by a recognizable premalignant lesion, although in many cases evident abnormality may have been present for some time (Table 10.2). The significance of leukoplakia as a premalignant lesion has been discussed above but it must be repeated that the clinical criteria by which a white patch may be judged as premalignant are far from clear, and that it is only after a study of the histological appearance of the lesion that any attempt at prognosis can be made.

The classical signs of a malignant condition, which should arouse immediate suspicion, are:

1. persistent ulceration: any unexplained ulcer that lasts for longer than 10 days should be treated with suspicion;

2. induration: thickening and hardening of the tissues;

3. proliferative growth of tissue above its normal level, often with changes in the surface texture and colour changes;

4. fixation of the affected tissue to the underlying structures.

Pain is not always present in the early stages of a carcinoma and the patient may be quite unaware of any abnormality until the lesion has become large and secondarily infected. If the affected area includes the teeth, these may become mobile due to the replacement of the periodontal membrane by tumour. Thus, unexplained rapid loosening of the teeth should be carefully investigated.

Lymph node involvement may occur early in oral carcinoma. However, enlarged regional lymph nodes may in fact show only non-specific inflammatory changes in some early cases. Unfortunately, this cannot be relied on and, in some cases, malignant deposits in the lymph nodes are found while the primary lesion is still small. It is certainly true that prognosis is more favourable if treatment is instituted before the lymph nodes are involved.

Lesions showing the signs outlined above are immediately suspect but such a lesion is at a relatively late stage (Fig. 10.5). In its early stages, a carcinoma may show none of these signs and may be detectable only by a change in colour or surface texture of the mucosa. It may be impossible to differentiate clinically between leukoplakia or erythroplakia and early carcinoma and, thus, biopsy examination is mandatory in every case in which the possibility of carcinoma may arise. Any prolonged ulcer, erythema, or unexplained white patch should be investigated in this way. A diagnosis of carcinoma should be followed as rapidly as possible by treatment and thus it is essential that the surgeon who carries out biopsy procedures should be in a position to arrange for immediate treatment if required. For this reason, it is often better for such investigation to be carried out in specialist centres rather than in the dental practitioner's surgery. Prognosis in late oral carcinoma is poor and much depends on the early detection of the lesion before the cervical nodes become involved, the overall 5-year survival rate being effectively doubled if the lesion is discovered early. It is also true that the prognosis becomes worse the further back in the oral cavity the lesion lies. Thus, it is quite clear that the patient's survival may depend on a thorough systematic examination of the oral mucosa. The use of toluidine blue dye has been advocated as an adjunct to the clinical diagnosis of suspicious oral lesions. Products such as OraTest® are now approved in the UK for oral screening, detection of second primary lesions, and defining margins of lesions for biopsy and surgery and are the subject of ongoing clinical trials. Suspicious oral lesions should always be biopsied regardless of the results of toluidine blue staining.

Carcinoma of the lip is a rather different lesion in that it is clearly visible and so is noticed early. It has a much better prognosis than intraoral carcinoma and early diagnosis often implies successful and relatively small-scale surgery. The lower lip is practically always affected, the patients being predominantly older males (Fig. 10.6). The carcinoma is often mistaken in its early stages for a herpetic lesion, but its persistent nature should arouse suspicion and the same criteria for investigation should be adopted as for intraoral lesions. Patients with actinic cheilitis are at increased risk of developing carcinoma of the lip (see Chapter 6).

Table 10.2 Oral carcinoma: suspicious clinical features

Persistent, unexplained ulceration
Induration
Proliferative growth
Changes in texture and colour
Fixation to underlying tissues
Sudden loosening of teeth
Lymph node involvement
Pain—often a late feature

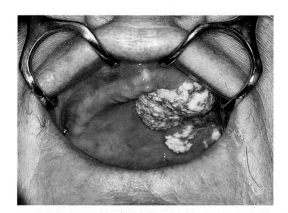

Fig. 10.5 Carcinoma of the palatal mucosa.

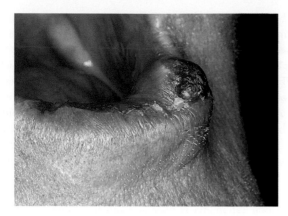

Fig. 10.6 Carcinoma of the lower lip.

Staging systems for oral carcinoma

In order to aid uniformity in studies of the epidemiology of oral carcinoma and the prognosis of those suffering from it, there have been a number of assessment methods introduced. These are generally known as staging systems. The most widely used is the TNM system (tumour, nodes, metastasis). In this system scores are given to each patient dependent on the size of the primary tumour, the extent of regional lymph node involvement, and the presence of distant metastases. Staging systems have been found of considerable value in selecting the most appropriate management and assessing the overall prognosis of patients in each group.

The management of oral carcinoma

The management of oral carcinoma should be coordinated by a multidisciplinary team, including maxillofacial surgeons, oncologists, radiotherapists, speech therapists, dedicated oncology nurses, and other personnel involved in rehabilitation. In some centres, a clinical psychologist may also be involved in the assessment and rehabilitation of patients undergoing treatment for oral cancer. Specialists in palliative care may also be involved in the management of these patients who have advanced disease or for whom treatment has proved unsuccessful. The treatment of choice depends on a number of factors including patient preference, biological age, general health, and site and staging of the tumour. Over the last 2 decades, there have been great advances in the reconstruction of patients who have undergone surgical treatment for oral carcinoma and these have led to a greatly improved quality of life.

> The management of oral cancer should be coordinated by a multidisciplinary team.

The treatment of oral carcinoma is clearly a complex matter, which in the majority of cases involves surgery (with reconstruction), radiotherapy, or a combination of both. Chemotherapy is not routinely used for the treatment of oral carcinoma at the present time. Management regimens for carcinoma must focus on longevity and quality of life.

> Management regimens for cancer must focus on longevity and quality of life.

Radiation mucositis

During the course of radiotherapy (which is likely to last for several weeks) the patient develops a progressive and generalized erythematous and ulcerative response of the oral mucosa (radiation mucositis) (see Table 10.3). Radiation mucositis generally starts about the second week and may be accompanied by a complaint about an altered taste. It is extremely painful, the problem being complicated by the fact that the salivary glands are also virtually always affected, with consequent lessening of salivary secretion and xerostomia. Secondary candidosis almost invariably occurs, and Gram-negative organisms may play a significant role. Following the course of radiation the mucositis gradually subsides leaving an atrophic oral epithelium on a relatively avascular submucosa. The salivary flow may be permanently reduced and the patient will develop signs and symptoms related to salivary gland dysfunction (see Chapter 8). In the long term, radiation therapy may result in trismus due to tissue fibrosis.

In the acute phase, simple non-astringent mouthwashes (for example, sodium bicarbonate or table salt) may have a soothing effect on the oral mucosa. Benzydamine hydrochloride mouthwash has anti-inflammatory, and antimicrobial properties and may reduce the severity of the mucositis. Miconazole gel may be used to combat candidosis. Patients may only be able to tolerate a soft, bland diet. In the long term, the combination of dry mouth and an atrophic mucosa may cause continuing discomfort for which artificial salivas (and saliva replacement gels) are the only available treatment, together with benzydamine hydrochloride rinse. Those containing added fluoride might well be considered. These patients become unusually susceptible to caries against which topical fluorides may be effective. Patients should be encouraged to maintain their oral hygiene as much as possible. Radiation caries should be managed by a combination of oral hygiene procedures, restoration of early lesions, and the application of topical fluorides. The management of salivary gland hypofunction has been discussed in Chapter 8.

Recent studies have shown that selective decontamination of oral flora with PTA (polymyxin E, tobramycin, and amphotericin) lozenges reduces the duration and degree of mucositis in patients irradiated for oral carcinoma—this should be started before and during radiotherapy (Table 10.4).

Osteoradionecrosis

Radiotherapy for oral malignancy also affects the vascularity of the bone, which becomes nonvital. It is, therefore, highly susceptible to infection and the effects of trauma. Osteomyelitis occurs as a consequence of infection and results in a painful necrosis (osteoradionecrosis) with sloughing of the overlying soft tissues. Modern methods of radiotherapy have reduced this complication. However, extractions in previously irradiated bone must be carried out with great care and consideration should be given to

Table 10.3 Oral complications of radiotherapy

Early onset	Later onset
Mucositis	Radiation caries
Altered taste	Osteoradionecrosis
Xerostomia	Trismus (fibrosis of muscles and other soft tissues)
Secondary infections	
Demineralization of teeth	
Hypersensitivity of teeth	

Table 10.4 Prevention and management of radiation mucositis

Maintenance of oral hygiene
Selective decontamination (e.g. lozenges containing polymyxin E, tobramycin, and amphotericin)
Dietary advice (bland, non-irritant foods and avoid alcohol)
Bland mouthwashes (e.g. salt/bicarbonate of soda)
Benzydamine hydrochloride (topical use)
Miconazole gel (oral candidosis)
Topical steroids*
Management of salivary gland hypofunction (Chapter 8)

* May predispose to oral candidosis.

Table 10.5 Prevention and management of osteoradionecrosis

Arrange extractions before radiotherapy commences
Avoid trauma to oral mucosa
Conserve teeth postradiotherapy—if possible
Extractions should be atraumatic and under antibiotic cover
Rinse with 0.2% chlorhexidine, prior to extraction
Consider the use of hyperbaric oxygen

antibiotic cover. Hyperbaric oxygen therapy is now being increasingly used to manage these patients. It appears that osteoradionecrosis after extractions is more likely when a longer time has elapsed since radiotherapy (Table 10.5).

The role of the dental team in the management of patients diagnosed with oral carcinoma

Clinical guidelines (see project 1 at the end of chapter) recommend that oncology protocols for patients diagnosed with oral carcinoma should include an early pretreatment oral assessment and the organization of oral care, including any dental treatment required. Ideally, a hospital dentist should be an integral part of the oncology team and can liaise with the patient's own dentist to organize dental treatment prior to, during, and after therapy for oral carcinoma. Any prophylactic requirements need to be instituted prior to radiation therapy. Essential dental procedures also need to be carried out as soon as possible, so not to delay cancer

therapy. Patients who have undergone radiotherapy may be at lifelong risk for oral disease, particularly dental caries and periodontal disease.

Input from a specialist prosthodontist is required for those patients who have undergone ablative procedures involving reconstruction. Endosseous implants may be used to retain bridges or dentures. The dental hygienist has an important role in assisting the patient with dietary advice, the maintenance of oral hygiene, and application of topical fluorides. Patients usually need to be monitored by the dental team at 2- or 3-monthly intervals after radiotherapy.

Prevention of oral carcinoma

This can be divided into primary, secondary, and tertiary prevention. The dental surgeon has a pivotal role in preventive aspects of oral carcinoma and is in an ideal position to give advice concerning lifestyle (for example, tobacco cessation and dietary advice) and to identify high-risk oral lesions (see Table 10.6).

Oral carcinoma as a genetic disease

Oral squamous cell carcinomas and those at other sites in the head and neck arise as a consequence of multiple molecular events. These are induced by the effects of various carcinogens from habits such as tobacco and influenced by environmental factors, possibly viruses in some instances, against a background of heritable resistance or susceptibility. Human cancers

Table 10.6 Summary of methods for the prevention of oral carcinoma*

Primary prevention
Advice on stopping (or reducing) smoking and chewing areca (betel) nut
Advise moderation of alcohol intake
Dietary advice (especially encouraging intake of fresh fruit and vegetables)
Secondary prevention (potentially malignant lesions)
Always screen entire oral mucosa
Recognize abnormalities (e.g. change of colour)
If candidal infection present, identify cause and treat
Refer any suspicious lesion to specialist, especially if there is no improvement within 2 weeks of removing possible causative factor
Tertiary prevention (prevention of recurrence)
Importance of routine extraoral and intraoral examination
Regular review
Low threshold for re-referral
Dietary advice (fresh fruit, vegetables)
Chemoprevention may play a role in the future

* Reproduced (with slight modifications) from Table 1 in Ogden, G.R. and Macluskey, M. (2000). An overview of the prevention of oral cancer and diagnostic markers of malignant change. *Dental Update* 27, 95–9 by permission of George Warman Publications (UK) Ltd.

develop by accumulating a range of somatic genetic changes throughout their progression; however, the molecular basis for these changes remains unclear in the majority of cancers. It has been postulated that genetic damage affecting the majority of autosomal chromosome arms, including activation of oncogenes and/or inactivation of tumour suppressor genes (TSGs) possibly working in conjunction with an impaired capacity of DNA repair mechanisms, may be a factor in the development of squamous cell carcinoma of the head and neck. It is generally accepted that there are three main classes of genes involved in tumourgenesis—TSGs, oncogenes, and DNA repair genes—although distinctions between the particular genes and their properties, and their classification within a certain group, are subject to controversy. Oncogenes includes growth factors, growth factor receptors, signal transducers, and nuclear proteins. However, mutations, amplification, or rearrangement of proto-oncogenes may result in the activation of oncogenes, which leads to malignant transformation. The range of oncogenes that have been studied in oral carcinoma (for example, myc and ras gene families and erB-1) and activated oncogenes produce either abnormal (mutated) proteins or aberrant expression of proteins at an inappropriate stage in the cell cycle. A second group of genes is involved in malignant transformation, TSGs. One of the most studied TSGs is p53, which is located on chromosome 17p. The p53 gene codes for a 53 kDa nuclear phosphoprotein that holds a key position in the complex network controlling genome stability, cell cycle, and apoptosis. p53 acts as a TSG by arresting cells carrying DNA damage in the G_0/G_1 phase, providing adequate time for the cell's DNA repair mechanism to function and, if unsuccessful, leads cells to apoptotic death. p53 mutations have been previously reported in many cancer studies including oral cancer and are considered to be the most frequent genetic event contributing to the molecular pathogenesis of oral cancer. Of crucial importance is the fact that abnormalities of p53 have been identified in oral cancer, associated with smoking and drinking, and in some dysplasic leukoplakias. The roles of oncogenes, TSGs, and DNA repair mechanisms are currently very active areas of research in oral cancer, as they are considered to be the basic mechanisms in the aetiology of the disease as well as having enormous potential as early detection markers and for use as targets for therapy.

> Oral carcinoma is a genetic disease.

One emerging concept, however, is that a number of activating and inactivating genetic events must occur for the initiation and progression of oral carcinoma and that these genetic changes most probably occur as a multistep process (Fig. 10.7).

> Genetic changes involved in the initiation and progression of cancer occur in a multistep process.

The potential role of viruses in oral carcinogenesis

There is considerable interest in the possible interactions in carcinogenesis between HPVs, simian virus (SV40), and large T

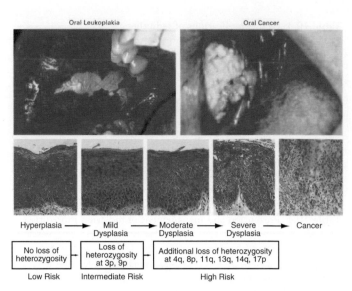

Fig. 10.7 Progression from leukoplakia to causes of the oral cavity. Reproduced from Lippman (2001). Molecular markers of the risk of oral cancer. *New England Journal of Medicine*, 344, p. 1323. Copyright © 2001 Massachusetts Medical Society. All rights reserved.

antigen. The reason for this renewed interest is based on the experimental evidence surrounding the p53 TSG's involvement in cancer and evidence that its aberrant expression may be altered by p53 gene mutations as a consequence of carcinogens, radiation, or other mutagens, or by other mechanisms, such as inactivation of the p53 protein by viral or other proteins. Significant in this respect may be viral proteins such as SV40, large T antigen, HPV type 16 E6 protein, as well as the cellular proteins such as MDM-2 (murine double minute-2). The presence of high-risk HPV types in squamous cell carcinoma of the head and neck may result in inactivation of p53 TSG function by nongenetic mechanisms. HPV has been found in p53 mutated oral carcinomas.

Molecular techniques to identify genetic changes/alterations in the oral mucosa

Genetic alterations can be studied in cellular DNA, RNA, and protein from tumour tissue specimens; biopsies; tissue scrapes; and also in plasma or serum from patients with premalignant and malignant disease.

Molecular techniques currently available for genetic analysis include: at the DNA level, allelic imbalance (loss of heterozygosity analysis), DNA sequencing, single-stranded conformational analysis, methylation profiling, and molecular–cytogenetic approaches; at the RNA level, Northern blotting and reverse transcriptase polymerase chain reaction (RT-PCR); and, at the protein level, Western blotting, immunohistochemical analysis, *in situ* hybridization, and peptide sequencing. The publication of the Human Genome Sequence now makes large-scale approaches to cancer genetics in patient groups applicable, by using expression chip analysis which contains most of all of the known human genes, as well as approaches such as CGH chip and methylation chip analysis. Furthermore, the identification of millions of single nucleotide polymorphisms (SNPs) in the human genome has made genotyping analysis a reality. Details of these techniques are clearly outside the scope of this book but it is important to gain an understanding of the scientific basis of these tests, their limitations, and applications.

Tumour markers

In future, molecular genetic markers of premaligancy and malignancy will be used alongside conventional histopathological techniques to aid in the diagnosis of oral cancer as well as being used in the management of these patients to optimize treatment. Many of these markers are only used as research tools at the present time but are currently being developed to become a part of routine diagnostic testing.

Molecular markers for malignant transformation of oral leukoplakia

There are currently no reliable clinical or histological features of oral leukoplakia that can be used to predict whether a lesion will regress or progress to carcinoma. The development of molecular markers that will determine the risk of malignant transformation is therefore of fundamental importance. Furthermore, molecular markers may make it possible to monitor cancer recurrence as well as providing the key for the development of effective chemopreventive and chemotherapeutic agents.

There have been recent important advances in the molecular assessment of the risk of malignant transformation in patients with oral leukoplakia. These studies have involved assessment of potentially predictive markers such as the establishment of ploidy status, detection of alleleic imbalance (or loss of heterozygosity), mutational profiling of TSGs such as p53, or determining aberrant expression of a range of genes involved in carcinogenesis However, it is now clear that a single genetic marker or class of markers cannot be used to predict the outcome of every case of oral leukoplakia. Complex models to predict the risk of cancer in patients with oral leukoplakia are therefore being developed.

Molecular assays may, in future, define patients who are at a low risk of oral cancer development and for whom non-invasive review of their oral leukoplakias and modification of lifestyle (for example, tobacco cessation) may be reasonable and based on scientific evidence. For those patients identified as 'high risk', resection of their lesions with verifiable clear resection margins may be the most appropriate management with or without chemoprevention. A wide range of new chemoprevention agents are currently being assessed and molecular biomarkers will be used as intermediate end-points to assess their validity. We are entering a new era of molecular diagnosis and targeted treatment modalities that will be based on the findings from the post-genomic revolution.

> Early detection and target drug therapy in oral carcinoma will be based on future genetic profiling.

Discussion of problem cases

Case 10.1 Discussion

Q1   What questions would you ask this patient?

The patient should be asked if he has noticed this ulcer and, if so, for how long and whether it has been sore. It is also important to find out if there has been any soreness and if he has a habit of biting his tongue or catching it with the denture. He should be questioned as to whether he has suffered from mouth ulcers in the past. You should recheck his medical history, with particular emphasis on skin, eye, genital, or gut problems and ascertain if he has generally felt well or suffered any weight loss. The patient's drug history should be reviewed to check for any prescribed or over the counter drugs. He should also be asked about his intake of alcohol.

Q2   What features of the ulcer are important to note?

The following significant features of the ulcer should be noted by visual inspection and palpation: induration; proliferative growth; changes in surface texture and colour; fixation to the affected tissue or underlying structures.

Q3   What is the most likely differential diagnosis in this particular case?

This patient appears to have presented with an asymptomatic ulcer but may, when specifically asked, report soreness or discomfort on eating. The broken denture could indicate the ulcer is traumatically induced, particularly if it has no clinical features suggestive of malignancy. An isolated aphthous ulcer is rarely symptom-free and the patient is likely to have given a history of RAS in the past. Drugs, such as nicorandil or NSAIDS can predispose to oral ulceration but lesions are usually painful and the patient would report a positive drug history. In the case of this patient who has one (or possibly more) significant risk factors (that is, he is a heavy smoker) and presents with an isolated, asymptomatic ulcer on the lateral border of the tongue (risk site), the likelihood of a squamous cell carcinoma is high.

Q4   How would you manage this patient?

If you suspect that the lesion is a traumatic ulcer and there is an obvious source of trauma, this should be eliminated by adjusting the denture. The patient must, however, be reviewed in 10–14 days, to check if there are any signs of healing.

This gentleman should be told at this stage why it is important for him to be followed up. If, however, the ulcer has any suspicious features, he should be referred to the nearest specialist centre (that is, oral medicine or oral and maxillofacial surgery) for further investigations, including biopsy. Biopsy of an oral lesion that you suspect may be a carcinoma, should be undertaken by the specialist who will decide on definitive treatment and not the general dental practitioner. A referral letter, describing the patient's history and full description of the ulcer, should be faxed (as well as posted) to the specialist centre, with a follow-up telephone call to check that this has been received. The patient should be advised of the importance of attending his specialist appointment. Patients may ask if their mouth ulcer could be a 'cancer' or 'malignant' or a 'tumour', and dentists may find this question awkward to answer. In the majority of cases it is better to inform the patient that this is a possibility and that it must be ruled out by further investigations. It may be helpful, at this stage, to point out that there are a number of different causes of mouth ulcers. If the patient's ulcer is found to be carcinoma, the dentist is likely to have a role to play in posttreatment rehabilitation.

Projects

1. Read the clinical guidelines, *The oral management of oncology patients*, published by the Faculty of Dental Surgery, Royal College of Surgeons of England.

2. What is meant by the term 'health-related quality of life'? How has this been measured in patients who have undergone surgery for the treatment of oral carcinoma?

11

Mucocutaneous disease and connective tissue disorders

Mucocutaneous disease

Lichen planus and lichenoid reactions

Immunobullous disease

- Pemphigus
- Pemphigoid
- Dermatitis herpetiformis
- Linear IgA disease

Epidermolysis bullosa

Erythema multiforme

Idiopathic oral blood blisters (Angina bullosa haemorrhagica)

Connective tissue diseases

- Lupus erythematosus
- Morphoea and systemic sclerosis
- Mixed connective tissue disease

Mucocutaneous disease and connective tissue disorders

Problem cases

Case 11.1

One of your edentulous patients, a 62-year-old lady, telephones the surgery requesting an urgent appointment because she is afraid she may have mouth cancer. Whilst cleaning her dentures the night before, she had noticed some white patches inside her mouth and remembers reading in a magazine that these can be a sign of mouth cancer. This lady had been unable to sleep due to worry. She is seen later that day and on examination you note a network of white 'lace-like' lesions on both buccal mucosae, which are painless. There are no other oral lesions. On further questioning the patient reports an itchy rash on her wrists.

Q1 What is the most likely diagnosis of this lady's oral lesions?

Q2 Are her skin symptoms related?

Q3 What investigations would you carry out?

Q4 What advice and treatment would you give to this lady?

Case 11.2

A 41-year-old Jewish man presents with a 9-month history of mouth ulceration, which has become persistent and considerably worse. It is also causing great discomfort on eating. He has noticed that large blisters occur inside his lips but these rapidly burst. Over the last few days he has developed skin lesions and he shows you some eroded skin lesions on his back. There are no ocular or genital symptoms. Examination of the mouth reveals widespread oral ulceration and the Nikolsky sign is positive.

Q1 How would you investigate and manage this gentleman?

Case 11.3

A 2-year-old boy is referred to you by a dermatologist for dental care. His parents tell you that he was diagnosed at birth as having epidermolysis bullosa (EB).

Q1 What are the orodental manifestations of this condition? Discuss the difficulties you might encounter when providing dental treatment for this boy.

Mucocutaneous disease

It was pointed out in Chapter 1 that the oral mucous membrane, although similar to other lining mucosae in structure and general behaviour, also resembles the skin in some ways. This is in keeping with the transitional position and function of the oral mucous membrane, lying as it does in an intermediate position between the skin and the gut mucosa proper. One result of this situation is that generalized diseases, both of mucosae and of skin, may affect the mouth. In such skin diseases, however, the oral lesions, because of the modifying effect of the environment, may bear little superficial resemblance to those of the skin. The continual presence of saliva, secondary infection by oral organisms, and the repeated traumas of the oral environment play their respective parts in the modification of the oral lesions. Particularly good examples of this form of modification are shown in the group of diseases (immunobullous) in which blisters or bullae are formed. When this occurs in the mouth the bullae rapidly break down to form ulcerated areas. Such behaviour affects the management of these conditions. It is often necessary to treat the secondary infection produced in this way before proceeding to more systemic treatment. A different form of modification in oral lesions occurs in some diseases (for example, lichen planus) in which the initial oral lesion may bear little morphological resemblance to the skin lesion, even though the basic histopathological changes are similar. These variants presumably depend on the differing structures of the skin and the oral mucosa rather than on the effect of the environment.

It is not easy to understand why some skin diseases commonly produce oral lesions while others do not. For example, psoriasis, one of the two most common skin diseases seen in European clinics (the other is eczema), produces oral lesions very rarely. In fact, there is some difference of opinion as to whether a characteristic oral lesion does exist. On the other hand, lichen planus produces oral lesions in a high proportion of the patients with skin involvement.

Oral lesions have occasionally been described in a very wide range of skin diseases, even though such behaviour may not be characteristic of the condition. Thus, in the diagnosis of oral lesions of doubtful aetiology, a history of skin diseases is always of interest. Perhaps the most important consideration in this context is the fact that, in some diseases of the skin (including some of the most serious such as pemphigus), the oral lesions may appear before those of the skin and may thus provide an opportunity for early diagnosis and the rapid initiation of treatment.

Definitive diagnosis of the oral lesions in skin diseases depends largely on biopsy examination and this should be carried out on any doubtful lesion. This is not, however, always an easy matter, particularly in the case of bullous lesions in which the manipulations of incisional or excisional biopsy may cause virtual disintegration of the lesion. If such a lesion cannot be removed intact for examination, then the edge of the lesion may often show the characteristic changes better than a central area where secondary changes may obscure the picture. A biopsy taken from an ulcerated area may show nothing but non-specific inflammatory changes. Immunofluorescent techniques and, in particular, direct immunofluorescent studies of biopsy material have revolutionized the methods of diagnosis of immunobullous skin diseases and their oral lesions. For this technique a perilesional biopsy is taken and fresh (unfixed) tissue sent to the pathology laboratory.

In this chapter the conditions chosen for discussion are those that are relatively commonly seen in the oral medicine clinic or those of particular interest or importance in the dental context. Other conditions that link oral medicine and dermatology include the genatodermatoses (Chapter 9), Peutz–Jegher's syndrome (Chapter 9), and Wegener's granulomatosis (Chapter 1).

Lichen planus and lichenoid reactions

Skin lichen planus

In this disease the skin lesions take the form of dusky pink papules that may occur in any site, but are most commonly found on the flexor surfaces of the wrists (Fig 11.1), on the genital skin, on the abdomen and lumbar regions, and on the ankles and shins. Fine white striations overlie the papules. These are the so-called Wickham's striae that are characteristic of the condition (Fig. 11.1). In general, the skin lesions are relatively short-lived, the average duration being of the order of 9 months. After this they fade, leaving behind a faintly pigmented patch that may take a considerable time to disappear. In a significant proportion of the patients, however, there may be a recurrence of the lesions. The

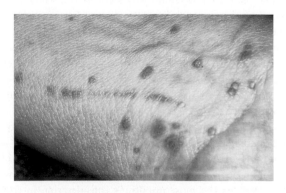

Fig. 11.1 Typical skin lesions of lichen planus.

majority of skin lesions cause little trouble apart from itching, which is very variable in its intensity—in some instances it is so insignificant that the lesions are not noticed by the patient. In a few cases the Köbner phenomenon may be seen with lesions distributed in a linear pattern along a scratch mark on the skin. Scalp lesions may also occur in a few patients (usually female). Often these are not papular, but are represented by patches of alopecia. There are widespread variations in the clinical picture, shown by occasional patients who may present with bullous, hypertrophic, or annular lesions, and, very rarely, the disease may first occur in an acute form with initial symptoms much more severe than those described above. The histology of a skin lesion is quite characteristic and, in all essentials, resembles that of the oral lesions. The most obvious feature is basal cell liquefaction and the presence of a narrow dense band of inflammatory cells, predominantly lymphocytes, within the dermis and lying just below the epithelium. In the skin the effect appears to be a pushing up of the epithelium to form the papules, although this may not, in fact, be the actual mechanism of papule formation. The overlying epithelium may undergo a variety of changes, hyperorthokeratosis being the most common finding in the case of the skin lesions.

> In the Köbner phenomenon individual skin lesions develop on a site of trauma or an operation scar. This is seen in a number of dermatological conditions including lichen planus and psoriasis.

Involvement of the nails is seen in about 10 per cent of patients and this manifests as fine ridging or grooving, severe dystrophy, and, in a few cases, destruction of the nail bed. The classic nail change of lichen planus is the pterygium, in which adhesion between the dorsal nail fold and the nail bed leads to the partial destruction of the nail.

> The flexor surfaces of wrists, ankles, and shins and lumbar regions are the usual sites of involvement in skin lichen planus.

The genital mucosa also can be involved in lichen planus but may be asymptomatic. The vulvovaginal gingival (VVG) syndrome is a rare variant of lichen planus, characterized by erosions of vulval, vaginal, and gingival mucosae with a predilection for scarring and stricture formation. This causes considerable problems to the patient and is difficult to manage.

> The vulvovaginal gingival syndrome is a rare variant of lichen planus, which is difficult to manage.

Aetiology of lichen planus

Lichen planus is an immunologically mediated disease but in the majority of cases does not appear to be consistently part of an autoimmune disturbance. A number of factors have been implicated in the aetiology of lichen planus and associations, often unsubstantiated, made with systemic diseases such as diabetes mellitus and liver disease. Lesions that clinically and histologically resemble those of oral lichen planus (lichenoid reaction) can be precipitated by an ever-increasing range of drugs. Lichenoid reactions will be discussed in the next section of this chapter.

Oral lichen planus

PREVALENCE

Oral lichen planus affects from 0.1 to 4 per cent of individuals depending on the population studied and is generally a disease of the middle-aged and elderly, with a female preponderance of 2:1. The age range is similar to that in patients reporting with skin lesions only, although, in the case of patients with oral lesions, there is a rather higher proportion of patients in the 60 year plus group. The authors have seen a small number of patients with confirmed oral lesions at a very early age, the youngest being 7 years old. This would be considered a great rarity in the case of skin lesions.

> Oral lichen planus affects 0.1 to 4 per cent of individuals, depending on the population studied.

Oral lesions occur in a considerable proportion of patients with lichen planus and are seen in the oral medicine clinic far more frequently than the oral lesions of other skin diseases. The true incidence of oral lesions is a little difficult to determine since the figures available vary widely, a significant factor being whether the patients are first seen in a dermatological clinic (in which case oral lesions are present in about 70 per cent of cases) or in a dental clinic. In these latter patients, presenting because of oral lesions, the incidence of skin lesions is of the order of 40 per cent. This variation is probably due to a number of factors, the most important being the asymptomatic nature of the oral lesions in many cases. A second important factor is the inconstant sequential relationship of the lesions—the oral lesions may occur before, after, or at the same time as the skin lesions. In general, however, oral lesions last much longer than skin lesions. A mean duration of 4.5 years has been suggested but there is no doubt that in many cases this period may be greatly exceeded.

CLINICAL PRESENTATION

The oral lesions are usually bilateral and involve the buccal mucosa in about 90 per cent of all cases. In descending order of frequency the tongue, gingivae, alveolar ridge, lips, and less commonly the palate may also be affected.

> In oral lichen planus, the buccal mucosa and tongue are the most common sites of involvement and lesions tend to be bilateral.

A range of clinical presentations can occur in oral lichen planus and may coexist in the same patient. There is, however, some confusion in the literature concerning the terminology used to describe the clinical variants of oral lichen planus (Table 11.1).

Reticular, plaque-like, and papular variants tend to be asymptomatic. In these variants the epithelial change is of

Table 11.1 Clinical variants of oral lichen planus

Reticular
Plaque-like
Papular
Atrophic
Erosive (ulcerative)
Bullous
Desquamative gingivitis

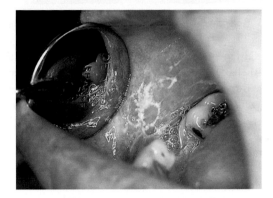

Fig. 11.2 Reticular, non-erosive lichen planus of buccal mucosa.

hyperparakeratosis or, occasionally, hyperorthokeratosis. There is no atrophy of the epithelium and, hence, no ulceration. The characteristic appearance is of white streaks on the oral mucosa, arranged in a reticular 'lace-like' pattern (Fig. 11.2). In some patients the lesions may be more confluent (plaque-like) and resemble a leukoplakia, whereas in others there may be papular, linear, or annular arrangements of the white areas. These are often described as being similar to the Wickham's striae of the skin lesions, but are, in fact, much more clearly defined. In the course of the disease the morphology of the lesions may change, and there may also be variations in their extent and intensity. In general, these lesions are often quite symptom-free and are often noticed incidentally by the patient, although a sensation of 'roughness' may be present. In the striated forms the diagnosis may initially be made with some confidence on appearance alone, but in the case of the confluent plaque-like lesions the diagnosis may be made only after biopsy.

In other forms of oral lichen planus, the oral epithelium undergoes atrophic changes and is easily lost from the weak and oedematous basal areas. This may result in the formation of ulcerative lesions on the mucosa, these often being associated with nearby areas in which reticular or atrophic lesions occur (Fig. 11.3). In a few patients the basal and subepithelial oedema may lead to separation of the epithelium with consequent bulla formation, but such bullae, developed in initially atrophic epithelium, are very fragile and rapidly disintegrate to produce the characteristic ulcerative lesions of the condition. In published studies of oral lichen planus the terms 'ulcerative' and 'erosive' have been used

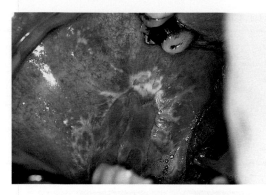

Fig. 11.3 Reticular and erosive lesions of oral lichen planus.

synonymously to describe a clinical appearance in which there has been epithelial loss. This variation in descriptive terminology used in oral medicine leads to confusion and does not necessarily reflect the histopathology of the lesion: in addition the results of clinical trials are difficult to evaluate. In this chapter, the clinically descriptive term 'erosive' will be used to describe the irregular areas of oral epithelial destruction (shallow or deep) which are covered in a yellow layer of fibrin. Atrophic lesions, in which there has been epithelial thinning, present as irregular areas of erythematous mucosa—both erosive and atrophic variants tend to be symptomatic. Unlike the situation in the reticular or plaque-like forms of the disease, there is often considerable discomfort to the patient, particularly when eating spicy or acid foods. The mucosa is also susceptible to mechanical irritation and the initial symptoms may occasionally appear as denture trauma before any other more characteristic lesions appear. Patients, often in older age groups, may present with extensive erosive lesions, covering large surfaces of the tongue and buccal mucosa. These lesions have a glazed appearance and tend to be separated from the adjacent mucosa by a clearly demarcated edge (Fig. 11.4). These areas of erosion can take months to resolve and are often replaced by

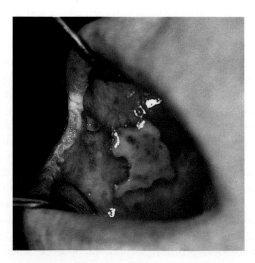

Fig. 11.4 Large erosive lesion of lichen planus with white plaque at commisure.

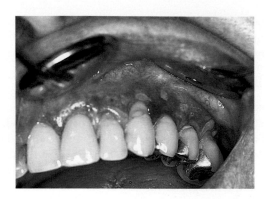

Fig. 11.5 Atrophic and erosive lichen planus affecting the gingivae.

white, confluent lesions, particularly on the tongue. Needless to say, this type of lichen planus causes a great deal of discomfort and patients have difficulty when eating.

All these clinical variants of oral lichen planus can affect the gingivae, with or without involvement of other oral sites. In about 10 per cent of cases gingival involvement alone occurs and can make the clinical diagnosis more difficult. In addition, gingival architecture can create problems when choosing a site to biopsy and the resulting histopathology is more difficult to interpret, particularly if there is a superimposed non-specific gingivitis. In patients with involvement of this site the gingivae often have a red, glazed appearance affecting their full width (Fig. 11.5). This clinical appearance is known as 'desquamative gingivitis' which may be difficult to clinically differentiate from involvement with other mucocutaneous diseases, particularly pemphigoid. The term 'desquamative gingivitis' is a clinical descriptive term and does not therefore infer any specific underlying pathology. Not all cases are due to lichen planus.

The definitive diagnosis of all types of lichen planus is by biopsy and histopathology should include periodic acid Schiff (PAS) staining for *Candida* species (see Chapter 4). Although the appearance of the lesions may give an indication of the diagnosis in some cases, this is not always so and the clinical features may sometimes be confused with those of immunobullous lesions or with patches of erythroplakia. The presence of skin lesions is a useful diagnostic pointer but, evidently, not a constant one.

HISTOPATHOLOGY

The essential histological change in these lesions is the same as in those of the skin—the presence of a subepithelial band of lymphocytes, predominantly of the T type, and some macrophages (Fig. 11.6)—but in the case of the oral mucosa there is a much wider range of epithelial response, with acanthosis or atrophy, orthokeratosis, or parakeratosis. However, the most common finding is of parakeratosis, the rete pegs being distorted to give a 'saw-tooth' or, more commonly, flattened appearance. Around the basement membrane there is oedema, associated with degenerative changes in the basal cells, an association that in some cases leads to virtual separation of the epithelium from the corium. The direct immunofluorescence findings in lichen planus are not

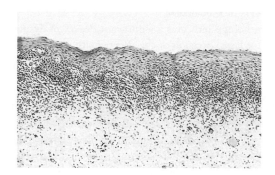

Fig. 11.6 Section of oral mucosa in lichen planus.

highly specific. A band of fibrin is shown up at the basal zone, but no immunoglobulin deposits. Cytoid 'civatte' bodies may be seen, however, both in the epithelium and in the dermis. These are non-disease-specific spherical structures that contain variable immunoglobulins and complement components. A high incidence of these is indicative, if not diagnostic, of lichen planus.

The pathogenesis of lichen planus is not fully understood but probably involves a cell-mediated immune response to antigenic changes in oral mucosa. This would be consistent with the predominantly T-lymphocyte infiltrate.

Lichenoid reactions

In a minority of cases (but still a substantial number) lichen planus is precipitated by drugs or other substances. A number of drugs have been implicated in lichenoid drug eruptions (LDEs) including nonsteroidal anti-inflammatory agents (NSAIDs), antihypertensive drugs (especially angiotension converting enzyme (ACE) inhibitors), antimalarials, and gold injections (Table 11.2). Withdrawal of the precipitating drug usually results in resolution of the LDE but not all lesions uniformly regress.

Localized lichenoid reactions have also been associated with hypersensitivity reactions to mercuric salts released from amalgam restorations. These characteristically occur where the oral mucosa is in contact with the offending restoration. Removal of the restoration frequently results in regression of the lesion and this would suggest a type IV hypersensitivity reaction, similar to that seen in contact dermatitis as a response to metals such as nickel. A few cases of lichenoid reactions have, however, already been reported in response to composite resins. Patients undergoing bone marrow transplantation can develop an oral lichenoid lesion as a manifestation of a graft-versus-host reaction.

> Lichenoid drug eruptions can be caused by a large number of drugs, including NSAIDs and antihypertensives.

LDE and idiopathic oral lichen planus are similar both *clinically and histologically*. Mucosal lesions in oral lichen planus tend to be bilateral, whereas LDEs have a tendency to occur unilaterally and may affect the palate. Histologically in LDEs, lymphoid follicles may be prominent and there may be a more mixed cell population including eosinophils and plasma cells.

Management of lichen planus and lichenoid reactions

INVESTIGATIONS

In addition to standard history taking and clinical examination, patients should be asked in detail about their drug history and possible involvement of other sites, including the skin and other mucous membranes. Microbiological sampling of mucosal sites may reveal candidal infection, which it may be advisable to treat prior to biopsy. Biopsy should be undertaken for all patients with suspected oral lichen planus and may need to be from more than one affected site. PAS staining of histological samples is essential.

THERAPY

Treatment of skin lichen planus is directed at controlling the itch and moderately potent topical steroids are probably the most effective agent for this. Sedating, systemic antihistamines may be helpful at night. Short courses of systemic steroids have been suggested for severe cases but long-term steroids should not be used for chronic cases. Retinoids and ciclosporin have been used in some reported cases, with mixed success.

Therapy for symptomatic oral lichen planus is aimed at providing relief of discomfort, healing of erosive lesions, and increasing epithelial thickness in areas of atrophy. It usually includes the use of an antiseptic mouthwash (to aid with plaque control and reduce secondary infection) and an analgesic mouthwash (to reduce discomfort) — see Table 11.3. Local steroids are the mainstay of treatment and assist in the healing of erosions and reduction of atrophy (Table 11.3). Hydrocortisone lozenges are of limited value in oral lichen planus and triamcinolone, in an adhesive paste, is difficult to apply to widespread erosive and atrophic lesions. These preparations, however, are unlikely to give rise to problems associated with systemic absorption. Other topical preparations (Chapter 3) include soluble betamethasone tablets, dissolved in water and used as a mouthwash, steroid sprays (for example, beclomethasone), potent steroid ointments (for example, fluocinonide) mixed with an adhesive base, and triamcinolone mouthwashes. In all these preparations, systemic absorption can occur and oral candidosis may occasionally complicate treatment. Topical antifungal therapy is often indicated for patients with

Table 11.2 Systemic drug groups commonly implicated in oral lichenoid drug eruptions

Nonsteroidal anti-inflammatory drugs (NSAIDs)
Angiotensin-converting enzyme (ACE) inhibitors
Oral hypoglycaemics
Diuretics
Antimalarials
Gold
Penicillamine

Table 11.3 Therapeutic options for oral lichen planus

Type	Examples
Antiseptic	Chlorhexidine gluconate (mouthwash)
Analgesics	Benzydamine hydrochloride (mouthwash)
	Lignocaine rinse
Antifungals	Nystatin pastilles (topical)
	Amphotericin lozenges (topical)
	Miconazole gel (topical)
	Fluconazole (systemic)
Topical corticosteroids	Hydrocortisone hemisuccinate (pellets)
	Triamcinolone acetonide (in adhesive paste)
	Fluocinonide (in adhesive paste)
	Betamethasone sodium phosphate (mouthwash)
	Triamcinolone mouthwash
	Beclomethasone dipropionate (spray)
	Budesonide (spray)
Systemic immunomodulators	Prednisolone
	Azathioprine
	Ciclosporin
Other reported therapies	Antimalarials (hydroxychloroquine)
	Topical tacrolimus
	Retinoids
	Dapsone

symptomatic oral lichen planus. Not only do topical steroids and other immunomodulators predispose to candidosis but several studies have shown an increased prevalence of *Candida* species—in both mycological and histological studies of oral lichen planus. Superimposed oral candidosis can exacerbate the oral symptoms of oral lichen planus and should be treated, in the first instance, by appropriate topical antifungal agents (Chapter 4). Nystatin pastilles or amphotericin lozenges are appropriate but topical nystatin may not be tolerated by patients with a sore, atrophic mucosa. Miconazole gel may be preferred and in some cases a systemic antifungal, such as fluconazole, is indicated. Care must be taken with the use of azoles because of their interactions with other drugs, notably warfarin.

In severe cases with major erosive lesions, short courses of systemic steroids can be effective to alleviate acute exacerbations of oral lichen planus but are contraindicated in the long term. High-concentration steroid mouthwashes in some cases appear to be equally effective. Azathioprine may be required as a steroid-sparing drug. Other systemic drugs, including ciclosporin, retinoids, antimalarials, and dapsone (Table 11.3), have been advocated for the treatment of severe oral lichen planus with varying reported results. There is, however, a paucity of evidence-based treatment protocols for this condition. Nearly all these systemic forms of medication have significant side-effects.

OTHER ASPECTS OF MANAGEMENT

If histopathology indicates a significant degree of dysplasia, then surgical (or laser) excision of the affected site may need to be considered. Lichenoid lesions due to drug therapy may be difficult to manage if the drug is required for a patient's general medical condition and an alternative cannot be submitted. Lichenoid drug eruptions can only be reliably confirmed if they resolve after withdrawal or return after re-challenge with the drug. In most cases, this is difficult or unethical to do. Dental restorations, particularly large, corroding amalgams in posterior molars, should be considered for replacement as this may result in resolution of an adjacent lichenoid reaction. Stress has been implicated as a factor in oral lichen planus but there are few studies that have proved a direct relationship. The chronic discomfort associated with symptomatic oral lichen planus is undoubtedly going to be a stressful factor and affect a patient's quality of life.

Patients should be encouraged to stop smoking and given advice about sensible drinking. Oral and denture hygiene should be addressed and attention paid to the patient's periodontal health. All these factors can deleteriously affect oral lichen planus and may predispose to oral candidosis.

LONG-TERM REVIEW OF ORAL LICHEN PLANUS

The great majority of oral lichen planus cases run a completely benign course and some will go into remission after a variable number of years. However, in a small proportion of cases (0.4–3.3 per cent in reported studies, over a follow-up period of 0.5–20 years), oral lesions undergo malignant change. For this reason, long-term reviews of all cases should be undertaken and re-biopsy performed if there are any suspicious clinical changes, such as a nodular, verrucous, speckled, or 'velvety-red' appearance of the mucosa. Patients should be advised to report any significant changes in their lesions or symptoms. Ideally, a photographic record of the patients' lesions should be taken at each follow-up visit. It has been suggested that it is the erosive/atrophic lesions of oral lichen planus that are more likely to transform and that these cases should therefore undergo more stringent follow-up. There are, however, no controlled studies to refute or substantiate this claim.

> A small proportion of oral lichen planus cases undergo malignant change. Long-term review is therefore essential.

Immunobullous disease

Pemphigus

Pemphigus is a group of immunobullous disorders that affect the skin and mucous membranes. It is characterized by the development of autoantibodies to antigens on the keratinocyte cell surface. The bullae are intraepithelial and therefore lie above the basal layer. Pemphigus is a disease of middle age with most patients between the ages of 40 and 60 years with an even gender distribution. There is a racial factor involved in that there is a high incidence of the condition among people of Jewish origin, although patients are by no means restricted to this group. The oral mucous membrane is involved in a high proportion of the patients and, in fact, half of all initial lesions are found in the mouth. Before the introduction of steroids the prognosis in this disease was very poor. The introduction of treatment by systemic steroids, however, has made the outlook considerably less gloomy, although pemphigus must still be considered a very serious condition. It is, therefore, particularly important that the oral lesions should be recognized early in order that treatment may be started at the earliest opportunity. There are four main varieties of pemphigus: pemphigus vulgaris, vegetans, foliaceus, and erythematosus. Pemphigus vulgaris is the most common variety and accounts for about 70 per cent of all cases. It usually begins with shallow erosions on the skin and ruptured blisters on mucosal surfaces. In pemphigus vegetans, the rupture of bullae is accompanied by exuberant granulation tissue, the 'vegetations' of the nomenclature. A rare hereditary form is known as familial benign chronic pemphigus (or Hailey–Hailey disease). In this condition the histology of the lesions closely resembles that of pemphigus proper, with marked acantholysis. The immunological findings are negative. This form is, however, a much less aggressive disease than pemphigus and runs a protracted chronic course. The oral lesions closely resemble those of pemphigus and the rare occurrence of this variant should be borne in mind in differential diagnosis.

> Oral mucosal involvement in pemphigus vulgaris is common and frequently precedes involvement at other sites.

Clinical presentation

The clinical picture in pemphigus is of widespread bullae formation on the skin and mucous membranes. The bullae, even of the skin, are fragile and break down rapidly to form crusted, eroded lesions (Fig. 11.7). The lesions of mucous membranes are even more fragile and rapidly break down with the formation of irregular ulcers, often with a ragged edge as a result of the split and fragile epithelium. The oral lesions may occur in any site within the mouth and oropharynx and may be accompanied by similar lesions of other mucosae. The vulva is often involved in this way.

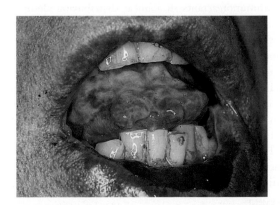

Fig. 11.7 Multiple ruptured bullae of the labial mucosa and tongue in oral pemphigus vulgaris.

Immunopathology (Table 11.4)

Bullae are produced as a result of acantholysis—the breakdown of the intercellular connections, usually in the stratum spinosum of the epithelium. Immunopathology shows the presence of autoantibodies directed against the epidermal and intercellular material. The autoantibody is usually an IgG and complement is also fixed at the site (Table 11.4). The target antigens are now recognized to be desmoglein I and desmoglein III, transmembrane glycoproteins belonging to the cadherin family of adhesion molecules.

Management

Patients frequently present with a severely ulcerated mouth with very little normal mucosa, between the lesions. Biopsy may prove to be difficult as the epithelium is readily detached from the underlying mucosa and it is important that perilesional tissue is obtained. The fragility of the epithelium may be confirmed in some patients by the positive Nikolsky sign; the epithelium can be detached by lateral pressure. Immunological methods are now employed for the diagnosis of pemphigus, as autoantibodies are found in both the affected oral (and skin) tissue and circulating in the patient's serum. Direct immunofluorescence (IMF) of the

Table 11.4 The immunopathology of bullous diseases

Disease	Direct IMF: site[†]	Indirect IMF[*] (circulating autoantibodies)	Target antigens
Pemphigus	Epithelial-bound, IgG, C3: Intercellular	Positive IgG (90%)	Desmoglein I and III
Bullous pemphigoid	Linear, IgG C3: BM zone	Positive IgG (75%)	Bullous pemphigoid antigens, BP180 and BP230
Mucous membrane pemphigoid	Linear IgG, IgA C3: BM zone	Positive IgG (75%), IgA (50%)	BP180 in the majority; laminin 5; β4 integrin
Linear IgA disease	Linear, IgA, C3: BM zone	Positive IgA (30% of adults)	A number of target antigens including BP180
Dermatitis herpetiformis	Granular, IgA, C3: tips of dermal papillae	Negative for epithelial autoantibodies	Unknown
Epidermolysis bullosa acquisita	Linear IgG, C3	Occasionally dermal binding IgG	Type 7 collagen

[*] The presence of circulating autoantibody depends on skin substrate used, i.e. monkey oesophagus for pemphigus and salt-split skin for pemphigoid and linear IgA disease.

[†] BM, basement membrane.

perilesional oral tissue demonstrates IgG-class antibodies binding to the intercellular substances and cell membranes in the stratum spinosum of affected epithelium. Positive direct IMF is essential for diagnosis. Circulating autoantibodies are demonstrated by indirect immunoflorescence in approximately 90 per cent of patients with pemphigus vulgaris.

The treatment of pemphigus is a multidisciplinary matter, involving oral physicians, dermatologists, and other medical specialities—as required. The particular role of the oral physician is, first of all, to enable early diagnosis by the recognition of the oral lesions and, later, to help in the management of the often very severe oral disease. The prognosis has been completely altered by the introduction of systemic steroids and many patients may lead reasonable lives maintained on substantial doses of prednisolone, often with the use of azathioprine as a steroid-sparing drug. Very high dosages are used initially to suppress bulla formation (of the order of 1 mg/kg prednisolone daily), but this may often be slowly reduced to a maintenance dose of 15 mg daily or thereabouts. Other steroid-sparing, immunosupressive drugs such as cyclophosphamide or ciclosporin have also been used to treat pemphigus—severe cases may require plasmapheresis. The titre of circulating antibodies reflects the disease severity and is therefore a useful guide for therapy.

Systemic steroid therapy may be supplemented by high-concentration steroid mouthwashes, since the oral mucosa is often less responsive to treatment than the skin. Just as the oral mucosa seems to be particularly prone to attack by the antibodies early in the course of the disease, it also often remains quite severely affected when the skin lesions are in remission. This may be the case even when the level of the antibody titre is unmeasurably low. Long-term, topical steroid therapy may be required, supplemented by such measures as antifungal therapy and the use of anaesthetic mouthwashes as necessary. Oral hygiene may present a great problem and care must be taken if the teeth are not to be lost, an important dental factor, since the wearing of dentures may be difficult, if not impossible.

Pemphigoid

This group of immunobullous disorders is characterized by the formation of subepidermal bullae and the presence of immunoreactants at the basement membrane zone. There are two broad clinical subtypes of this conditon: the first, which predominantly affects the skin with occasional mucosal involvement, is referred to as bullous pemphigoid (BP). There is a further cutaneous subgroup occurring in pregnancy known as pemphigoid gestationis. The second subtype predominantly involves the mucous membranes with only occasional skin involvement and is now referred to as mucous membrane pemphigoid (MMP)—this was formerly referred to as benign mucous membrane pemphigoid or cicatricial pemphigoid.

Bullous pemphigoid

CLINICAL PRESENTATION

The patients with pemphigoid are, in the main, elderly, most being over the age of 60 years, although some very few may be

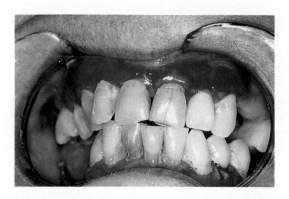

Fig. 11.8 Desquamative gingivitis in a patient with bullous pemphigoid.

considerably younger. As in pemphigus, the gender distribution is even. There is no racial factor involved. Bullous pemphigoid is the most common immunobullous disease in Western Europe.

The condition starts with a pruritic, sometimes urticarial rash, often on the limbs but it may also involve the trunk. Within these erythematous areas develop tense bullae at an interval varying from a few days to a few weeks. Bullae may remain localized to the limbs or may become more generalized. They are fluid-filled but may later become haemorrhagic. Mucous membrane lesions are usually confined to the mouth and occur in up to 20 per cent of patients—in some cases the gingivae are involved (Fig. 11.8). Intraorally, in contrast to pemphigus vulgaris, blisters may occasionally be seen. The clinical course of BP is usually less severe than that of pemphigus with many patients having a resolution within 2 to 5 years. Nevertheless, while patients with localized disease may be controlled adequately with topical corticosteroid creams, patients with more widespread lesions will require systemic immunosuppression. In this elderly population, patients are at a particular risk from the complications of systemic drug therapy.

IMMUNOPATHOLOGY

The blisters in bullous pemphigoid are subepidermal and may therefore remain intact for a number of days. Direct immunofluorescence on biopsy material should demonstrate IgG or C3 immunoreactants in a linear distribution along the basement membrane zone (Fig. 11.9). Circulating anti-basement membrane zone IgG autoantibodies (75 per cent of patients) and occasional IgA may also be detected by indirect immunofluorescence techniques to bind on to the basement membrane of the epithelium (Table 11.4). Linear deposition of IgA antibodies alone, in the context of a predominantly cutaneous blistering disease, is more suggestive of linear IgA disease. The main target antigens in bullous pemphigoid are the BP230 and BP180 antigens. These are considered to be important proteins in maintaining the structural integrity of the basement membrane, that is, in providing cohesion of the dermis to the epidermis.

MANAGEMENT

Diagnosis is based upon a combination of clinical signs (skin and oral) and immunofluorescent findings. To improve the success of

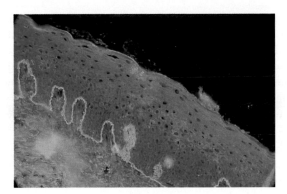

Fig. 11.9 Immunofluorescent demonstration of IgG-group antibody complexes along the basal zone in pemphigoid.

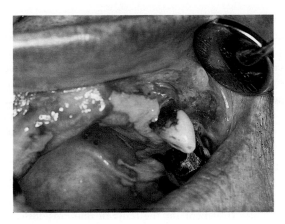

Fig. 11.10 Ruptured gingival bullae in mucosal pemphigoid.

IMF techniques, a perilesional biopsy is essential. With the use of systemic and topical steroids most patients can be kept in reasonable comfort. Steroids can, in most cases of bullous pemphigoid, be reduced to a minimum or completely tailed off, as most patients will eventually achieve remission, tailed off after 3–6 years (unlike pemphigus). For long-term use of steroids, additional immunosuppressive agents such as azathioprine should be added as steroid-sparing agents. Dapsone may be an alternative first-line agent in BP. Topical steroid preparations and analgesic mouthwashes may be beneficial for oral lesions.

Mucous membrane pemphigoid (MMP)

This comprises a heterogeneous group of disorders that may be distinguished from classical bullous pemphigoid by having a predilection for mucosal sites and a tendency to result in fibrosis.

CLINICAL PRESENTATION

Mucous membrane pemphigoid is a clinically heterogeneous disease, which may present to a wide range of specialists including oral physicians, dermatologists, ophthalmologists, gynaecologists, and ENT specialists. While the majority of patients have oral lesions, with additional mucosal sites frequently involved, there are subgroups of patients with disease limited to one site, for example, pure ocular pemphigoid or pure oral pemphigoid. Skin lesions are infrequent and are present in 10–25 per cent of cases, usually appearing on the face, neck, or scalp.

Intraorally, intact bullae may sometimes be present, for example, on the gingivae or soft palate. More often patients present with ulcerated areas of mucosa involving the buccal, palatal, or occasionally lingual or lip mucosa (Fig. 11.10). Desquamative gingivitis is a frequent presentation and may be localized or generalized. The differential diagnosis of this includes lichen planus and pemphigus. Intraoral scarring may occur in MMP but it may be a significant finding in other mucosal sites such as the conjunctiva or in the skin. The term 'cicatricial' pemphigoid has thus been favoured in the past for this subgroup of pemphigoid and remains the preferred term in the ophthalmology literature.

Onset of MMP varies from under 30 years of age to over 70, but is more common in late middle to old age (50–70 year age group). There is a 2:1 preponderance of female patients. The frequency and extent of blistering vary from virtually continuous and multiple, to intermittent and single. The bullae, when established, are in general painless, but there may be discomfort when the bulla is forming and after rupture.

Mucous membrane pemphigoid may present as a desquamative gingivitis.

In a considerable proportion of patients (as much as 75 per cent) the conjunctiva are eventually involved and, since the lesions in this site heal with scarring, vision may be affected. A combination of subconjunctival fibrosis leading to adhesions of the conjunctiva, symblepharon formation (adhesion of bulbar conjunctiva to the eye-lid), and loss of the tear film results in opacification of the cornea and blindness.

All patients diagnosed as having mucous membrane pemphigoid should be referred to an ophthalmologist, as early treatment of ocular involvement, which may be asymptomatic, is essential.

Ocular involvement in mucous membrane pemphigoid is common and may lead to blindness. All patients should be referred for ophthalmological assessment.

Other mucous membranes such as vulval, nasal, pharyngeal, laryngeal, oesophageal, and anogenital may be affected. Patients should therefore be asked about symptoms (such as hoarseness, dysphagia, and genital discomfort) that might indicate involvement of other mucous membranes.

IMMUNOPATHOLOGY

As in bullous pemphigoid, the oral blisters are subepithelial. Direct immunofluorescence on unfixed, fresh biopsy material shows IgG, IgA, or C3 in a linear distribution along the basement membrane zone. Not all patients with the clinical disease have positive immunofluorescence.

Immunopathological findings concerning the detection of circulating anti-basement membrane zone autoantibodies in MMP have shown wide variation in the past and in many previous studies autoantibodies were infrequently detected. However, with the use of a battery of skin substrates and, in particular, with the use of salt-split skin substrate, detection of both IgG and IgA circulating antibodies in MMP has considerably increased (see Table 11.4). Molecular techniques have recently demonstrated that autoantibodies target specific proteins in the basement membrane. The majority of sera react to the bullous pemphigoid antigen, BP180. However, additional subgroups react to alminin 5 and β4 integrin (ocular subgroup).

MANAGEMENT

Treatment of oral involvement is initially on a local basis, using topical steroids in a mouthwash, spray or incorporated in a paste. Symptomatic treatment for the relief of oral erosions caused by the perforation of the bullae may also be necessary. Patients with recurrent multiple bullae may need long-term steroid mouthwashes. Often, however, control, even with high concentrations of local steroids, is inadequate. Dapsone has been advocated as a second-line treatment for mild to moderate mucosal pemphigoid. It is, in general, a well-tolerated drug, but may cause a haemolytic anaemia. Therefore, careful monitoring of the patient's blood count is required. In the most severe cases of mucosal disease, for example, in the presence of active conjunctival inflammation and scarring, systemic steroids combined with a steroid-sparing agent such as azathioprine or cyclophosphamide may be required.

The clinical course of MMP is variable but for the majority of patients it is a chronic disorder that relapses and remits over many years. For those with mild disease limited to the oral mucosa, the condition may 'burn out' after a few years. Among these patients in whom, for example, minimal desquamative gingivitis or bullae occur once every few months, oral discomfort may be relieved by the intermittent use of topical steroids and antiseptic or analgesic mouthwashes alone. For the remainder of patients attending oral medicine clinics with multisite disease or severe oral disease, long-term dapsone may be required with occasional additional short courses of systemic steroids. It is important to appreciate that some of these patients may require multidisciplinary management to achieve optimal care.

Oral immunobullous diseases: summary

It should perhaps be added that the concept of rigid classifications of bullous diseases, clearly defined on clinical and histological grounds, is to some extent giving way to the idea that overlap conditions may occur. This recognition by dermatologists of a spectrum of presentation of bullous skin disease is paralleled by similar observations in the case of oral lesions. Although the great majority of these may be classified with some degree of confidence into one or other of the accepted disease patterns, there remain some lesions that both clinically and histologically seem equivocal.

Dermatitis herpetiformis

Dermatitis herpetiformis is an uncommon bullous skin disease, invariably associated with gluten enteropathy. The cutaneous presentation is of groups of itchy vesicles that characteristically affect the knees, elbows, and buttocks. Two types of oral lesion have been described—one consisting of fragile vesicles and the second of keratotic patches clinically somewhat resembling lichen planus. However, skin and oral lesions share the same characteristic immunopathological features—of granular IgA deposits localized to the apex of the papillae of the lamina propria (Table 11.4).

Linear IgA disease

A mention should be made of linear IgA disease, a rare bullous disease of skin that clinically overlaps with dermatitis herpetiformis and bullous pemphigoid. There are two types of linear IgA disease: one affecting children (chronic bullous disease of childhood) and the other adults (adult linear IgA disease). Skin lesions are classically seen as tense bullae on the trunk, limbs, or scalp, sometimes arranged in groups known as 'rosettes'. In many patients the clinical picture is distinguishable from that of bullous pemphigoid. Oral lesions appear to be uncommon but are similar to those seen in pemphigoid. As the name suggests, the characteristic immunohistological feature is of linear deposits of IgA at the basement zone (Table 11.4). The IgA antibodies are directed at a number of target antigens, including the bullous pemphigoid antigen, BP180. This finding emphasizes the broad overlap between the subepidermal blistering diseases. Dapsone is the systemic drug of choice for the treatment of linear IgA disease.

Epidermolysis bullosa

In these groups of disorders there is skin and mucosal fragility with blistering following mechanical trauma—hence they are sometimes referred to as 'mechanobullous diseases'.

Inherited forms

Inherited forms of epidermolysis bullosa (EB) comprise a rare but serious group of blistering disorders, of which over 20 types have been reported. They are, however, highly unlikely to be diagnosed on the basis of oral symptoms alone but may be of great significance to dental treatment.

The various types of EB have been divided into three main subgroups, based on the histological level of bulla formation, the molecular basis of the defect, and mode of inheritance (Table 11.5).

The predominating feature is extreme fragility of the epithelium, the result of bullae formation occurring either spontaneously or as a response to minimal degrees of trauma. In the 'simplex' form of the disease there is less severe bulla formation and the mucous membranes and teeth are rarely involved. Many patients only have blisters on the soles of their feet. In the lethal junctional and dystrophic type of EB, there is extensive involvement of mucous membrane and the oral mucosa is extremely fragile. Bullae break down to form painful erosions and there is scar formation. In the junctional type of EB the affected child at birth presents with an extreme degree of fragility of the skin and mucous membranes that is incompatible with life, and death is

Table 11.5 Subgroups of epidermolysis bullosa

Clinical features	Site of blister	Inheritance
Simplex epidermolysis bullosa		
Skin blisters at birth, mainly induced by friction. Oral involvement absent or mild. Teeth normal	Basal cells	Mainly autosomal dominant
Junctional epidermolysis bullosa		
Herlitz (lethal) form results in extensive skin and mucosal involvement, dental abnormalities and often with death in infancy. The nonlethal form produces widespread skin and variable mucosal involvement	Lamina lucida	All autosomal recessive
Dystrophic epidermolysis bullosa		
Dominant form is often mild. Recessive form is very severe with extensive blisters and scarring of skin, loss of nails, severe oral mucosal blistering and scarring, and hypoplastic teeth	Immediately below the lamina densa of the basement membrane	Dominant and recessive forms

common in infancy. In the nonlethal junctional type, there is extensive skin and mucosal blistering but scarring is much less severe than in recessive dystrophic EB.

In recessive dystrophic EB, bullae are seen at, or soon after, birth. The lesions are produced in response to the most minor degrees of trauma and eventually heal with scar formation, this leading eventually to gross tissue deformity, particularly of the extremities. The oral mucous membrane is equally susceptible to damage and, as a result of the repeated scar formation, opening of the mouth may become greatly restricted and the tongue bound down. The essential pathology in this form of the disease is dermal; the fragility of the tissues is due to deficient collagen formation in the subepithelial structures. This situation is paralleled in the teeth, there being abnormalities in dentine formation that lead to hypoplasia and a high susceptibility to caries. Since conservative dental treatment or even effective oral hygiene measures may be almost impossible in these patients, the resulting grossly carious teeth, associated with a restricted access and extreme mucosal fragility, present a major problem to the dental surgeon. It has also been reported that the oral scars have, in some patients, been followed by the onset of leukoplakia and, finally, carcinoma, but this cannot be regarded as a characteristic of the disease.

> In epidermolysis bullosa the oral mucosa and teeth may be affected.

Epidermolysis bullosa acquisita

Epidermolysis bullosa acquisita is a rare autoimmune subepidermal bullous disorder involving the skin and mucous membranes. There are two broad clinical subgroups—an inflammatory type reminiscent of BP and a mechanobullous subtype in which bullae occur in response to trauma and lesions are therefore most prominent on the knees elbows, hands, and feet. Oral lesions, where present, may vary in severity from mild desquamative gingivitis to severe generalized ulcerative and often scarring mucosal involvement. Direct immunofluorescence is positive for linear basement membrane IgG and C3. On salt-split skin, circulating IgG antibodies bind to the base of the split corresponding with the target antigen, type 7 collagen. Treatment is often very unsatisfactory despite systemic immunosuppression, and patients frequently develop prominent mucosal and skin scarring.

Erythema multiforme

Erythema multiforme (EM) is an acute vesiculobullous disease of skin and mucous membranes with a wide range of clinical presentations—hence the term 'multiforme'. It may be precipitated by a range of factors, including infections (particularly viral), drugs of various kinds, neoplasia, and pregnancy (Table 11.6). In less than half of the cases no such inducing factor is found. In the most fully developed form (alternatively known as the Stevens–Johnson syndrome), there is widespread involvement of the skin and mucous membranes but, in the more usual restricted form, the oral mucous membrane is mainly involved, with no more than minor lesions in other sites. The patients are predominantly young adults, males being affected more frequently than females.

> Erythema multiforme is an acute vesiculobullous disease of skin and mucous membranes.

The main feature of an attack is the sudden development of widespread erosions of the oral mucosa, characteristically involving the lips. The erosions are produced by the disintegration of subepidermal bullae, lesions that only rarely last long enough to become a diagnostic feature. The erosions on the lips (especially the lower lip) are accompanied by crusting and bleeding and are, if not absolutely diagnostic, strong pointers to the nature of the condition (Fig. 11.11). There is often a cervical lymphadenitis with

Table 11.6 Some precipitating factors in erythema multiforme

Infections
Herpes simplex viral (HSV) infections
Mycoplasma pneumonia (rarely)
Drugs
Sulfonamides
Anticonvulsants
Pregnancy

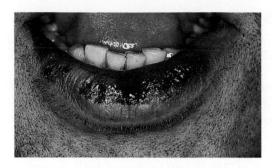

Fig. 11.11 Crusted lesions of the lips in erythema multiforme.

pyrexia and the patient feels unwell. The accompanying skin lesions, when present, may have a characteristic 'target' (or 'iris-like') appearance that is diagnostic. Ocular involvement, if present, may result in conjunctival damage but this is unusual. An attack gradually subsides after some 10 days, but there is a considerable likelihood of recurrence of EM after a period varying from no more than a few weeks to a year or so. This is more likely if EM is associated with recurrent herpes simplex virus (HSV) infection.

> Recurrent erythema multiforme is associated particularly with HSV infection and patients may require long-term prophylactic aciclovir.

The initial diagnosis is entirely clinical, the important differential diagnosis being from a primary herpetic stomatitis. In the case of a recurrent attack, however, herpetic stomatitis may be confidently excluded since this is an isolated event in immunocompetent individuals. Similarly, a history of recurrent herpes simplex renders the diagnosis of herpetic stomatitis unlikely. The involvement of the lips is a strong indication of the diagnosis of erythema multiforme and the presence of 'target' lesions of the skin can be taken as almost conclusive evidence for the diagnosis. Biopsy of the oral lesions shows a rather non-specific histological picture with degenerative changes in the epithelium and subepithelial bulla formation. Because of the acute clinical features, however, the diagnosis does not often depend on the histological appearance of the lesions. Other immunobullous diseases may need to be excluded by immunofluorescence studies.

Treatment of the cases restricted to the mouth depends on the use of local or systemic steroids, to which there is usually a rapid response. A steroid mouthwash is likely to give symptomatic relief and effectively reverse the process in a few days. In the more severe cases (particularly when other mucous membranes are involved), when the skin or oral lesions are severe or when the eyes are affected, a short course of systemic steroids may be necessary to shorten the attack. The use of systemic steroids for EM remains controversial. However, a course of 40 mg prednisolone daily for 1–4 weeks, rapidly reducing over the next few weeks, may be beneficial for symptomatic relief. A topical or systemic antifungal agent may also be required. Such patients may be sufficiently ill to require hospital admission, particularly if they become dehydrated. Patients with recurrent EM require long-term prophylactic aciclovir.

Some authorities have suggested that EM and Stevens–Johnson syndrome are distinct clinical disorders, on the basis of their clinical features and specific causes. However, others have challenged this concept as some patients with EM and mild symptoms may subsequently develop severe attacks, necessitating hospital admission.

Idiopathic oral blood blisters (angina bullosa haemorrhagica)

Some patients develop spontaneous blood-filled bullae ('blood blisters') of the oral mucosa from time to time. These have been described under the rather unfortunate and inappropriate title of 'angina bullosa haemorrhagica'. The usual pattern is that the patient feels a sharp pricking sensation in the mouth (most usually on the palate) and finds that a blood-filled blister has suddenly developed. This most commonly occurs when the patient is eating. The bullae may be quite large (up to 2–3 cm in diameter) and the patient may be in considerable fear of obstruction. The blister eventually ruptures or is perforated by the patient and healing occurs uneventfully.

These patients have no demonstrable abnormality of the blood-clotting mechanism, although patients with thrombocytopenia may also develop blood blisters. Both male and female patients have been described, over a wide age range. The method of formation of the blisters is not known. It is speculated that the basic mechanism is of bleeding from the capillary bed below a basal zone that is for some reason weakened. This may indeed be the mechanism, but the reasons for it are far from clear.

The patient's history is often suggestive of the diagnosis, but it is important to exclude an immunobullous condition and also to carry out a full blood count and clotting screen.

Perforation of a large, intact, blister to release the contents may be necessary and antiseptic or analgesic mouthwashes can be prescribed. Often, however, only a ruptured bulla is presented for examination, the patient having perforated it as a first measure. No preventive treatment is known.

Connective tissue diseases

This is a compendium term used to describe a number of diseases with a similar, but by no means identical immunological background. They are not skin diseases, but there are skin lesions in a number of them, and it is common practice to group them with the skin diseases for descriptive purposes. The group includes Sjögren's syndrome and rheumatoid arthritis, which do not have specific skin lesions. These are discussed in Chapters 8 and 15. Apart from these two conditions, lupus erythematosus has important oral manifestations as do mixed connective tissue disease and systemic sclerosis, although these last two are relative rarities.

Lupus erythematosus

The group of diseases included under this heading presents with a wide range of symptoms, but all result from abnormalities of the connective tissues brought about by an autoimmune process. Two main clinical entities are recognized, although there are many variations. These are systemic lupus erythematosus (SLE) and discoid lupus erythematosus (DLE).

Systemic lupus erythematosus

SLE tends to occur in adult life and females are affected much more than males. In this condition, there are widespread changes in the connective tissues with secondary effects in the cardiovascular, musculoskeletal, and other systems, as well as in the skin. Cutaneous LE classically presents as a photosensitive eruption of the face (butterfly-pattern) and hands. The course of the disease varies from a relatively mild chronic condition to a rapidly fatal process, and an equally wide range of skin reactions may occur. These are paralleled by an equally diverse range of oral symptoms, the most commonly described being superficial erosions and erythematous patches on the mucosa. It would seem very unlikely that the initial diagnosis of the disease would be made on the grounds of oral lesions alone, but the possibility of such an aetiology for unrecognized oral lesions should be borne in mind. In particular, it should be remembered that most clinical descriptions of the oral lesions of lupus variants resemble those of lichen planus. Histologically, also, there is a close resemblance between these conditions. The final diagnosis of SLE is likely to be made as a result of the immune abnormalities present—in particular, a wide (and variable) range of antinuclear autoantibodies may be found in the serum. In SLE, circulating antibodies to DNA are almost always present and this is the most significant immunological screening test. If there are skin lesions, the histology and immunofluorescent findings on biopsy are as in discoid lupus erythematosus (below).

Just as a lichenoid reaction may occur as a response to drugs, SLE may be precipitated in the same way and by an equally wide range of drugs. Hydrallazine, used in the management of refractory hypertension, is the most quoted example, but other drugs include beta-blockers, anticonvulsants, and quinidine.

> SLE may be precipitated by drugs.

Treatment of SLE is essentially with steroids, often required in high doses, and with the addition of steroid-sparing drugs such as azathioprine. The oral lesions may be both very painful and difficult to treat. High-concentration steroid–antibiotic mouthwashes may be useful, together with such supporting measures as analgesic mouthwashes.

Discoid lupus erythematosus (DLE)

This is a much more restricted form of the disease, which presents as a skin disorder and without the widespread generalized abnormalities found in the systemic form. The skin lesions, which result from degenerative changes in the subepithelial connective tissues, present as scaly red patches that later heal with scar formation. The face is the area most commonly affected, and circumscribed lesions occur bilaterally. Alopecia can occur if the scalp is involved. Follicular plugging of the skin is an important cutaneous feature to elicit the diagnosis. The patients are predominantly female (female:male, 2:1), the age of incidence being widely distributed, but having a peak in the fourth decade of life. The first appearance of the lesions may follow some form of trauma (such as an unusual degree of exposure to sunlight) and later exacerbations may follow repeated trauma of this kind. Oral lesions are found in a considerable proportion of patients with DLE, although the estimated incidence varies very widely from 3 to 50 per cent according to the source quoted. Although lesions may be found on any part of the oral mucosa, the characteristic site is on the lips. The lesion starts as an area of erythema that develops to a thickened, rather crusted, lesion with a white margin. The histological appearances are of epithelial atrophy at the centre of the lesion with hyperkeratosis at the margins with a close resemblance to the changes in lichen planus. The fundamental difference between the histological findings in lichen planus and in LE (and other connective tissue diseases with skin and mucosal lesions) is that the subepithelial band of lymphocytes, relatively evenly distributed in lichen planus, has a tendency to a follicular distribution in DLE. Direct immunofluorescence in LE gives variable results with homogeneous or granular deposits of IgG, sometimes with IgM and complement components, at the dermo-epidermal junction or below the basal zone. Circulating autoantibodies are found in approximately one-third of patients with skin lesions of DLE.

Treatment of DLE is often symptomatic with the use of potent topical steroids to suppress the lesions. Parenteral treatment, oddly enough, is with the antimalarial drugs, such as hydroxychloroquine, which may completely suppress the symptoms but which may also introduce a wide range of side-effects, some minor and some more serious, for example, the production of corneal deposits and retinopathy. The most significant consideration, so far as the oral lesions are concerned, is the possibility of malignant change. It is difficult to assess the incidence of this from the published figures, but there is no doubt that cases involving malignant transformation in lip lesions have been documented. It is, therefore, necessary to observe the lesions on a long-term basis.

Morphoea and systemic sclerosis

Morphoea is a purely cutaneous disease, in which there is a spontaneous appearance of a scar-like band or plaque. Systemic sclerosis is a multisystem disease in which there is widespread fibrosis of the skin and gut, together with other organs. There may also be other elements of connective tissue disease present, such as SLE and occasionally Sjögren's syndrome (see Chapter 8). Females are more commonly affected and the earliest feature is usually Raynaud's phenomenon. Involvement of the perioral tissues can lead to restricted mouth opening and difficulties with oral hygiene and dental treatment. Patients may develop an expressionless 'mask-like' facial expression.

In systemic sclerosis there may be restricted mouth opening due to involvement of the perioral tissues.

Widening of the periodontal membrane space, particularly in posterior teeth is the characteristic radiological dental finding. A variant of systemic sclerosis has been named the CRST or CREST syndrome (C, calcification; R, Raynaud's phenomenon; E, oesophageal dysfunction; S, sclerodactyly; T, telangiectasia). Most patients with systemic sclerosis have high titres of antinuclear antibody (ANA), usually of the speckled variety, although other types can also be found. Treatment of systemic sclerosis is essentially symptomatic.

Widening of the periodontal membrane space is a characteristic radiological feature of scleroderma.

Mixed connective tissue disease

Mixed connective tissue disease is an overlap condition in which a number of the characteristics of other diseases in the group are found in a single patient. Patients are predominantly female and may have features of SLE, systemic sclerosis, dermatomyositis, and polymyositis. It is a rare condition, but of interest in the present context since there are a number of oral diagnostic indicators of the disease. The first is a 'lichen planus-like' lesion of the oral mucosa, but with a histological appearance resembling that of LE. The second is the involvement of the trigeminal nerve in the neurological changes that may occur in mixed connective tissue disease. This may lead to a complaint of facial anaesthesia, due to a trigeminal neuropathy. In addition, mixed connective tissue disease may be associated with secondary Sjögren's syndrome (Chapter 8). The most important immunological indicator in this condition is the presence of antinuclear antibodies of the speckled type and high levels of a specific antibody to RNAase-sensitive, extractable nuclear ribonucleoprotein (RNP) antigen.

Discussion of problem cases

Case 11.1 Discussion

Q1 What is the most likely diagnosis of this lady's oral lesions?

Q2 Are her skin symptoms related?

Q3 What investigations would you carry out?

Q4 What advice and treatment would you give to this lady?

The most likely diagnosis of this lady's oral condition is lichen planus in its non-erosive, reticular form. She should be specifically asked about medication, as lichenoid eruptions can be drug-induced, although these may be unilateral. Female patients may be reluctant to report genital involvement, if present. The flexor surfaces of the wrists are classical sites for skin lichen planus. Incisional biopsy of the oral mucosa is advisable to confirm the

clinical diagnosis. This lady should be reassured about the diagnosis but advised about the need for long-term follow-up. The oral lesions are asymptomatic and, therefore, no treatment is required. A topical steroid preparation can be prescribed for her skin.

Case 11.2 Discussion

Q1 How would you investigate and manage this gentleman?

The history and clinical examination are suggestive of an immunobullous condition with involvement of the skin and oral mucosa. Oral biopsy, with direct immunofluorescence of perilesional tissue should be arranged and blood taken for indirect immunofluorescence. Biopsy of the oral mucosa may be difficult because of the extreme tissue fragility and extensive involvement of the oral mucous membrane.

Pemphigus vulgaris is the most likely diagnosis in this case and there is a higher incidence amongst the Jewish race. The patient's age and history of oral lesions, preceding involvement of the skin, together with a positive Nikolsky sign are more suggestive of pemphigus than bullous pemphigoid. Mucous membrane pemphigoid tends to affect an older age group, particularly women, and does not commonly involve the skin. The protracted history of oral ulceration and clinical appearance of skin lesions is not consistent with erythema multiforme, which tends to be episodic and manifest as target lesions on the skin.

The clinical diagnosis of pemphigus vulgaris is confirmed by the presence of autoantibodies directed against epidermal intercellular substance of the epithelium. Routine histology in pemphigus reveals bullous formation with acantholysis. Positive direct IMF will demonstrate intercellular deposition of IgG and usually C3 in the epithelium (the so-called 'fishnet' or 'chicken wire' appearance). Urgent treatment is required and the patient is managed in conjunction with a dermatologist. Admission to hospital is usually required. Initially high doses of steroids are given, with the later addition of a steroid-sparing drug, if necessary. Antifungal medication is usually required. Analgesic mouthwashes, containing lignocaine, provide symptomatic relief and help the patient maintain fluid and nutritional intake. Skilled nursing care is essential if there is widespread skin involvement. Attention should be paid to long-term maintenance of oral hygiene. Dental treatment is often difficult.

Case 11.3 Discussion

Q1 What are the orodental manifestations of this condition? Discuss the difficulties you might encounter when providing dental treatment for this boy.

Oral mucosal involvement occurs in the dystrophic and junctional types of epidermolysis bullosa (EB). In children with the junctional type, there are often severe dental abnormalities. Hypoplastic teeth have been described in patients with dystrophic EB. Minimal trauma from toothbrushing and eating causes oral bullae and scarring, as does suckling in neonates. As a result of repeated scarring, mouth opening becomes restricted and the tongue and lips may become immobile. Cracking at the corners of the mouth frequently occurs.

Oral hygiene is difficult for these children and inadequate plaque control, superimposed on defective teeth and a restricted diet often results in rampant caries. Physical access for dental treatment becomes difficult because of scarring. Due to excessive tissue fragility affecting all mucous membranes, local and general anaesthesia are problematical and extractions must be carried out with extreme care. Parents of affected children need to be given preventive advice concerning diet, oral hygiene, and fluoride supplementation before the deciduous teeth erupt. Regular dental reviews and empathetic support for parents are essential. Most cases are treated by a specialist paedodontist.

Project

1. Find out about the short- and long-term effects of systemic steroids and how these may be prevented and/or managed. Discuss the implications of providing oral and dental care for patients who are taking systemic steroids.

12

Gastrointestinal disease

Coeliac disease (gluten-sensitive enteropathy)
- Oral manifestations of coeliac disease

Inflammatory bowel disease (IBD)
- Crohn's disease
- Oral Crohn's disease
- Orofacial granulomatosis
- Ulcerative colitis
- Stomatitis and inflammatory bowel disease

Gastro-oesophageal reflux disorder (GORD)

13

Blood and nutrition, endocrine disturbances, and renal disease

Disorders of the blood
- Anaemias
- Oral signs and symptoms in anaemia
- Management of patients with anaemias and haematinic deficiencies
- Leukaemia
- Leukopenia
- Myelodysplastic syndromes
- Platelet abnormalities
- The selection of patients for haematological examination

Disorders of nutrition
- Nutritional deficiencies
- Scurvy

Endocrine disturbances
- Normal endocrine changes
- Adrenocortical diseases
- Thyroid disease
- Diabetes mellitus

Renal disease
- Chronic renal failure
- Renal patients undergoing dialysis
- Renal transplant patients

Blood and nutrition, endocrine disturbances, and renal disease

Problem cases

Case 13.1

A 40-year-old lady reports to her dentist with a 2-month history of spontaneous bleeding from her gums, which also bleed excessively when toothbrushing. Her mouth has become very sore over the previous 2–3 weeks. She complains of feeling tired and looks very pale. On closer questioning the patient reports frequent attacks of sinusitis and chest infection. In addition, she has noticed that she tends to bruise easily. She is not taking any medication.

Q1   What diagnosis must be excluded in this lady's case? What other oral manifestations of this condition might you find on examination?

Q2   How would you manage this lady?

Case 13.2

A 45-year-old male patient with a history of chronic renal failure presents with severe toothache. He is not a regular dental attender. This gentleman undergoes regular haemodialysis and has an indwelling arteriovenous shunt. He looks very tired and has come directly from the renal dialysis unit, where he had been given some analgesics to take for his dental pain. On examination there is a grossly carious maxillary first molar that requires extraction. There is no associated soft-tissue swelling but you notice white plaques on the tongue and buccal mucosae. These do not wipe off and the patient reports that 'they come and go'.

Q1   How would you manage the dental extraction of this medically compromised patient?

Q2   What is the most likely diagnosis of the white plaques on the patient's oral mucosa?

Disorders of the blood

It is well known that lesions of the oral mucosa may occur in patients with abnormalities of the blood. In particular, the appearance of glossitis or angular cheilitis in anaemic patients has often been described. However, it has more recently become recognized that such oral symptoms may be the result of rela-

tively minor changes in the condition of the blood and that they may occur early in the disease process, even before abnormalities can be demonstrated by a simple blood examination. Thus, an early diagnosis of the blood disorder may depend on a recognition of the significance of the oral symptoms. The great majority of these patients are suffering from anaemias of various kinds and, hence, the major interest is centred on this group of conditions, but it must be borne in mind that abnormalities of the white cell and platelet components of the blood may also be reflected in oral changes.

Anaemias

The characteristic feature of anaemia is a reduction in the level of haemoglobin, which is usually accompanied by a decreased number of erythrocytes. The red cells (erythrocytes) are the circulating cells predominantly concerned with the transport of oxygen to the tissues by means of the iron-containing substance haemoglobin within them. They are normally regular, biconcave discs but, if disturbances of formation occur, they may become quite irregular in size and shape. Such irregularity is often a sign of impaired function. The formation of the erythrocytes within the bone marrow is stimulated by a number of nutritional factors, the two of greatest significance being vitamin B_{12} and folic acid. Both these substances are absorbed from the gut and must be present in balanced quantities for normal red cell production to take place, even when sufficient iron is available for the synthesis of haemoglobin. Iron, folic acid, and vitamin B_{12} are known as haematinics and are essential for normal erythropoiesis. Absorption depends on normal mucosa in the small intestine and, in particular, on the presence of intrinsic factor, which is synthesized in the gastric mucosa and which must be present before absorption of vitamin B_{12} can take place. If there are abnormalities that lead to failure of intrinsic factor synthesis, vitamin B_{12} cannot be absorbed from the gut and must be replaced parenterally. Lack of either vitamin B_{12}, folic acid, or intrinsic factor will therefore affect red cell production in the bone marrow. The erythrocytes formed under these conditions are larger than normal (macrocytic) and their function is severely disturbed. The resultant clinical conditions are known as megaloblastic anaemias.

Megaloblastic anaemias

Vitamin B_{12} or folic acid deficiency are the most common causes of anaemias with macrocytosis. Pernicious anaemia is an autoimmune condition causing atrophy of the gastric mucosa (atrophic gastritis) and consequent failure to secrete intrinsic factor due to an anti-intrinsic factor antibody. Therefore, in patients with this condition antibodies to intrinsic factor may be detected in the blood. More complex malabsorption syndromes may also occur, involving failure to absorb not only vitamin B_{12}, but also folic acid and iron compounds. The term megaloblastic anaemia refers to the change in size and structure of the basic marrow cell from which the erythrocytes are derived—the large circulating erythrocytes formed from these abnormal stem cells are macrocytes. Similar large circulating red cells may be found in other anaemias that are not dependent on abnormalities of the vitamin B_{12}/folic acid metabolism (for instance, in some iron deficiency anaemias) and such macrocytic anaemias form a separate group that, evidently, will not respond to treatment with vitamin B_{12} or folic acid. Other causes of vitamin B_{12} and folate deficiency include malabsorption and dietary deficiency. Folate deficiency can be due to drugs (for example, phenytoin) or the result of the increased physiological demand during pregnancy.

The situation is complicated by the fact that, in multiple deficiencies, the tendency to microcytosis as a result of iron deficiency may be counteracted by a tendency to macrocytosis caused, say, by folate deficiency. The result may be a normal mean corpuscular volume (MCV) in a patient with both deficiencies present. In these circumstances a routine blood count will be returned as normal. It is also clearly established that patients with folate or B_{12} deficiencies may well develop oral signs and symptoms before the erythrocytes are affected and before anaemia develops. Again, this is an argument for the necessity for a full haematological examination in these patients. It may well be that the patients developing oral signs at an early stage of a haematological abnormality represent a selected group with an unusually sensitive mucosal response to the changes.

Iron deficiency anaemia

A much more common cause of anaemia than failure to absorb vitamin B_{12} or folic acid is iron deficiency, which leads to inadequate haemoglobin synthesis. The deficiency may be due either to inadequate intake of iron or to excessive blood loss as in menstrual abnormality or gastrointestinal bleeding. In iron deficiency anaemia, the essential feature observed is a reduction in the haemoglobin concentration within the erythrocytes (hypochromic). They appear pale on microscopic examination, and there may be variations in size and shape. In iron deficiency the erythrocytes are usually small (microcytic). However, the number of erythrocytes per unit volume may not vary greatly from its normal value. The erythrocyte count is not considered to be a particularly important diagnostic test in most cases.

Of the total iron content of the blood, by far the greater proportion is combined in the form of haemoglobin within the red blood cells. A small fraction is present in the plasma, bound to a specific protein, transferrin, and represents the transport iron made available from the body reserves to replace haemoglobin losses. If the stores become exhausted, there is a period of latent iron deficiency in which the haemoglobin concentration is within normal limits and the erythrocytes are of normal size and form, but the serum iron concentration is reduced. This is sideropenia, an iron deficiency that may affect the tissues and is capable of causing oral symptoms, but which does not produce anaemia since the haemoglobin remains unaffected. When the serum iron is depleted in this way, the degree of saturation of the transferrin by the iron will evidently be reduced. This forms the basis of a valuable diagnostic test. In more complex conditions than iron deficiency, there may also be a reduction in the circulating transferrin and so the degree of saturation may remain high in spite of a low serum iron value. As was pointed out in Chapter 2, the test for serum ferritin levels is now regarded as the best general indicator of body iron stores.

The stages of iron deficiency are summarized in Table 13.1. The serum ferritin levels, as a measure of the overall body iron status, would be expected to fall over these three stages. Oral symptoms may appear in the second and third of these stages.

Haemolytic anaemias

There is a further group of anaemias, the haemolytic anaemias, in which the essential abnormality is an increase in the rate of erythrocyte destruction. Under normal conditions, the red cells last for about 100 days, but in haemolytic anaemias their life may be reduced to only a few days. Haemolytic anaemias may be due to an intrinsic defect or may be acquired—an important, although relatively uncommon, cause of the acquired form being the effect of some drugs (Table 13.2). However, the most important haemolytic anaemia in terms of dental practice is sickle-cell anaemia, although this condition is somewhat different from the others under consideration in that its major significance to the dentist is not in the production of oral lesions.

SICKLE–CELL DISEASES

The sickle-cell diseases are a group of genetically determined conditions in which the red cells contain an abnormal haemoglobin, HbS. When HbS loses oxygen it undergoes changes that

Table 13.1 Stages of iron deficiency

1 Pre-latent iron deficiency, in which the body stores of iron are depleted, but the circulating haemoglobin and serum ferritin remain within normal limits
2 Latent iron deficiency, in which the body stores are exhausted and the serum ferritin reduced. The haemoglobin concentration remains unaffected
3 Latent iron deficiency, in which the body stores are exhausted and the serum ferritin reduced. The haemoglobin concentration remains unaffected

Table 13.2 Oral signs and symptoms of haematinic deficiencies

Glossitis
Smooth, depapillated tongue (iron deficiency)
Raw, beefy tongue (vitamin B_{12} and folate deficiencies)
Oral candidosis (including angular cheilitis)
Exacerbation of RAS
Plummer–Vinson (Patterson–Kelly) syndrome (iron deficiency)

produce distortion of the cells, the sickle effect. HbS is inherited as an autosomal recessive condition prevalent in those with Black African/Caribbean ancestry and in some families from the Middle and Far Eastern countries. The carrier state (in which the patient inherits the condition from only one parent) is known as the sickle-cell trait and is by far the more common condition. In this trait the proportion of HbS in the red cells is low and sickling does not take place under normal circumstances. However, sickling may occur in conditions of low oxygen tension and, if this change does take place, the oxygen-carrying capacity of the blood is greatly reduced with the consequent possibility of anoxia in the patient. The fully developed sickle-cell anaemia is the result of the presence of two HbS genes, one from each parent. In this case, the proportion of HbS is high and sickling occurs under normal body conditions. In these patients, the oxygen-carrying capacity of the blood is poor, there is impairment of vascular flow, and a haemolytic anaemia results from the shortened life of the abnormal erythrocytes. This is a severe condition and the symptoms of general ill health are so marked as to make it very unlikely that a patient would present for dental treatment undiagnosed. However, there is no such guarantee in the case of the sickle-cell trait and the only way to identify these patients is to carry out a test for the presence of HbS. Fortunately, the initial screening test for this condition is relatively simple and is easily performed in the laboratory. It is also true that modern techniques of anaesthesia, designed to avoid even transient and minor degrees of hypoxia, are much less likely to cause problems in these patients than previously was the case.

Orofacial manifestations of sickle-cell anaemia have been reported and include prominence of the maxilla and mandible and orofacial pain. These occur as a result of marrow hyperplasia and expansion of the marrow space due to a longstanding haemolytic anaemia. Destructive osteomyelitis is a recognized complication of dental infection in sickle cell disease. Peripheral neuropathies associated with sickle cell crisis have also been reported, including mental anaesthesia.

Normocytic anaemias

Normocytic anaemias may be secondary to systemic diseases, such as scurvy (see below) or associated with primary or secondary bone marrow aplasia and neoplasia. Aplastic anaemias can be caused by a number of cytotoxic drugs.

Oral signs and symptoms in anaemias

A wide range of oral signs and symptoms may appear in anaemic patients but these are due to the underlying deficiency of iron, vitamin B_{12}, or folic acid—for mucosal pallor to be noticeable in the mouth the patient's haemoglobin needs to be low (< 8 g/dl). The oral signs and symptoms are a result of basic changes in the metabolism of the oral epithelial cells, which are particularly susceptible to minor variations in the quality of the blood supply. These changes give rise in their turn to abnormalities of cell structure and of the keratinization pattern of the oral epithelium, the end result often being atrophy. This atrophy seems particularly to affect the complex filiform papillae of the tongue, which may be almost completely lost. However, the changes are by no means restricted to the tongue and ulceration or generalized soreness may occur over the whole of the oral mucosa. Apart from this type of symptom, the patient with anaemia or latent iron deficiency is particularly susceptible to infection by *Candida albicans* and angular cheilitis or thrush may occur. In addition to these changes, the patients may complain of disturbances of taste sensation. It has been suggested that this is due to atrophy of the tongue epithelium with resulting disturbance of the underlying nerve endings, but such a disturbance of taste has been observed in patients with apparently clinically normal tongue epithelium. A number of reports have described the results of the investigation of oral lesions in anaemic patients and it has become evident that there is no clear correlation between the oral symptoms and the basic aetiology. Sore tongue, taste disturbance, generalized stomatitis, candidosis, angular cheilitis (Fig. 13.1), gingivitis, and an exacerbation of recurrent aphthous stomatitis (RAS) may occur in any of these patients (see Table 13.2).

The same considerations apply in relation to folate and B_{12} deficiency. It has been pointed out above that very early deficiencies of either of these factors may result in oral mucosal changes. These are certainly not due to secondary anaemia since none may be present. The precise reason for these changes is not known.

In the Plummer–Vinson (Patterson–Kelly) syndrome, patients present with dysphagia, caused by an oesophageal web, iron

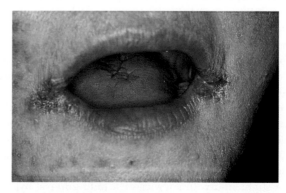

Fig. 13.1 Bilateral angular cheilitis and a generalized stomatitis in uncontrolled pernicious anaemia.

deficiency anaemia (hence the term sideropenic dysphagia), and glossitis. They may also develop oral candidosis and are predisposed to the development of postcricoid and oral carcinoma (see also Chapter 10).

The relationship between RAS and coeliac disease was discussed in Chapter 5. It is generally accepted that RAS is not directly associated with iron deficiency (as may occur in coeliac disease), although pre-existing RAS may well be exacerbated by it. It is less easy to define the role of folate or B_{12} deficiencies—some deficient patients with RAS show an immediate response to supplementation whilst, quite clearly, those with coeliac disease respond primarily to the gluten-free diet. This, however, results in the correction of the malabsorption process and the restoration of deficient levels. It is, therefore, difficult to tell precisely what part each component plays in the reversal of the RAS.

Further uncertainty is introduced by the fact that some patients with advanced haematological disturbances do not show oral changes. Some patients, for example, those with advanced megaloblastic anaemia, the result of folate deficiency, may have no oral complaints and the mucosa may appear to be within normal clinical limits. It would seem reasonable to revise the long-held view that clear-cut oral signs and symptoms may be ascribed to specific blood deficiencies, and to adopt the alternative view point that a wide range of oral changes may arise from any of the conditions under discussion.

Management of patients with anaemias and haematinic deficiencies

In the majority of the patients described, treatment of the underlying haematological deficiency leads to a rapid resolution or improvement in the oral symptoms. In patients with longstanding latent iron deficiency, however, the response may be a slow one. Such refractory behaviour is well recognized and may indicate poor drug compliance or impaired patient absorption of replacement therapy.

Leukaemia

Leukaemia represents a malignant proliferation of white cells, replacing their normal development in the bone marrow. This process may affect any of the white cell strains, but the most usual forms are lymphocytic, monocytic, and myeloid, depending on whether lymphocytes, monocytes, or granulocytes are involved. Each of these forms of leukaemia present either in an acute or a chronic form (see Table 13.3).

It is not uncommon for oral signs and symptoms to be the first indication of the presence of leukaemia, particularly of one of the acute types (see Table 13.4). The gingivae are frequently involved with a hyperplastic gingivitis. The hyperplastic gingivitis results in fragile red spongy gingivae that bleed spontaneously or following slight injury. In a few cases, a mild gingival hyperplasia may be the first indication of an acute leukaemia (Fig. 13.2). In acute monoblastic leukaemia (a subgroup of acute myeloblastic

Table 13.3 Classification of leukaemias

Acute	Chronic
Lymphoblastic*	Lymphocytic
Nonlymphoblastic (myeloblastic)[†]	Myeloid

* Most common acute leukaemia in children.
[†] Most common acute leukaemia in adults

Table 13.4 Orofacial manifestations of acute leukaemia*

Spontaneous haemorrhage for gingivae (reduction in platelets)
Oral purpura and petechiae
Gingival swelling (leukaemic infiltration)
Oral ulceration (leukaemic deposits, infections, haematinic deficiencies)
Mucosal swelling and loosening (exfoliation) of teeth (leukaemic deposits)
Opportunistic infections (e.g. herpes, *Candida*)
Lymph node enlargement

* N.B. Chemotherapy to treat leukaemia may also produce oral side-effects.

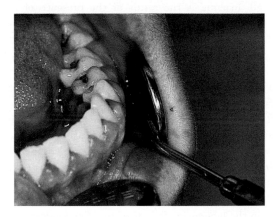

Fig. 13.2 Mild gingival hyperplasia—the first indication of acute myeloblastic leukaemia.

leukaemia), the monocytes are known to infiltrate sites of inflammation such as the gingiva. In more acute cases, the hyperplastic nature of the gingivitis may not be evident and the condition may show as spontaneous haemorrhage from the gingival margins (Fig. 13.3). The gingivae are highly susceptible to infection and a secondary acute ulcerative gingivitis is common. This susceptibility to infection occurs also in more chronic cases when the oral symptoms may consist of recurrent attacks of acute ulcerative gingivitis. These may occur without any of the hyperplastic changes mentioned above and so may appear to be not of great significance. Unexplained or repeated recurrence of acute ulcerative gingivitis should be treated with suspicion and blood examination arranged in order to eliminate the possibility of the blood dyscrasia. The orofacial manifestations of chronic

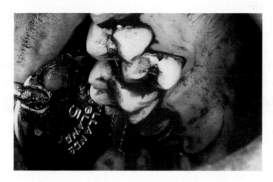

Fig. 13.3 Spontaneous haemorrhage from the gingival margin in acute leukaemia.

leukaemias are similar to those of acute leukaemias but are often less florid and may present in an insidious manner. In chronic lymphocytic leukaemia there is invariably lymph node involvement. Leukaemic infiltration of the salivary and lacrimal glands is occasionally seen.

In more advanced cases of leukaemia, oral ulceration is very common. The ulcers, produced by the breakdown of the tissues overlying deposits of leukaemic cells, may be large, painful, and difficult to treat. The maintenance of oral hygiene may be of great help in reducing the distressing oral symptoms in these patients. Covering agents and antiseptic mouthwashes are also helpful in easing the painful symptoms during the late stages of the disease.

Leukopenia

Leukopenia represents a fall in the white cell content of the blood. This may be a spontaneously arising condition, but may occur also as a response to drug therapy. Carbamazepine has been associated with severe haematological effects, including leukopenia and aplastic anaemia. Leukopenia may also occur as a transient stage in the development of leukaemia and other diseases affecting the bone marrow. It may also result from autoimmune disorders such as systemic lupus erythematosus (SLE) and viral infections; particularly HIV/EBV infections.

Although it is not a particularly common condition, the most usual clinical presentation is of agranulocytosis. This represents a reduction in the number of granulocytes formed in the marrow and circulating in the blood. The effect of this is to increase the susceptibility of the patient to infections of various kinds. In the case of the oral mucosa this may lead to widespread infection and ulceration of all parts of the mucosa. These changes may not be dissimilar to those occurring in leukaemia. The aetiological process is similar in that the protective function of the white cell component of the blood is reduced, in the one case by the excessive production of abnormal cells and, in the other case, by an inadequate production of normal cells.

In cyclic neutropenia, a rare condition in which neutrophil production is intermittently deficient, gingivitis and RAS-like ulceration may occur during the neutropenic episodes (see Chapter 5).

Myelodysplastic syndromes

This is a group of stem cell disorders in which there is a suppression of one or more cell lines in the bone marrow. In some cases this leads to bone marrow failure and in others to leukaemia. Myelodysplastic syndromes are more common in males over 60 years of age and may be detected in the oral medicine clinic when patients undergo routine haematological screening. An abnormal blood count in an elderly patient should therefore suggest the possibility of a myelodysplastic syndrome. Oral ulceration and gingival infiltration have been reported in a few cases.

Platelet abnormalities

When the function or the number of the platelets in the circulating blood is reduced, there is a tendency for spontaneous haemorrhage to occur within the tissues. This may well show initially in the form of petechial haemorrhages on the oral mucosa and these are, in fact, a well-known sign of early immune thrombocytopenia. In leukaemias of various kinds, both platelet function and numbers are greatly reduced, and haemorrhages of mucosa and skin may therefore be an early warning sign. It is advisable to carry out a full blood screen, including a platelet count, on any patient with otherwise unexplained areas of haemorrhage affecting the oral mucosa. It should be remembered, however, that transient haemorrhages of this kind may occur on the soft palate in patients with a severe cold. Idiopathic oral blood blisters (without any associated haematological defect) were described in Chapter 11. Similar blood-filled blisters may also be produced in thrombocytopenia, particularly on the palate, although they may occur elsewhere on the oral mucosa.

The selection of patients for haematological examination

Patients with the symptoms described in Table 13.5 form a considerable proportion of those referred to the oral medicine clinic for investigation and, as a consequence, a full haematological examination must be carried out in all these cases. The accepted routine 'blood screen', consisting of a full blood cell count (haemoglobin (Hb), differential white cell count (WCC), and platelet estimation) and the examination of a blood film, is sometime insufficient to demonstrate anaemias in their early or latent stages but it is important to extend the investigation further in selected patients (Table 13.5). The rationale for this has already been discussed in Chapter 2. When an extended investigation is decided upon, a reasonable scheme of investigation is that shown in Table 13.6.

It is evident that further, more specialized tests may be necessary for a full diagnosis of some of the patients involved. A number of these were discussed in Chapter 2.

It is essential that the presence of some haematological abnormality should be followed up with appropriate investigations according to the clinical circumstances. Simple replacement therapy for a deficiency is unacceptable unless attempts are made

Table 13.5 Oral medicine patients who should be considered for an extended haematological examination

Patients with recurrent aphthous stomatitis (RAS)
Patients with a persistently sore and/or dry mouth
Patients with oral lesions with an atypical history or unusually resistant to treatment
Patients complaining of a sore or burning mouth or tongue, or abnormal taste sensation, even though no mucosal changes can be seen
All patients with persistent oral and orofacial candidosis
Patients showing abnormalities following an initial screening

Table 13.6 Haematological investigations for oral medicine patients

- Full blood count and film examination. This is the routine screen procedure, and from it evident anaemias are demonstrated by variations in red cell morphology and lowered haemoglobin values. Abnormalities of the white cells and platelets are also shown
- Estimation of serum ferritin as an indicator of full-body iron status. This has replaced the previously used serum iron/iron binding capacity/saturation tests when used for this purpose. This latter group of tests, however, is still used in the investigation of complex iron deficiency states
- Serum B12, serum folate, and red cell folate estimations. The necessity for carrying out both folate estimations has been discussed in Chapter 2
- As an additional test an erythrocyte sedimentation rate (ESR) measurement is useful as a non-specific guide to underlying pathological processes such as chronic inflammatory conditions or neoplasia—alternatively, measurement of C-reactive protein (CRP) may be used as a marker for pre-existing disease

to define the underlying cause. It must be said, however, that, even after carrying out full investigations, a small number of patients presenting with oral symptoms attributed to deficiencies remain a diagnostic puzzle in terms of the aetiology of the deficiency.

Disorders of nutrition

The integrity of the oral mucous membrane is maintained by a wide-ranging complex of factors, including those dependent on adequate nutrition. The significance of iron metabolism and associated factors was previously discussed, as was the relationship between gastrointestinal disease and nutrition.

Nutritional deficiencies

A wide range of conditions that depend on the absence or reduction of certain specific nutritional factors, particularly vitamins, has been described in the past. With a few exceptions these specific conditions are now rarely seen under European conditions, although this may certainly be far from the case in other situations. It should be remembered that a nutritional deficiency may occur in three ways: (1) as a result of reduced intake; (2) as a

result of faulty absorption or metabolism; and (3) as a result of increased excretion. The relationship of iron deficiency anaemia to these three factors is a good and simple example.

Most patients seen in the oral medicine clinic with folate deficiency have this as a result of some form of malabsorption rather than poor intake. It should be remembered, however, that a high alcohol intake may result in low folate levels, as may some drugs—phenytoin in particular. Only rarely, and then usually in strict vegans, is vitamin B_{12} deficiency a result of poor dietary intake. On the whole, those patients who adopt unusual diets do so on a reasonably informed basis and are found to have satisfactory haematological indices.

There has recently been considerable interest in the role of other nutritional elements in the integrity of the oral mucosa—the B complex of vitamins and a number of trace elements (particularly zinc) have been the subject of investigations. Serum zinc levels have been investigated in patients with burning mouth syndrome (BMS) and 'geographic tongue', but there is no convincing evidence that zinc deficiency is involved in the pathogenesis of these conditions.

It was previously pointed out that, in patients with nutritional deficiencies, secondary effects may follow. Predominant amongst these is the suppression of the normal immune response. This was described in Chapter 4 in the case of nutritionally deficient children affected by cancrum oris. Nutritional deficiencies dependent on faulty diet are rarely simple ones and the patient suffering from any specific deficiency should be considered a candidate for a more complete investigation of nutritional standards.

A special case is that of the anorexic patient—most commonly, but not exclusively, young and female. Such patients may come to the oral medicine clinic as a result either of general nutritional deficiencies, which may result in stomatitis or some other mucosal problem, or of the parotid swelling that is a feature in some patients. The acid-induced erosion of the teeth that may occur in patients with the bulimic form of anorexia is discussed in Chapter 17.

Scurvy

Scurvy (ascorbic acid deficiency) is now an uncommon disease in Europe, but is not by any means unknown, being the most commonly recognized condition associated with a single vitamin deficiency. Although the disease occurs more often in old and neglected patients, there are occasional cases of much younger individuals who adopt such a restricted form of diet that clinical signs of ascorbic acid deficiency appear.

The predominant oral symptom in a severe vitamin C deficiency is a hyperplastic gingivitis, the gingivae becoming swollen and friable and purple-red in colour. There is marked false pocketing and this, together with general lack of tissue resistance, may lead to secondary infection. There may be, therefore, a superimposed acute gingivitis. Generalized symptoms include tiredness and malaise. Capillary fragility is a feature of this condition and may lead to the appearance of spontaneous haemorrhage and widespread bruising, particularly around the joint areas.

Investigation of such a patient must include a blood examination in order to eliminate the possibility of a blood disease, since the most important differential diagnosis is from leukaemia. The main blood change in scurvy is the presence of a secondary anaemia. The positive diagnosis is by laboratory tests for leukocyte or plasma ascorbic acid levels. However, a satisfactory clinical diagnostic test is derived from the response of the symptoms to therapeutic doses of vitamin C, a response that occurs within a few days and that is accompanied by a dramatic reversal of all the symptoms.

The treatment of scurvy is a general medical and, sometimes, social problem. Although the administration of a high dose of ascorbic acid (1 g daily) for a few days may improve the condition of the patient remarkably, the further management must be a matter for the general medical practitioner. Not only the deficiency state itself, but also the conditions leading to its appearance must be corrected. It should also be remembered that, although the symptoms presenting may be of ascorbic acid deficiency, there is every likelihood that, in fact, multiple dietary defects exist.

> Scurvy (vitamin C deficiency) is rare. In advanced cases there may be a marked gingivitis with swelling or bleeding.

Endocrine disturbances

In general, changes in the oral mucosa dictated by endocrine abnormalities are not common. Perhaps the most frequently cited changes are those due to the endocrine disturbances found in normal life—especially during pregnancy, and at the menopause. However, a few well-established oral changes occur in some endocrine pathologies and these will be outlined below. It should be remembered that endocrine disorders are highly complex and often involve a number of systems because of the feedback mechanisms that control the endocrine system as a whole. It is, therefore, often difficult to determine the exact effect of a single endocrine abnormality on any structure. Endocrine disorders affecting bone and teeth (gigantism, acromegaly, and hyperparathyroidism) are discussed in Chapter 18. Hypoparathyroidism resulting from parathyroid or thyroid surgery has no particular effects on the orofacial tissues but results in a low serum calcium. Tetany is the clinical manifestation of reduced serum calcium. Tetany may also be encountered in anxious dental patients who hyperventilate—this results in alkalosis and a reduced plasma ionized calcium.

Normal endocrine changes

Pregnancy

During pregnancy, the hormonal changes that occur may have the effect of exacerbating a previously existing chronic gingivitis that may have been previously symptom-free and unrecognized. The resulting gingivitis is essentially hyperplastic, although there is minimal proliferation of fibroblasts. The most marked proliferation is of capillaries and this leads to the typically purple coloration of the gingival papillae (Fig. 13.4). These papillae tend

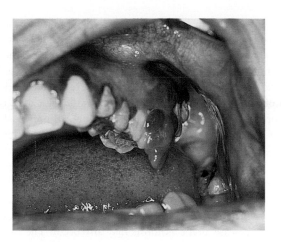

Fig. 13.4 Pregnancy gingivitis, including the formation of a pregnancy epulis.

to be fragile and may bleed at the least injury. Because of the presence of false pocketing and bleeding, stagnation and secondary infection may occur, and may lead to halitosis.

Occasionally, a single papilla may become considerably enlarged and present as an epulis. This is the so-called 'pregnancy epulis' (Chapter 9). The clinical characteristics and timing of the occurrence of these pregnancy lesions are sufficient to give a strong presumptive diagnosis. However, should any doubt occur as to the nature of the condition, full investigation is essential, including excisional biopsy of any doubtful overgrowth. Pregnancy is, in itself, no contraindication to such a biopsy, but it should be remembered that the lesion is likely to be extremely vascular and profuse bleeding is to be expected. On balance, it is often better, if a confident clinical diagnosis has been made, to avoid biopsy, since the condition is likely to regress considerably, if not completely, after pregnancy. The relationship of RAS to pregnancy and the menstrual cycle has not yet been established.

Treatment during pregnancy should consist of the application of strict oral hygiene measures. This, in itself, is often sufficient to halt the progress of the gingivitis. However, oral hygiene measures alone are unlikely to lead to the complete resolution of a discrete 'epulis-like' mass and eventual excision may be necessary.

Menopause

There is no substantive evidence that the hormonal changes occurring during and after the menopause directly affect the oral mucosa. The question of oral symptoms of various kinds with no identifiable physical cause or abnormality is further addressed in Chapter 17. These have a tendency to occur in menopausal women.

Adrenocortical diseases

Addison's disease

Addison's disease is the result of lack of function of the adrenal cortex, usually the result of an autoimmune disorder, but with other possible aetiologies. As a result of this destruction, the feedback mechanism between the adrenals and the pituitary is disturbed and a wide-ranging series of endocrine changes results. The oral change of significance in Addison's disease is melanotic pigmentation of the oral mucosa, which may include the buccal mucosa, gingivae, and palate. It should be remembered that this form of pigmentation is by no means specific, but none the less the appearance of such signs in a patient known previously to be free of pigmentation should always be considered as of significance. The mechanism of melanin production in this way is not clearly known. Although a melanin-stimulating hormone is secreted by the pituitary gland, it seems that the actual onset of pigmentation may be associated with variable adrenocorticotrophic hormone (ACTH) levels. In more fully developed Addison's disease, oral candidosis may also occur. The association of oral melanotic pigmentation with candidosis is evidently a further, more marked indication for endocrine studies. Investigation of a patient with suspected Addison's disease is shown in Table 13.7.

Although Addison's disease is a well-known cause of oral mucosal pigmentation, it is, in fact, very unusual for the disease to be recognized in this way. There are many much more common causes of melanin pigmentation, which were considered in Chapter 9.

Cushing's syndrome

This is due to hyperfunction of the adrenal cortex, usually as a result of an ACTH-secretory pituitary adenoma. Corticosteroid therapy, particularly if prolonged, can have physiological effects similar to those of Cushing's syndrome (see Chapter 2).

Phaeochromocytoma and the adrenal medulla

Phaeochromocytoma is a tumour of the adrenal medulla, which secretes catecholamines. It can be associated with neurofibromatosis and the multiple endocrine adenoma syndrome (type III). Neurofibromas of the oral mucosa or lips should alert the clinician to the rare possibility of a phaeochromocytoma.

Thyroid disease

Hyperthyroidism

Excessive production of thyroid hormones (hyperthyroidism) does not appear to have any direct effect on the oral mucosa but may cause problems of dental management. Dental practitioners may be the first to observe patients with exophthalmos who may also appear hyperexcitable and report weight loss—they may also have a tremor and tachycardia. Treatment is usually by drugs such as carbimazole or use of radioactive iodine. Partial thyroidectomy is rarely required unless the thyroid is causing compression symptoms.

Hypothyroidism

Hypothyroidism in adults is often autoimmune but may occur as a consequence of excessive removal of the thyroid gland to treat hyperthyroidism. Acquired hypothyroidism (myxoedema) manifests as weight gain, inability to tolerate cold, dry skin, loss of hair, and a slowing down of activity and mental processes. Hypothyroidism is associated with an impaired immune mechanism and oral candidosis may be the result. There is often a relationship between pernicious anaemia and hypothyroidism—possibly in the family if not in the individual.

Congenital hypothyroidism (cretinism) is characterized by dwarfism and mental retardation. Orofacial signs include enlargement of the tongue (see Chapter 6), defective facial development, and delayed eruption of the teeth.

Diabetes mellitus

Diabetes mellitus is a common endocrine disorder that occurs as a result of a deficiency of insulin or resistance to insulin. Two clinical types are recognized: juvenile onset (insulin-dependent, type 1) and maturity onset diabetes (type 2).

Diabetes mellitus has no specific oral signs or symptoms. However, possibly because of the general lack of resistance to infection of the diabetic patient, periodontal disease processes may become exaggerated (Table 13.8). It is not uncommon to find that an undiagnosed diabetic presents with advanced periodontal disease. The principles of treatment of this are simply those of periodontal treatment in the nondiabetic patient. However, in this and in all other treatment, the dental surgeon must always remember that the diabetic patient is more than normally susceptible to infection. The frequent occurrence of oral candidosis in diabetic patients was discussed in Chapter 4. Patients with undiagnosed or poorly controlled diabetes may report xerostomia, which is due to dehydration, secondary to polyuria. Oral hypoglycaemic drugs may cause lichenoid drug

Table 13.7 Investigation of patient with melanotic pigmentation due to possible Addison's disease

Impaired adrenal response to synthetic analogue of ACTH (Synacthen® test)*
Measurement of serum electrolytes (Na ↓, K ↑)†
Measurement of plasma cortisol (↓) and ACTH(↑)†
Blood pressure measurement (↓hypotension—especially postural)

* Definitive test for Addison's disease.
† May be normal.

Table 13.8 Oral features of diabetes mellitus

Dry mouth
Compromised periodontal health*
Oral candidosis
Glossodynia—BMS
Lichenoid drug reactions (oral hypoglycaemic drugs)

* Depends on oral hygiene.

reactions and, occasionally, patients present with swelling of the salivary glands (sialosis). Glossodynia (burning mouth syndrome, BMS) may be an early manifestation of undiagnosed diabetes (Chapter 17).

The patient with undiagnosed or inadequately treated diabetes may have a generalized stomatitis and, in particular, a sore tongue. This is probably at least partly due to dehydration and partly due to candidal infection. The possibility of latent diabetes should be considered, amongst others, in the patient with non-specific glossitis or a candidosis. A family history of diabetes is of particular significance. Just as in the case of the sore tongue due to anaemia, a sore tongue resulting from diabetes may occur early in the disease process, before substantial amounts of glucose are passed into the urine. In order to provide a sufficient screening procedure, it is necessary in these patients to carry out a blood glucose estimation, preferably fasting, rather than a simple urine screen (see Chapter 2).

Renal disease

Renal disease is of great significance in oral medicine and general dental practice. Oral changes occur not only as a result of chronic renal failure but also as a consequence of the medical management of renal disease. The dental management of patients with renal disease may also need to be modified to prevent complications.

Chronic renal failure

Chronic renal failure (CRF) is irreversible deterioration in renal function. When plasma creatinine persistently exceeds 300 μmol/l (normal range 80–120 μmol/l), there is progressive deterioration in renal function, irrespective of aetiology. When the plasma creatinine reaches 1000 μmol/l, dialysis will be required. The glomerular filtration rate (GFT; normal, 120 ml/min) measures renal function. Progressive impairment in function of the kidneys leads to the development of the clinical syndrome of uraemia.

Orofacial manifestations of chronic renal failure

Chronic renal failure and its resultant uraemia cause a number of physiological changes that can cause oral symptoms (Table 13.9). In addition, restricted fluid intake, as part of the medical management of this condition, can cause oral dryness and, in some patients, infections of the parotid glands. In chronic renal failure, uraemic stomatitis occurs either in the form of widespread and painful oral ulcerations (ulcerative uraemic stomatitis) or as white plaques affecting the oral mucosa. The latter are pain-free and transient. Once the underlying metabolic dysfunction is treated, the oral mucosa reverts back to normal. In patients with anaemia, pallor of mucosa may be evident and purpura or haemorrhage can occur as a result of platelet deficiencies. Oral candidosis is frequently a problem and contributes to oral symptoms in patients with chronic renal failure.

Giant cell lesions of the jaws may occur as a result of hyper-parathyroidism secondary to renal failure (or prolonged dialysis) and give rise to oral lesions or osteolytic lesions in the bone. Patients with CRF are now treated with potent alpha-hydroxylated vitamin D supplements to prevent secondary hyperpathyroidism.

Great care must be taken when prescribing drugs for patients with renal failure and the safest drugs to use are those that are metabolized primarily by the liver. Dosages of other drugs need to be adjusted to compensate for decreased renal excretion.

Renal patients undergoing dialysis (Table 13.10)

When patients reach a stage of renal failure in which the kidney function is inadequate, they are assessed for dialysis. Haemodialysis is a technique whereby the patient's blood is detoxified by passing it through a machine. Access to the patient's circulation is achieved by fashioning an arteriovenous shunt, usually on the forearm. Patients undergoing haemodialysis are heparinized and dental extractions are best delayed until at least 12 hours afterwards. The optimum time for dental procedures is 12–24 hours posthaemodialysis. Immediately after dialysis, patients also tend to be extremely tired. Indwelling arteriovenous shunts may become infected and many authorities consider that antibiotic prophylaxis is advisable for orodental procedures likely to produce a bacteraemia in dialysed patients. As for those with chronic renal failure, care must be taken when prescribing drugs for these patients. Haemodialysed patients have been reported as having an increased carriage rate of hepatitis B and C. However, following fatal outbreaks of hepatitis B amongst staff and patients in renal units, dialysed patients are regularly screened for hepatitis B. Universal precautions for cross-infection control should, however, be instituted for all dental patients, regardless of their medical or 'risk' status.

Table 13.9 Orofacial manifestations of chronic renal failure

Dry mouth
Mucosal ulceration
Bacterial and fungal plaques
Pallor of the mucosa (anaemia)
Oral purpura
White plaques (uraemic stomatitis)
Giant cell lesions—osteolytic lesions in jaws

Table 13.10 Dental management of haemodialysed patients: some important considerations

Impaired excretion of drugs by kidney
Bleeding tendency
Heparinization prior to dialysis
Arteriovenous shunts susceptible to infection
Anaemia
Increased carriage of hepatitis B and C
Hypertension

The optimum time for renal patients to undergo dental procedures is 12–24 hours posthaemodialysis.

An alternative form of dialysis is CAPD (continuous ambulatory peritoneal dialysis), which does not require hospitalization. Individuals on CAPD should be treated as haemodialysed patients but do not have the problems associated with arteriovenous shunts and heparanization. CAPD patients are, however, at risk from peritonitis.

Renal transplant patients

Renal transplantation, either from a tissue-matched cadaver or close relative, offers the best hope of a normal life. However, it is not without problems, mainly due to the side-effects of immunosuppressive regimens given to prevent rejection of the transplanted kidney (Table 13.11). In the past large doses of corticosteroids gave rise to considerable short- and long-term problems (see Chapter 3). Renal transplant patients pose a number of dental and medical management problems.

Ciclosporin A is widely used in all branches of transplant surgery yet, paradoxically, this is a nephrotoxic drug. Gingival overgrowth is a well-recognized complication of ciclosporin (Fig. 13.5), but can also occur with calcium channel blockers, such as nifedipine, which may be prescribed for concomitant hypertension in renal patients (see Chapter 14). Recent studies have shown that pretransplant gingival hyperplasia appears to be potentiated by ciclosporin therapy, resulting in severe posttransplant overgrowth.

Table 13.11 Oral complications of renal transplantation

Drug-induced gingival overgrowth (hyperplasia)
Bacterial and fungal plaques
Increased incidence of oral malignancy (reported)
Oral candidosis
Herpes simplex infections (secondary)

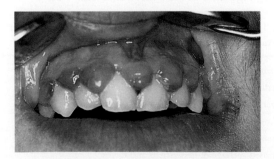

Fig. 13.5 Gingival hyperplasia induced by ciclosporin in a renal transplant patient.

Immunosuppressives, given to prevent tissue rejection, may cause a number of oral complications including the development of bacterial (or candidal) plaques, widespread oral candidosis, herpes simplex virus infections (secondary), susceptibility to dental infections, and, less commonly, 'hairy leukoplakia'. Lesions presenting as superficial plaques on the oral mucosa may resemble acute pseudomembranous candidosis (thrush) and can be wiped off when firmly scraped. However, it is now recognized that the infective organism may be bacterial (for example, staphylococci, streptococci, coliforms) and will not respond to anti-fungal therapy. These plaques grow in virtually pure culture and in adherent plaque-like lesions. Treatment of these lesions depends on culture and sensitivity of putative bacteria. There is also a reported increased incidence of oral carcinoma in renal patients taking immunosuppressive drugs. Carcinoma arising in ciclosporin-induced gingival overgrowth has also been reported.

Controversy still exists as to whether renal transplant patients should be given antibiotic cover for orodental procedures likely to generate a bacteraemia. It is essential that the dentist liaises with the patient's renal transplant team, many of whom advise prophylactic antibiotic cover. Antimicrobials and other drugs that are potentially nephrotoxic to the transplanted kidney should be avoided. Every attempt must be made to keep these patients dentally fit and free from infections.

Discussion of problem cases

Case 13.1 Discussion

Q1   What diagnosis must be excluded in this lady's case? What other oral manifestations of this condition might you find on examination?

The most likely diagnosis in this lady's case is an acute form of leukaemia. If she presented on medication, it would be important to consider a drug-induced agranulocytosis. Pallor and fatigue are both manifestations of iron deficiency and a history of susceptibility to recurrent infections would be consistent with leukaemia. A secondary platelet deficiency (thrombocytopenia) will predispose to spontaneous bruising of the skin and bleeding from the gingivae. Spontaneous gingival haemorrhage, as reported by this lady, is unusual even in those patients with poor oral hygiene and reinforces the clinical suspicion of leukaemia. Other oral signs to check for include: oral purpura and petechiae, gingival swelling or infection, oral ulceration, mucosal swelling, and evidence of opportunistic infections, such as candidosis (Table 13.4). There may also be cervical lymphadenopathy, either as a result of a lymphadenitis secondary to oral infection or (less commonly) leukaemic infiltration.

Q2   How would you manage this lady?

This patient must be immediately referred for full blood count. If this is consistent with your clinical diagnosis of leukaemia, then the patient must be referred to a haematologist for further investigation and appropriate treatment. As an interim measure this patient should be given appropriate therapy for her oral condition. This lady has reported soreness of the mouth, which may be helped by using an analgesic or antiseptic mouthwash, particularly if plaque control is poor. Candidal infection should be treated by appropriate topical antifungal therapy. Systemic antibiotics are probably best avoided at this stage as these might complicate this lady's medical management. The haematologist should, however, be informed if there is evidence of orodental infection that may need treating before definitive therapy for the leukaemia is commenced. If any extractions are needed, these must be carried out in a hospital environment because of potentially serious complications, such as excessive postextraction bleeding.

Case 13.2 Discussion

Q1   How would you manage the dental extraction of this medically compromised patient?

Arrangements should be made for this patient to have his extraction carried out at least 12 hours posthaemodialysis, when potential bleeding problems associated with heparinization are likely to be less (the half-life of heparin is 4–6 hours). A recent full blood count should be checked to exclude thrombocytopenia. If there is no established local protocol for preoperative antibiotic prophylaxis in haemodialysed patients, then the patient's renal unit should be contacted for advice. Routine local anaesthesia should be employed for this patient. After the extraction it is advisable to suture the socket and/or insert a haemostatic gauze and check that there is no postoperative bleeding. This preventive measure is important as the patient may have a tendency to bleed after the extraction. The patient should be reviewed and arrangements made for regular dental care.

Q2   What is the most likely diagnosis of the white plaques on the patient's oral mucosa?

These transient white plaques are likely to represent uraemic stomatitis and require no treatment. If the plaques rub off they may be due to oral candidosis, in which case the patient requires a systemic antifungal agent (for example, fluconazole) or a bacterial infection. Culture and sensitivity of putative microorganisms will indicate the therapy of choice.

Project

What drugs should be avoided for patients undergoing haemodialysis?

14

Immunodeficiency, hypersensitivity, autoimmunity, and oral reactions to drug therapy

Immunodeficiency

Hypersensitivity

Angioedema

C1 esterase inhibitor deficiency

Autoimmunity

Oral reactions to drug therapy
- Spectrum of adverse reactions
- Oral reactions to antibiotics
- Oral reactions to steroids
- Drug therapy and the periodontal tissues
- Fixed drug eruptions

field, at the present time, is in the profound immunosuppression that may accompany HIV infection, associated with the acquired immune deficiency syndrome (AIDS). The oral manifestations of AIDS are discussed in Chapter 4.

Hypersensitivity

In contrast to the diseases caused by immune deficiencies, there are others that depend on an overactive or exaggerated response of some aspect of the immune system. The conditions known as hypersensitivity reactions are of this type, and they depend on an enhanced response of either the humoral or the cell-mediated mechanisms, consequent upon a second contact with an antigen to which the host has previously been sensitized. These reactions include some in which a severe toxic effect may be produced in the host. The term 'allergy' is now used to describe adverse reactions that result from a patient being immunologically hypersensitive to an exogenous agent, that is, an allergen.

Hypersensitivity reactions were classically defined into four groups by Coombs and Gel (Table 14.2). It is, however, convenient to consider two main types: immediate and delayed reactions. Type I hypersensitivity reactions are immediate and mediated by IgE antibodies. Clinical manifestations of this type of reaction range from systemic anaphylaxis to angioedema, asthma, allergic rhinitis, and generalized or localized urticaria. Type IV reactions are delayed hypersensitivity reactions and mediated by sensitized T lymphocytes. The clinical manifestations usually occur after 48 hours, and examples include contact dermatitis due to nickel allergy and organ transplant rejection.

The significance of these hypersensitivity reactions in oral medicine is that the oral mucosa may be directly involved or the oral tissues affected as part of a generalized reaction. An allergic angioedema (type I reaction) frequently presents as swelling of the lips (see below). A localized contact stomatitis (type IV reaction) can occur on the oral mucosa as a response to a wide range of allergens, including toothpastes, topical anaesthetics, and resins in composite materials.

There are a number of conditions encountered in oral medicine in which 'allergy' has been implicated but convincing evidence for these associations has yet to be produced. These include recurrent aphthous stomatitis (RAS), orofacial granulomatosis (OFG), erythema multiforme, lichen planus, and plasma cell gingivitis.

Table 14.2 Hypersensitivity reactions

Type	Description
I	Anaphylactic type
II	Cytotoxic reactions
III	Serum sickness
IV	Delayed hypersensitivity

Angioedema

Angioedema (soft-tissue swelling) can be allergic or non-allergic in aetiology and may occur with or without urticaria (raised wheals or plaques on the skin, as in 'nettle rash' and often referred to as 'hives'). Most cases of angioedema (and urticaria) are non-allergic and idiopathic.

Acute angioedema can, however, occur as an allergic response to a wide range of stimulae, including food stuffs (for example, peanuts), drugs (for example, penicillin), insect bites (for example, wasp stings), and natural rubber latex. Attacks of acute angioedema can result in widespread and often dangerous soft-tissue swelling that may affect the facial, oral, and pharyngeal regions and compromise the airway. Urticaria can accompany soft-tissue swelling. These manifestations are the result of a type I hypersensitivity reaction that is IgE-mediated. Degranulation of mast cells leads to the liberation of histamine and 'histamine-like' substances that cause an increase in vascular permeability and result in soft-tissue swellings. Respiratory occlusion is life-threatening and patients must be given adrenaline (epinephrine), supplemented by steroids and antihistamines as appropriate (see Chapter 19, 'Medical emergencies in dentistry').

> Allergic angioedema affecting the face and neck can be life-threatening.

Some patients present with angioedema (with or without urticaria) that is non-allergic and intermittent in nature. Angioedema is a well documented adverse side-effect of angiotensin converting enzyme (ACE) inhibitors and can occur for the first time even after prolonged treatment. Symptomatic episodes of angioedema may also follow the ingestion of a nonsteroidal anti-inflammatory drug (NSAID), such as ibuprofen or aspirin. Patients with a history suggestive of non-allergic angioedema should be checked for C1 esterase inhibitor deficiency (see below). Oral antihistamines are the mainstay of treatment for non-allergic angioedema (and urticaria). Relatively non-sedating preparations are now available.

> Angioedema is a well documented adverse, side-effect of ACE inhibitors and can occur for the first time even after prolonged treatment.

C1 esterase inhibitor deficiency

C1 esterase inhibitor deficiency can be hereditary or acquired and presents as angioedema. Hereditary angioedema is a rare autosomal dominant genetic disease. As a result of C1 esterase inhibitor deficiency, the action of the complement system is uncontrolled and activation of kinins leads to increased capillary permeability. In its fully developed form it is a serious and life-threatening condition that may be precipitated by minimal local trauma, such as dental treatment. C1 esterase inhibitor and complement components C3 and C4 levels can be measured. Prophylaxis and management of hereditary angioedema is by use of a synthetic androgen (for example, stanazole) or, in an emergency, fresh frozen plasma.

> C1 esterase inhibitor deficiency can be hereditary or acquired and presents as angioedema.

Autoimmunity

In an autoimmune reaction the immune response is directed against the host's own tissues, which, for some reason, have become antigenically active. Both the cell-mediated and the humoral responses may be involved in the process. It is not known how the facility to recognize 'self' is destroyed, and many different theories have been proposed.

A number of diseases of accepted autoimmune origin affect the oral tissues secondarily. Thus, in pernicious anaemia (Chapter 13), although the primary autoimmune process directly affects the gastric parietal cells, the haematological changes induced by the resulting inability to absorb vitamin B_{12} may cause marked abnormalities in the oral mucosa. These are the result of instability of the epithelium induced by the deficiency. Apart from these and similar secondary effects, however, a number of diseases of established or suspected autoimmune origin affect the oral tissues directly, producing oral lesions as a primary symptom. These include: immunobullous skin diseases (Chapter 11) and Sjögren's syndrome (Chapter 8). The detection of autoantibodies in patients with suspected autoimmune disease is discussed in Chapter 2.

Oral reactions to drug therapy

Spectrum of adverse reactions

There is a large number of drugs that can cause adverse effects on the oral mucosa and these include oral ulceration (Chapter 5) and lichenoid drug eruptions (Chapter 11). Localized reactions to topical therapy, including irritant substances, can also occur (Table 14.3) and the oral tissues may be affected as a manifestation of a systemically induced drug reaction (Table 14.4). One of the common adverse reactions of the oral mucosa to drugs is that of chemical trauma following contact with aspirin or an aspirin-containing tablet of some kind. Patients frequently use this form of therapy for the relief of toothache and the association of a carious tooth causing toothache and an acutely presenting white patch of

Table 14.3 Topical therapy: localized oral reactions

Therapy	Example
Aspirin	—
'Toothache' solutions	Oil of cloves
Irritant chemicals	Hydrogen peroxide used as root canal irrigant
Topical antibiotics	Chlortetracycline
Topical steroids	Betamethasone rinse

Table 14.4 Systemically induced drug reactions with oral manifestations

Drug reaction	Example of drug
Lichenoid eruptions	NSAIDs
Erythema multiforme (Stevens–Johnson syndrome)	Sulfonamides
Lupus erythematosus	Hydrallazine
Type I hypersensitivity reactions	Penicillins
Fixed drug eruptions	Salicylates
Drug-induced bone marrow suppression	Methotrexate
Immunosuppressive drugs	Ciclosporin
Salivary gland hypofunction	Tricylic antidepressants

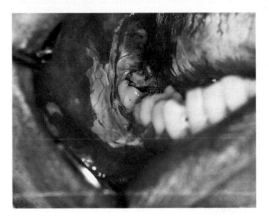

Fig. 14.1 Aspirin burn of the buccal mucosa.

the adjoining buccal mucosa should bring this possibility strongly to mind (Fig. 14.1). The appearance of the affected area may be quite spectacular and only the history will provide the diagnosis. The condition is, quite evidently, self-limiting and requires no treatment except for the toothache. Xerogenic medication is discussed fully in Chapter 8 and drugs causing discolouration of the oral mucosa are discussed in Chapter 9. Oral reactions to antibiotics and steroids are discussed in this chapter, together with drug-induced gingival overgrowth and fixed drug eruptions.

Oral reactions to antibiotics

It is well known that hypersensitivity reactions may occur during antibiotic therapy. These are commonly generalized reactions involving the whole metabolism. Their severity may vary from a mild and transient rash to the extremely severe reaction of angioneurotic oedema, in which oedema and swelling of the tissues of the head and neck may extend to the tongue and larynx and result in dangerous respiratory obstruction. Such a condition represents an extreme medical emergency and must be treated as such.

Hypersensitivity reactions may occur occasionally following the repeated use of tetracycline mouthwashes. The reaction may occur either early in the initial course or after many treatments. The reaction often takes the form of a localized angioneurotic oedema with swelling of the eyelids and the facial tissues in general. If this reaction occurs, it indicates that the patient has acquired a hypersensitivity to the tetracycline and must be warned that future use of the drug may be dangerous. The possibility of this type of reaction is yet another argument against the indiscriminate use of antibiotic therapy. Occasionally, a localized form of hypersensitivity reaction may be seen in the oral tissues following tetracycline mouthwash therapy. This is relatively limited in nature and leads to multiple vesicle formation. Again, the appearance of these symptoms should lead to the immediate cessation of the use of the antibiotic, together with warnings as to further use. The incidence of hypersensitivity reactions due to the use of tetracycline mouthwashes is, however, remarkably low. Treatment of hypersensitivity reactions depends on the severity and acuteness of the symptoms. In a mild reaction it may only be necessary to discontinue the use of the drug and to observe the patient carefully. In other cases, the use of antihistamines alone will be sufficient to suppress the symptoms. In a fully developed angioneurotic oedema, immediate treatment with intramuscular adrenaline (epinephrine) often combined with hydrocortisone may be necessary (see Chapter 19).

Apart from these manifestations of hypersensitivity, there are a number of minor reactions to antibiotics that may be localized to the mouth. Black hairy tongue occasionally follows treatment with either wide- or narrow-spectrum antibiotics. As the essential feature of black hairy tongue is elongation of the filiform papillae and this is associated only with secondary bacterial changes, it is difficult to understand why antibiotic therapy should induce this particular form of reaction. Following the cessation of the therapy the tongue may return to normal either quickly or, occasionally, very slowly. This form of reaction may occur after either systemic or local antibiotic therapy, although most cases of black hairy tongue are of unknown aetiology.

It might well be thought that the use of antibiotic mouthwashes to treat oral lesions would lead to symptoms arising from the widespread local overgrowth of resistant organisms and, in particular, *Candida* spp, but, in fact, this is not often so. Precisely as general physicians have found it unnecessary to incorporate antifungal antibiotics with wide-spectrum antibiotics in order to avoid gastrointestinal infestations by yeasts, so it has been found unnecessary to combine antifungal antibiotics with wide-spectrum antibacterials in mouthwash therapy for oral ulceration. This does not mean, however, that such an overgrowth is not possible and it must always be remembered that any localized use of an antibiotic may leave behind resistant strains of organisms, even if no clinical overgrowth occurs. It is, therefore, worth reiterating that the use of antibiotic mouthwashes should be reserved for situations in which there are positive indications.

Oral reactions to steroids

There are now many patients taking systemic steroids on a long-term basis, and often this treatment results in susceptibility to infection and general loss of tissue resistance. In the mouth, this takes the form of acute erythematous candidosis in most cases, although acute or chronic pseudomembranous candidosis may also occur. Although the palate is most often affected, the whole of the oral and pharyngeal mucosa may become involved, as may the mucosa of the larynx. Secondary infection by *Candida albicans* is almost invariably present, and treatment of these patients by local antifungal therapy is often satisfactory in reducing symptoms. In severe cases a systemic antifungal agent may be required. This, however, can be no more than a temporary solution since these patients are, in general, destined to maintain steroid therapy for an indefinite period. It may, therefore, be necessary to repeatedly treat this candidal infection. In these persistent cases of candidal infection the long-term use of a topical antifungal preparation is required.

Steroid mouthwashes and other topical preparations are advocated for a number of conditions in oral medicine and may obviate the need for systemic steroids. This form of therapy might be expected to be a prolific source of candidosis but, in fact, this complication is relatively unusual. If it does occur, long-term antifungal measures must accompany the antibiotic–steroid therapy. Miconazole gel is often very helpful in these circumstances, particularly if the patient has a sore mouth and cannot tolerate nystatin pastilles or amphotericin lozenges. Patients who regularly use a steroid inhaler for respiratory disease, such as asthma, are predisposed to developing oral candidosis, particularly of the palate and oropharynx. They should always rinse their mouth after use of the steroid and, in some cases, a spacer device may be indicated (Fig. 14.2).

Drug therapy and the periodontal tissues

Drug-induced gingival hyperplasia (overgrowth) is a well recognized complication and the drugs most commonly implicated are phenytoin, ciclosporin, and calcium-channel blockers (nifedipine, verapamil, diltiazem). Oral contraceptives have been associated with a hyperplastic oedematous gingivitis but it is likely that this response is a secondary reaction to plaque and is therefore dependent on the standard of plaque control.

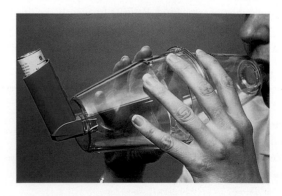

Fig. 14.2 Steroid inhaler with a spacer device.

Gingival overgrowth and sodium phenytoin (Epanutin)

Sodium phenytoin is the most commonly used drug for the treatment of epilepsy and, in approximately 50 per cent of the patients taking it, there is a marked chronic hyperplastic gingivitis. The hyperplastic reaction is typically papillary and the interdental papillae become swollen, sometimes grossly so. This is essentially a fibroblastic reaction and the tissue is generally firm and much less haemorrhagic than in the case of pregnancy gingivitis. In view of the marked false pocketing that may occur, there are great difficulties in maintaining oral hygiene and secondary inflammatory changes are almost invariably present. The nature of the reaction to the drug is not clear since there is evidence that the hyperplasia represents an exaggerated form of chronic gingivitis, which does not occur if immaculate standards of oral hygiene are maintained. Although withdrawal of the drug is, in itself, sufficient to halt the progress of the condition, the difficulties of stabilization in an epileptic patient may make it impractical to suggest its withdrawal as a treatment for the oral condition. Stringent oral hygiene and regular scaling, preceded, if need be, by gingivectomy, must be carried out. In severe cases, the gingivectomy should be performed under hospital conditions. Although the proliferation is essentially fibroblastic, the secondary infective processes often result in the production of very vascular tissue, and blood loss may be considerable if surgery is undertaken during this phase. Histologically, none of the drug-induced gingival changes show true hyperplasia, but there is an increase in collagen and ground substance.

Gingival overgrowth and ciclosporin

Ciclosporin is an immunosuppressive drug that is now widely prescribed in all branches of transplant surgery and increasingly used for systemic diseases such as rheumatoid arthritis. Ciclosporin-induced gingival overgrowth (Fig. 13.5) in renal patients was discussed in Chapter 13.

Gingival overgrowth and calcium-channel blockers

These drugs are used extensively for the management of cardiovascular disorders, including angina, hypertension, and cardiac arrhythmias. Nifedepine, one of the dihydropyridines, has been reported as causing gingival overgrowth in 10 to 15 per cent of dentate patients. Renal patients may be taking ciclosporin to prevent rejection of their transplanted kidney and a calcium-channel blocker to control hypertension.

Drugs commonly implicated in drug-induced gingival overgrowth

- Phenytoin
- Ciclosporin
- Calcium-channel blocking drugs

Fixed drug eruptions

The immunological mechanism involved in fixed drug eruptions has yet to be elucidated but it would appear that these represent a type of delayed hypersensitivity reaction. The oral mucosa is rarely affected and most lesions occur on the skin. Fixed drug reactions occur at the same site each time the precipitating drug is administered. Oral lesions can occur on the palate, lips, or tongue and they frequently start as vesicles or bullae, which rapidly break down to form ulcers. Drugs commonly implicated in fixed drug eruptions include: salicylates, dapsone, tetracyclines, and sulfonamides. Barbiturates have been reported as causing oral lesions in the absence of skin involvement.

Discussion of problem cases

Case 14.1 Discussion

Q1 What is the significance of this lady's atopic history and her previous occupation?

Atopy (that is, a history of asthma, eczema, hay fever) is a risk factor for developing NRL allergy. Other patients identified as 'at risk' include those with long-term exposure to NRL-containing items, that is, health-care workers (latex gloves) and patients with spina bifida (urinary catheters).

Q2 Why is the reported allergy to fruit of relevance?

There is a reported cross-sensitivity between NRL and certain fruits (for example, bananas, kiwi fruits, avocados).

Q3 What special precautions need to be taken when providing dental treatment for this lady?

This lady needs to be treated in a latex-controlled, dental environment. Non-NRL gloves must be worn by all staff directly involved in her care and items such as NRL dams and polishing cups must not be used. Non-NRL dental and medical equipment can be substituted. Local anaesthetic cartridges with synthetic (non-NRL) bungs are available to avoid the potential risk of contamination of the local anaesthetic solution. Emergency equipment with non-NRL must also be available (see local and national guidelines for further advice).

Case 14.2 Discussion

Q1 What information do you need to answer this lady's enquiry?

You will obviously require a list of this lady's current medication, which can then be checked against a national drug formulary and manufacturers' drug data sheets. Both list potential side-effects of the drugs.

Stable angina usually results from atherosclerotic plaques in the coronary arteries. Most angina patients will have a nitrate (glyceryltrinitrate (GTN) or isosorbide nitrate) for use during an acute attack, either as a tablet or a spray for sublingual use. GTN is also available as a fast-release tablet that is placed between the upper lip and labial mucosa and left to dissolve. Many patients with angina may require regular drug therapy and will have been prescribed prophylactic aspirin. Maintenance drugs for the treatment of angina include beta-blockers, calcium-channel blockers (for example, nifedipine), and nicorandil (a potassium-channel blocker).

The potential oral (dental) side-effects of these drugs include the following.

- Glyceryltrinitrate—rapid release 'buccal preparation' that contains lactose; this causes a pronounced drop in pH, which predisposes to dental caries.

- Beta blockers—xerostomia (saliva flow reduced—see Chapter 8).

- Calcium-channel blockers (nifedepine)—gingival overgrowth.

- Nicorandil—oral ulceration.

Your patient should be reassured that the potential oral and dental side-effects of medication for angina are minor and can be managed. It is important that this lady adheres to medical advice concerning her medication and the correct dosage. Most patients suffering from angina receive dental treatment in general practice but it is essential that appropriate drugs and equipment are available if they develop an angina attack. It is also important that staff are adequately trained to deal with all medical emergencies (see Chapter 19).

Projects

Dentists and doctors are required to report any adverse reactions that they suspect are due to drugs that the patient has been prescribed.

1. What mechanisms are in place for the reporting of adverse drug reactions?

15

Facial pain and neurological disturbances

Facial pain: an overview
- The nerve supply to the face
- The evaluation of facial pain

Neuropathic pain
- Trigeminal neuralgia
- Glossopharyngeal neuralgia
- Postherpetic neuralgia
- Neuropathic pain secondary to other conditions

Migraine

Cluster headache (periodic migrainous neuralgia/ migrainous neuralgia)

Tension-type headache

Facial pain: miscellaneous conditions
- Giant cell arteritis (temporal arteritis/cranial arteritis)
- Auriculotemporal syndrome (Frey's syndrome)

Neurological disturbances
- Facial nerve deficits
- Anaesthesia and paraesthesia
- Bell's palsy
- Multiple sclerosis
- Extrapyramidal syndromes

Facial pain and neurological disturbances

Problem cases

Case 15.1

A distressed 60-year-old patient with facial pain presents to the oral medicine clinic. After taking a history and carrying out an examination, you exclude a dental cause for the pain and make a clinical diagnosis of trigeminal neuralgia. You discuss the medical and surgical options for the management of this condition—in the first instance the patient requires some medication.

Q1   What is the usual drug of choice for this patient and what starting dose would you prescribe?

Q2   What warnings and information would you give to the patient?

Q3   What investigations do you need to carry out before starting on this drug?

Q4   If your patient had presented taking warfarin, would you envisage any management problems?

Case 15.2

A 25-year-old, healthy female patient is receiving treatment in your surgery. After administration of a local anaesthetic mandibular nerve block (for crown preparation of the mandibular first permanent molar), your patient reports that the left side of her face feels strange. She is unable to close her left eye or smile. You have prepared less than half of the crown.

Q1   How would you manage this situation?

Facial pain: an overview

Patients with a complaint of facial pain are seen daily in the dental practitioner's surgery. They are often diagnosed and treated with relative ease, but there remain some few patients in whom the origin of the pain symptoms remains obscure and who are referred to specialist clinics of various kinds for diagnosis. Apart from these patients with symptoms of pain, very few patients present with other neurological disturbances around the mouth and face. The diagnosis of these may be a complex matter and outside the province of dentistry, but it is important that the dental practitioner is able to recognize significant changes and initiate fur-

ther action. Table 15.1 gives some of the conditions that might give rise to facial pain.

The matter may be further complicated by the difficulties that may be met by the patient in describing his or her symptoms accurately. On the whole, however, the terms used by patients to describe pain—'stabbing', 'throbbing', 'dull ache', and so on—are fairly constant and related to the aetiology of the pain.

The reaction of the patient to pain depends on two factors that are independent of the strength of the pain stimulus. These are the pain threshold for the patient (the degree of stimulation necessary for the patient to perceive pain) and the individual's sensitivity to the pain when perceived. These two factors vary greatly from patient to patient and, in the case of the individual sensitivity, may vary from time to time in the same patient, depending on general health and other psychological factors. Pain cannot be separated from an emotional response.

Table 15.1 Conditions that may cause facial pain

Dental pain
Pulpitis, cracked tooth, periradicular pathology, pericoronitis, dry socket
Temporomandibular pain disorders
Neuropathic pain disorders
Trigeminal neuralgia, glossopharyngeal neuralgia, postherpetic neuralgia
Pathology in associated local structures (i.e. salivary glands, paranasal sinuses, eyes, cervical spine disorders, nasopharynx, ears)
Vascular disorders
Headaches: migraine, cluster headache, tension-type headache
Giant cell arteritis
Psychogenic facial pain
Atypical facial pain
Intracranial lesions
Neoplasms
Multiple sclerosis
Referred pain from a remote site
Angina pectoris

Facial pain

Pain is a common and frequent occurrence experienced by most patients. Pain may be acute or chronic. Pain not only has consequences to the patient and his or her quality of life, but it can also have an impact on the patient's social circle and on the society and economy of a nation. Pain is responsible for a large proportion of missed days of work.

The majority of patients with facial pain are suffering from some easily detectable pathological process in the teeth, their supporting tissues, or associated structures. Whatever the nature of the pain and however unusual its presentation, the first step must be the elimination of the pains of local origin—such as abnormal pulps, buried teeth and roots, periapical lesions, or acute periodontal lesions. Odontogenic pain may be readily diagnosed by clinical and radiographic examination. Unfortunately, every dental practitioner knows that this is not always so straightforward. Facial pain of dental origin may be difficult to recognize and referred or projected pain may make localization difficult. Clinical and radiographic examination may be inconclusive. Vitality testing of the teeth and the use of diagnostic local anaesthetic injections may be useful aids. Pulpitis may be difficult to localize, especially in a heavily restored quadrant—sometimes restorations have to be removed and teeth dressed in a systematic manner. This is frustrating for both the clinician and the patient. In particular, the pain associated with temporomandibular joint dysfunction may be very puzzling and may simulate a number of other conditions.

The diagnosis of facial pain can be difficult due to the multifactorial nature of the problem.

The nerve supply to the face

The sensory nerve supply to the face and oral tissues is shared among a number of nerves: the trigeminal nerve; the glossopharyngeal nerve; and the branches of the cervical plexus (see Fig. 15.1). However, the great majority of pain symptoms in the face are felt in the area covered by the trigeminal nerve. There is usually a clear-cut distinction between the zones supplied by the various terminal branches of the trigeminal nerve, with very little overlap, but there is often considerable overlap between the trigeminal and cutaneous branches of the cervical plexus where these are adjacent. Apart from areas of overlap there is also a complex series of interconnections between the trigeminal, facial, and glossopharyngeal nerves and the nerves arising from the autonomic nervous system, in particular, the sympathetic fibres associated with blood vessels serving the area. These sympathetic fibres may play some part in the transmission of deep impulses. It has been shown that such pain can be produced by the stimulation of the superior cervical sympathetic ganglion.

The great majority of patients complaining of pain in and about the face are suffering from some form of toothache. However, there

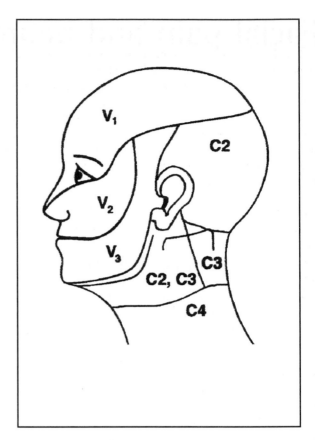

Fig. 15.1 Sensory dermatomes of the trigeminal and upper cervical nerves.

are many other possible causes of such pain (Table 15.1). The structures related to the mouth that might give rise to pain symptoms are so complex, and the innervation of these structures so interrelated, that errors in diagnosis are easily made. The main sensory nerve of the area, the trigeminal nerve, eventually divides into a large number of small terminal branches supplying the skin of a large part of the face and scalp as well as the majority of the oral tissues and many deeper structures. Although the superficial limits of the trigeminal nerve can be accurately determined with little overlap, the deeper limits are much less well defined and understood. It is often difficult to determine the point at which a facial pain becomes a headache (for example, in the temporal region) and there may be consequent difficulties in communication between the patient and the clinician.

Another possible source of confusion when diagnosing orofacial pain is that of projected and referred pain.

Projected and referred pain

If a pain pathway is subjected to stimulation at some point along its course, it is possible for pain to be felt in the peripheral distribution of the nerve. This is projected pain. An example of this is the facial pain that may occur in patients with intracranial neoplasms.

If the source of a pain and the site of the pain (the location) are one and the same, the pain is considered to be primary pain. This must be distinguished from referred pain in which the pain is felt in an area distant from that in which the causative pathology is located. Pain referral is a common occurrence in the orofacial region and clinicians must appreciate this phenomenon—otherwise erroneous diagnoses and management may ensue. In referred pain the practitioner must be able to identify the true source of the pain from the site (location) of the pain. In the dental field, perhaps the most common example of referred pain is that in which pain is felt, for instance, in the maxillary teeth due to a lesion in a mandibular tooth. In this case the pain impulses originate in the diseased tooth and, if the pathway from this tooth is blocked, for example, by a local anaesthetic, then the referred pain will cease. Thus, in our dental example, anaesthesia of the mandibular branch of the trigeminal nerve will relieve the pain felt in the area supplied by the maxillary branch. This is the basis of a most useful test for the investigation of suspected referred pain.

Although pain is frequently referred between differing branches of the trigeminal nerve, pain referred to the face from a distant area is relatively uncommon. The only referred pain of this type seen with any degree of frequency is that in coronary insufficiency, when pain may radiate over the left side of the mandible. Angina pectoris has also been described as presenting as a pain of the soft palate, but this is unusual. This accompanies other well-recognized symptoms of the condition, but a very few instances have been reported in which pain over the left mandible has been the first complaint of a patient who subsequently developed symptoms of myocardial infarction.

The mechanism of projected pain is fairly clear, but that of referred pain is more contentious. There is still considerable debate as to the theories of pain referral and the site at which the 'cross-over' or neural convergence occurs leading to the sensory misinterpretation of the impulses transmitted from the diseased site.

Referred pain

> Pain of dental origin can be referred to the opposing dental arch.

The evaluation of facial pain

Pain is extremely subjective and in many instances there are few clinical signs. Pain needs to be assessed on two dimensions—as a disease, using a medical model, and as an illness that inevitably has an effect on the quality of life. The response of patients to pain is extremely variable and it is this that makes assessment of pain so difficult. Some pain acts as an early warning system and so is crucial for survival, whereas other pains have outlived their usefulness. Many of the clinical conditions seen by the dental surgeon seem to fall into a category in which minor (or even quite unrecognizable) pathological changes elicit a quite dispro-

portionate response leading to great distress in the individual concerned.

The assessment and diagnosis of orofacial pain require the clinician to have knowledge and understanding of the anatomy, physiology, and pathology of the head and neck and, in particular, of the orofacial structures. The clinician should be able to undertake a systematic clinical assessment as shown in Table 15.2. The investigation of a patient complaining of facial pain may be thought of as having two stages. In the first stage an assessment of the pain is made relative to the dental apparatus (teeth and supporting tissues) and the closely related structures, such as the maxillary antra and the temporomandibular joints. If, after full examination, no abnormalities are found in these areas, the investigator is justified in considering other possibilities. If the essential first step of eliminating dental causes of the pain is omitted, confusion is bound to follow in many cases. When all these localized causes of pain are eliminated by careful investigation, there remains a number of conditions of less evident origin for consideration in a possible diagnosis.

History

A detailed pain history is crucial for patients with facial pain and in 70–80 per cent of cases a diagnosis is made on history alone. The clinician can gain valuable information by observing the patient when he or she is describing the features of the pain. It is also important that the patient is initially allowed to describe the pain in his or her own words—without prompting from the dentist. A pain history should be undertaken in a systematic fashion and all the features listed in Table 15.3 should be explored. Some form of more objective assessment of pain is important in order to measure not just intensity but the disability it is causing. The use of a linear pain scale and the McGill pain questionnaire may be helpful. The history should include the effects that the pain has on the lifestyle of the patient. Social, cognitive, emotional, and behavioural factors become very important in chronic pain and these are discussed further in Chapter 17. The social and family histories are crucial as a patient's pain impacts on those with whom they are living.

Examination

The examination of the orofacial tissues should include a gross sensory and motor evaluation of the cranial nerves (listed in Table 15.4). Abnormal functioning of the cranial nerves should indicate to the clinician that referral to a neurologist or other appropriate specialist is required. The fifth and seventh nerve need to be examined with care and alterations in sensory function are anaesthesia, paraesthesia, dysaesthesia, and heightened sensitivity to pain (hyperalgesia). Motor dysfunction is evident from paralysis, gross muscle weakness, muscular atrophy, or spasticity.

Neuropathic pain

According to the International Association for the Study of Pain, the definition of neurogenic pain (also known as neuropathic

Table 15.2 The assessment and management of facial pain

History
- Complaint
- Pain history

  Onset, periodicity, location and radiation, duration, frequency, character, and intensity of pain

  Modifying factors (initiating, aggravating, and alleviating factors)

  Effect on lifestyle

  Effect on mood—depression, anxiety

  Outcome of previous investigations and therapies (e.g. medication)

  Consider use of a visual analogue linear pain scale and a pain questionnaire
- Dental history
- Medical history (including alcohol and drug use)
- Social history

Examination
- Odontogenic structures

  Dental status, pulp vitality tests, static and dynamic occlusal relationships;
- Related structures

  Muscles of mastication, temporomandibular joint, salivary glands, sinuses
- Cranial nerve function

  Gross test of selected or all cranial nerves

  Sensory deficits
- Investigations

  Radiography and other imaging techniques

  Haematology and clinical chemistry (eg ESR, vitamin B$_{12}$)

  Virology

  Diagnostic occlusal appliance

  Biopsy

  Psychometric questionnaires

  Nerve conduction tests
- Diagnostic, local anaesthetic nerve block

  This may help define the distribution of pain, and can eliminate or confirm referred pain
- Request further information

  From general practitioner, specialists, hospital casenotes

Management
- Establish patients' treatment goals and likely adherence to therapy
- Elimination of odontogenic pain

  Investigate or dress a restored tooth, occlusal adjustment, extraction
- Medical treatment

  Drug therapy (carbamazepine, antidepressants)
- Refer to appropriate specialist

  Further investigations (e.g. to neurologist for nerve conduction tests)

Table 15.3 Pain characteristics to be evaluated when taking a pain history

Duration	Periodicity
Location	Character
Radiation	Severity
Provoking factors	Relieving factors
Associated factors	

Table 15.4 The cranial nerves

Number	Name	Number	Name
I	Olfactory	VII	Facial
II	Optic	VIII	Acoustic vestibular (vestibulocochlear)
III	Oculomotor	IX	Glossopharyngeal
IV	Trochlear	X	Vagus
VI	Abducens	XI	Accessory
V	Trigeminal	XII	Hypoglossal

Some useful neurological terms

Alogenic	Causing pain
Allodynia	Pain from a stimulus that does not normally provoke pain, e.g. light touch
Analgesia	Absence of a pain response to a painful stimulus
Anaesthesia	Complete loss of sensation
Dysaesthesia	Altered unpleasant sensation; may be spontaneous or in response to a stimulus
Hyperalgesia	An increased response to a stimulus that is normally painful
Neuropathic pain	Pain initiated or caused by a primary lesion, dysfunction, or transitory problem in the peripheral or central nervous system

pain) is *pain initiated or caused by a primary lesion, dysfunction, or transitory pertubation in the peripheral or central nervous system*. This definition is all-inclusive and encompasses nerve-injury-related conditions.

The term neuropathic pain will be used in this chapter. Chronic neuropathic pain includes disorders such as trigeminal and glossopharyngeal neuralgia, postherpetic neuralgia, diabetic neuropathy, and peripheral nerve damage due to HIV infection and alcohol. Trauma or inflammatory change affecting the extra- or intracranial course of the nerve, for example, spinal nerve injury or multiple sclerosis, can also result in neuropathic pain. Benign or malignant neoplasms either compressing or infiltrating a nerve can give rise to neuropathic pain.

This chapter discusses neuropathic pain that is likely to be encountered in the oral medicine clinic. It may present with or without other symptoms of neurologial disturbances (such as paraesthesia, hyperalgesia, allodynia, and motor nerve dysfunction).

Neuropathic pain does not usually respond to conventional analgesics such as aspirin, paracetamol, and nonsteroidal anti-inflammatory drugs (NSAIDs). The medical management of this pain is best achieved using other pharmacological agents such as anticonvulsants and sometimes antidepressants. Treatment should be initiated, where possible, using single drug therapy. This will limit the side-effects.

> Neuropathic pain is pain initiated or caused by a primary lesion, dysfunction, or transitory perturbation in the peripheral or central nervous system.

Trigeminal neuralgia

> Trigeminal neuralgia: sudden, usually unilateral, severe, brief, stabbing, recurrent pains in the distribution of one or more branches of the fifth cranial nerve.

Trigeminal neuralgia is a disease of such characteristic intensity that it has been known and described over a long period of history. In spite of this, the true nature of this extremely painful condition is not known. In some patients there is a vascular abnormality (venous or arterial) that causes compression of the trigeminal root—adjacent to the pons in the posterior cranial fossa. This results in areas of demyelination and abnormal conduction. Elimination of this compression has led to long-term pain relief in most patients. The association between multiple sclerosis (MS) and trigeminal neuralgia is well known and is discussed later in this chapter.

A small proportion (approximately 2 per cent) of patients with posterior fossa tumours (for example, acoustic neuromas or benign tumours) present with typical trigeminal neuralgia. Painful symptoms may precede or accompany sensory or motor deficits in these cases.

The pathophysiology of trigeminal neuralgia has yet to be elucidated but one theory is that the paroxysms of pain in this condition may represent discharges in selected neurones whose threshold for repetitive firing has been altered, possibly by focal nerve injury. Such firing may then be initiated by innocuous tactile stimuli (this would explain 'trigger zones'). Cross-excitation of neighbouring nerves could then result in the recruitment of sufficient discharging cells for a nociceptive signal to be perceived as pain. However, none of the current theories fully explain the clinical features of trigeminal neuralgia.

Pretrigeminal neuralgia

This condition is described as a dull ache, similar to toothache, and the patients subsequently develop trigeminal neuralgia. It is thought to occur in up to 20 per cent of patients who develop trigeminal neuralgia. Therapeutic options for trigeminal neuralgia are effective for this condition. The clinician must first, how-ever, ensure that there is no pain of dental origin responsible for these symptoms. It is at this time that the patients are most often seen by the dental surgeon for the investigation of what may be highly perplexing pain symptoms. Pretrigeminal neuralgia is a diagnosis made in retrospect.

Clinical presentation of trigeminal neuralgia

The incidence of trigeminal neuralgia is around 150 per 1 million and more patients are female (female:male ratio approximately 2:1). The prevalence of the condition is 1 in 1000. The peak onset is in the fifth to seventh decades and symptoms usually occur after the fourth decade.

The pain distribution is almost always unilateral in the first instance, with only 3 per cent of cases subsequently developing bilateral involvement. Pain may affect one, two, or even three divisions. The first division on its own is only rarely affected. The pain is of great intensity, is described as sharp and stabbing in nature (lancinating), and lasts for only a few seconds. This transient attack may be repeated in a matter of minutes or hours. There may be no apparent precipitating factor, but many patients have a 'trigger zone', a point on the face or in the mouth (often outside the area of pain distribution) where the lightest contact may initiate an attack. Stimuli may include touching, washing, draughts of cold air, toothbrushing, eating, or smiling. Between the paroxysms of pain there may be a dull background ache in the area or no pain at all. These attacks rarely occur at night. The so-called 'frozen face' is an attempt by the patient to defer attacks by limiting movement, hence avoiding the triggering of the pain. Spontaneous remission for a matter of weeks or months may occur, but this is rarely permanent. Patients in severe pain lose weight, are unable to socialize, and often become depressed.

> Descriptors of pain in trigeminal neuralgia:
> - sharp
> - stabbing
> - 'electric shock-like'

Investigation of patients with trigeminal neuralgia

Trigeminal neuralgia is diagnosed principally from the pain history. There is no specific diagnostic test, but a full clinical examination, including assessment of the cranial nerves, should be carried out to exclude other causes of pain. Very few patients have subtle sensory changes, and trigger points can usually be elicited. The dental surgeon has a pivotal role in the diagnosis of patients presenting with trigeminal neuralgia. He/she must always exclude a dental cause for the patient's painful symptoms.

Patients with trigeminal neuralgia may ascribe the pain to toothache in what may appear to be an entirely sound tooth. Following the extraction of this tooth the pain may then be described as coming from a nearby tooth and extraction of this may also be demanded by the patient. It is not rare to find patients made virtually unilaterally edentulous in this way. Many eventual difficulties can be avoided if it is recognized that any patient presenting with possible trigeminal neuralgia symptoms

Trigeminal neuralgia—key features

- Brief paroxysms of sharp, stabbing pain
- Trigger zone(s)
- Provoking factors include eating, talking, shaving, washing face
- Pain usually confined to one division of trigeminal nerve
- Usually unilateral
- Usually pain-free during sleep
- Drug therapy with carbamazepine is the medical treatment of choice
- Peripheral or central surgical treatments are management options
- May have extended remission with completely pain-free periods

should be considered as worthy of full investigation before further extractions are considered.

> The dental surgeon has a pivotal role in the diagnosis of patients presenting with trigeminal neuralgia—a dental cause for the patient's painful symptoms must always be excluded.

Conversely, the situation may arise in which pain closely resembling trigeminal neuralgia may arise from some quite ordinary dental pathology such as a retained root or a cracked tooth or even from unsatisfactory dentures. If there is any abnormality of this kind present, it should be treated as the essential first step in the management of the patient.

> Younger patients (< 50 years of age) presenting with trigeminal neuralgia, particularly if there is bilateral involvement, should be referred to a neurologist for appropriate diagnostic testing to exclude multiple sclerosis.

As has been pointed out, trigeminal neuralgia tends to occur in later life. The onset of symptoms of trigeminal neuralgia in a patient under the age of 40 years should be treated with some suspicion as a possible first warning of the onset of multiple sclerosis (see next section). In this condition the neuralgia-like pains are often the first symptoms. It has been suggested that patients of this age group should possibly be referred for a specialist neurological assessment. When assessing the need for a neurological opinion on a patient with suspected trigeminal neuralgia, it should always be remembered that there are no diagnostic indicators other than the pain itself. Any other associated neurological features, such as muscle weakness, blurring of vision, dizziness, paraesthesia, or the possible involvement of other cranial nerves, should be taken as absolute indications for a full neurological assessment and cerebral imaging.

> Central nervous system imaging should be undertaken if there is sensory loss.

Table 15.5 The differential diagnosis of trigeminal neuralgia

Dental pain, especially 'cracked tooth syndrome'
Sinus pain
Postherpetic neuralgia
Trigeminal neuralgia secondary to nerve injury, tumour, or other pathological condition
Cluster headache
Atypical facial pain
Temporomandibular pain dysfunction syndrome

There are a number of conditions to be considered in the differential diagnosis of trigeminal neuralgia (Table 15.5) but in many of these the pain symptoms reported by the patient are not characteristic of trigeminal neuralgia (that is, brief, shooting, paroxysmal pain). Trigeminal neuralgia may be the first manifestation in a small number of patients with MS. These are younger than the trigeminal neuralgia population as a whole and their neuralgia is often bilateral. Conversely, trigeminal neuralgia is diagnosed in 1–5 per cent of patients with MS.

Medical management of trigeminal neuralgia

Pharmacological therapy is still considered the most appropriate management for most patients with trigeminal neuralgia, but recent results from large neurosurgical series would justify surgical intervention early on, particularly in the younger patient. All patients should be given a dispassionate account of the medical and surgical options available.

- The medical treatment of trigeminal neuralgia is primarily with the use of anticonvulsants
- Carbamazepine is currently the drug of choice
- The initial dose of carbamazepine is 100 mg, twice daily; this is increased gradually, by 100 mg each day, until the pain is controlled
- A maximum daily dose of 800–1000 mg should not be exceeded

Pharmacological treatment of trigeminal neuralgia depends largely upon the use of anticonvulsants and the drug of choice has traditionally been carbamazepine (Tegratol). Response to carbamazepine is reportedly diagnostic for trigeminal neuralgia; however, it is worth mentioning that carbamazepine can occasionally reduce (or abolish) pain of odontogenic origin. Dental causes of facial pain should, therefore, have been eliminated prior to the commencement of drug therapy. Other anticonvulsant drugs are occasionally used, but carbamazepine remains the 'gold standard' therapeutic agent for trigeminal neuralgia and has been evaluated in randomized placebo-controlled trials. The initial dosage of carbamazepine is kept low and started at 100 mg, twice daily, and gradually increased in daily increments of 100 mg until control of pain is attained. A maximum dose of 800–1000 mg daily should not be exceeded. The medication should be taken about

30 minutes before meals, thus maximizing pain control for mastication. About 70 per cent of patients with trigeminal neuralgia are estimated to benefit from carbamazepine. All patients will have minor side-effects, which vary and are dose-dependent. Some patients experience drowsiness or dizziness, whereas some report gastrointestinal reactions. In a very few patients, however, the much more serious side-effect of agranulocytosis may occur. The elderly are particularly susceptible to side-effects. The white cell count may be monitored by repeated blood tests, but it would appear that, when this reaction occurs, it may do so suddenly and without prior warning. Other, less serious, haematological effects have been recorded including anaemia, neutropenia, thrombocytopenia, and hyponatraemia. For these reasons it is generally recommended that haematology and blood chemistry testing is carried out at the commencement of treatment, and at 1 month and 3 months, and thereafter depending on circumstances. It is important to reiterate, however, that a sudden, potentially fatal, fall in the white cell count may occur as a very rare event, and may be entirely missed by long-term blood-testing regimes. It is also generally recommended that liver function tests should be part of the drug monitoring programme, as carbamazepine is active in liver enzyme induction. Hyponatraemia (a reduced serum level of sodium) has also been reported with carbamazepine. When prescribing carbamazepine the clinician should always be aware of possible drug interactions—some drugs may become ineffective because therapeutic serum levels are not achieved or maintained due to the increased rate of metabolism. Warfarin is one such drug.

Monitoring for patients on carbamazepine therapy

Full blood count, liver function tests, and electrolytes should be monitored:

- prior to therapy
- at 1 month
- at 3 months

A further side-effect of carbamazepine, which occurs in approximately 7 per cent of patients, is the occurrence of a severe rash. Just as in the case of agranulocytosis, this may occur quite unexpectedly after a long period of treatment with the drug.

As a response to the problems associated with carbamazepine therapy, a related drug, oxcarbazepine, was introduced. This has essentially the same properties as carbamazepine but is reputed to be better tolerated. This is not, however, always the case. Oxcarbazepine has yet to establish its place as a substitute for carbamazepine as up to a quarter of patients experience cross-sensitivity.

There are other drugs that may be used in the treatment of trigeminal neuralgia for patients who cannot tolerate carbamazepine. These include phenytoin, lamotrogine, baclofen, and

Side-effects of carbamazepine therapy

- Drowsiness, dizziness, confusion
- Vertigo
- Nausea
- Skin reaction—rash
- Leukopenia (anaemia, neutropenia, thrombocytopenia, and aplastic anaemia occur rarely)
- Hepatic microsomal enzyme induction (and consequent drug interactions)
- Hyponatraemia

clonazepam. None of these drugs are as effective as carbamazepine in the control of trigeminal neuralgia, although phenytoin in conjunction with carbamazepine may be valuable in some patients unresponsive to carbamazepine alone. The starting dose for phenytoin is usually 300 mg/day (in divided doses) although this drug alone is rarely successful in controlling pain. Phenytoin has a number of side-effects including a severe rash. Considering the morbidity and prevalence of trigeminal neuralgia, very few controlled studies have been carried out on drugs available for treatment. A recently introduced drug, gabapentin, has been evaluated for use in postherpetic neuralgia and diabetic neuropathy and may be useful for trigeminal neuralgia. It appears to be comparatively free of serious side-effects and can be used in combination with carbamazepine.

Surgical treatment of trigeminal neuralgia

A minority of patients are unsuitable for drug therapy, either because they are—or have become—unresponsive to it or cannot tolerate the side-effects. Others are keen to explore the surgical options in the hope of a permanent cure. There a number of different surgical approaches available for the treatment of trigeminal neuralgia and these vary in complexity from relatively simple peripheral procedures (for example, cryotherapy) to high-frequency selective coagulation of the nerve fibres in the region of the ganglion and open intracranial procedures in the posterior fossa for microvascular decompression of the trigeminal nerve (Table 15.6). Full details of these procedures are, however, outside the scope of this book (see Project 3 at the end of this chapter). When considering a surgical approach to treatment, the following factors must be considered: postoperative pain relief; recurrence rates; general health; risks; and adverse effects.

Microvascular decompression of the trigeminal nerve is now considered the surgical treatment of choice by a number of centres, provided that the patient is in reasonable health and evidence of vascular decompression has been identified, as it is the only procedure that is non-destructive. A specific imaging technique, magnetic resonance tomographic angiography (MRTA), is

Table 15.6 Surgical treatments in current use for trigeminal neuralgia

Surgical therapies	Procedure	Morbidity	Recurrence after surgery (average)
Peripheral			
Cryotherapy, neurectomy, alcohol injections	The peripheral nerve branch is either directly exposed or injected under local anaesthesia	Low and local, mainly mild sensory loss	Up to a year
Gasserian ganglion			
Radiofrequency, thermocoagulation	Short-acting, intermittent general anaesthesia used to penetrate foramen ovale. The Gasserian ganglion is subjected to cycles of thermal lesioning (temperature varying from 60° to 80°C)	Sensory impairment to the trigeminal nerve, anaesthesia dolorosa (rare), corneal anaesthesia (with subsequent risk of keratitis). Mortality rate low.	3–5 years
Glycerol injection	Local anaesthesia (± sedation) can be used. Meckel's cave is filled with glycerol	Dysaesthesia within the trigeminal area	Up to 3 years
Microcompression (balloon compression)	Full general anaesthesia used. The Gasserian ganglion is compressed by a balloon for a few seconds	Dysaesthesia can be problematic. Motor component often involved	3–5 years
Posterior fossa			
Microvascular decompression	Full general anaesthesia used. Any vessels lying on the trigeminal nerve at the point of entry to the cranium are moved aside or removed	8th cranial nerve damage may occur. Mortality rates of up to 0.7% reported. Serious morbidity, 10%	8 years
Stereotactic radiosurgery	Local anaesthesia (± sedation) can be used. Using stereotactic techniques the posterior fossa is identified and a gamma knife is directed at the proximal trigeminal root near the pons	Long-term effects of radiation unknown. Sensory loss of slow onset	Mean 15 months

* Adapted with permission from T.J. Nurmikko, Pain Research Institute, University of Liverpool, and P.R. Eldrige, The Walton Centre for Neurology and Neurosurgery NHS Trust, Liverpool, UK.

used to optimally image the trigeminal nerve and blood vessels in its vicinity.

> Surgical treatment of trigeminal neuralgia—factors to be considered:
> • pain relief
> • recurrence rates and their management
> • complications—morbidity and mortality

Glossopharyngeal neuralgia

Glossopharyngeal neuralgia is similar to neuralgia affecting the trigeminal nerve, but much less common. The pain is of the same nature as that of trigeminal neuralgia and is unilaterally felt in the oropharynx, sometimes with pain referred to the ipsilateral ear. Although the main component of the pain is described (as in

trigeminal neuralgia) as stabbing or shooting in nature, there may also be an appreciable residual ache that may last for some time after the paroxysmal attack. It is less severe than trigeminal neuralgia. The pain is often precipitated by swallowing, chewing, or coughing, and there may be a trigger zone. Cardiac arrhythmias and syncope have been described during attacks. Glossopharyngeal neuralgia may be secondary to a tumour of the throat, posterior cranial fossa, or jugular foramen.

> Glossopharyngeal neuralgia is a rare condition characterized by a paroxysmal, sharp, lancinating pain that affects one side of the throat and base of the tongue. It is usually triggered by swallowing.

Treatment is the same as for trigeminal neuralgia. Spontaneous remission of this condition is possible but first-line treatment is usually with an anticonvulsant and carbamazepine is successful in most cases. A positive response to this helps confirm the diagnosis. A surgical approach may be required if drug therapy becomes ineffective or problematical.

Postherpetic neuralgia

Herpes zoster (shingles) is the reactivation of a latent infection with the varicella zoster virus (see Chapter 4). This virus is usually reactivated once in a lifetime, with fewer than 5 per cent of patients having a second attack. Herpes zoster is more likely to occur in later life and in patients who have T-cell immunosuppression. Pain may occur before, during, or after an attack of facial herpes zoster. The first warning of such an attack may be a severe burning pain occurring in the area of the eruption, up to 2 days before the vesicles appear. The pain in herpes zoster is much more severe than that in herpes simplex, in which the symptoms are largely due to the secondary infection of ruptured vesicles (Chapter 4). The pain associated with herpes zoster usually subsides within weeks. In some patients a neuralgia-like pain persists for months or even years. The pain has an intense burning component and may be accompanied by stabbing sensations—there is typically hyperalgesia or paraesthesia and allodynia. The distribution of pain follows the distribution of the original infection. This neuralgia tends to be a persistent as opposed to a paroxysmal pain. In addition, the pain has a more variable character and severity than trigeminal neuralgia. The incidence of trigeminal postherpetic neuralgia is uncertain, but older patients with herpes zoster are particularly susceptible to postherpetic neuralgia—60 per cent of patients over 60 are affected by this distressing condition. It is relatively uncommon in those under the age of 50 years. The risk of postherpetic neuralgia is also thought to be greater if patients have severe pain or rash during the acute phase and also if the patients experience pain prior to the appearance of the rash.

Treatment of established postherpetic neuralgia can be very difficult—it is often resistant to treatment. It does not appear to respond to carbamazepine and analgesics may also be ineffective. Steroids have been advocated but there is no confirmation of their value in preventing postherpetic neuralgia. Tricyclic antidepressants have been associated with pain relief in some patients and gabapentin has been shown, in clinical trials, to be effective for postherpetic neuralgia. Antiviral treatment combined with antidepressants in the elderly in the acute phase has been found to reduce the duration and prevalence of postherpetic neuralgia, by as much as 50 per cent. The use of transcutaneous electrical stimulation is thought to be effective for some patients.

To summarize, prophylaxis offers the best hope of preventing the distressing pain of postherpetic neuralgia affecting the trigeminal nerve. All patients with herpes zoster should be vigorously treated with systemic antiviral agents such as aciclovir. These should be commenced as soon as possible after the onset of the rash. Multicentre clinical trials have established that success-

ful treatment of the primary infection considerably reduces the risk of the subsequent development of neuralgia.

> - Pain may precede, accompany, and persist after the acute vesicular phase of herpes zoster
> - Pain persisting after herpes zoster is called postherpetic neuralgia
> - The main risk factor is increasing age

Neuropathic pain secondary to other conditions

Facial pain and headache may be symptoms of a wide variety of intra- and extracranial lesions such as neoplasms or vascular abnormalities. Facial pain may arise through involvement either by pressure or by malignant infiltration of the trigeminal ganglion of the peripheral branches of the nerve. Primary and secondary intracranial neoplasms, nasopharyngeal tumours, aneurysms, and cerebral epidermoid cysts are among the most commonly recorded lesions of this type causing facial pain. Similarly, the lesions left following brain damage of any kind may be the source of facial pain. In cases of this type, facial pain is only rarely the only symptom, although it may well be the earliest. Involvement of other cranial nerves and the presence of unusual symptoms such as anaesthesia or paraesthesia should at once raise the suspicion of the possibility of a lesion of this kind.

Another cause of facial pain arising from compression of the trigeminal nerve occurs in Paget's disease affecting the base of the skull (see Chapter 18). Some degree of closure of the foramina is common, and the consequent stricture of the nerve may lead to a variety of pain symptoms. A further cause of trauma to the trigeminal nerve in Paget's disease may be the deformation of the skull as a whole, causing compression of the sensory root of the nerve where it crosses the petrous bone. The pain often simulates trigeminal neuralgia, although aching pains may sometimes be reported. A similar compression of the auditory nerve may give rise to deafness, and changes in the cervical spine may also lead to pain in the area served by the sensory nerves of the cervical plexus.

Migraine

There are many variants of migraine and a full description of the different types is outside the scope of oral medicine. The dentist should, however, be familiar with the symptoms of migraine. Patients with migraine and cluster headache (migrainous neuralgia) occasionally present in the oral medicine clinic. Although migraine is essentially a headache, it may also have a facial component, usually over the maxilla, and this may cause confusion. In most cases, however, the patients complain of an intense headache, intermittent in nature and usually (but not invariably) unilateral—hence the term 'hemicrania'. Each attack of headache may last for several hours or even a number of days, and is often associated with various symptoms such as nausea and visual disturbance. The systemic upset is considerable and many patients need to take bed rest in a quiet dark room until the attack subsides. In classic migraine patients have an aura where the headache is preceded by neurological symptoms and deficits—visual, sensory, speech, or motor disturbances may occur and usually last around 15 minutes. Migraine without aura is, however, well recognized. The history of the condition with its associated disturbances often gives a strong clue to its nature, as does the frequent presence of a family history. Some patients recognize a precipitating factor—sometimes of stress, sometimes of a foodstuff. The onset of migraine may occur at any age, but is most common during adolescence. In migraine there are no symptoms between attacks.

The cause of migraine has generally been attributed to instability of the cranial arteries. The response of migraine to drug therapy is variable. Simple analgesics, anti-emetics, propranolol, and ergotamine can be successful. First-line drug treatment for the acute phase should be a simple analgesic such as paracetamol, aspirin, or a NSAID. An anti-emetic may be helpful in some patients when vomiting is a problem—the administration of drugs by suppository is beneficial for such patients. 5-hydroxy-tryptamine (5-HT_1; serotonin) agonists (for example, sumatriptan or newer analgesics) may be given by the oral, intranasal, or subcutaneous route. Historically, the most widely used group of drugs have been derived from ergot, these are now best avoided in view of their powerful side-effects.

Migraine prophylaxis may be valuable for patients who have two or more severe attacks each month. Beta-blockers, such as propranolol, and 5-HT_1 antagonists (Pizotifen) may be beneficial. Methysergide is used only occasionally because of the risk of unwanted side-effects, including the very serious one of retroperitoneal fibrosis. Methysergide should only be administered under hospital supervision. Sodium valproate and tricyclic antidepressants may be considered. Clonidine, a drug that has been used in larger doses for the treatment of hypertension and which has a vascular stabilizing effect, has been used for the control of migrainous attacks. This drug has considerable side-effects, it may aggravate depression and produce insomnia, and is not now recommended routinely for prophylaxis of migraine.

The diagnosis of migraine is made on basis of the clinical history, but a physical examination of the patient and a careful assessment of the history is required to exclude other causes of headache. There is no evidence that occlusal problems cause migraine. The use of a nocturnal acrylic occlusal splint, which significantly increases the vertical occlusal dimension, has been advocated by some to help patients who wake up in the morning with migraine or develop migraine shortly after waking but the evidence is not based on randomized controlled trials. Pain of a migrainous type may also be associated with Melkersson–Rosenthal syndrome (see Chapter 12).

Cluster headache (periodic migrainous neuralgia/migrainous neuralgia)

This condition, closely associated with migraine, may also appear as a diagnostic problem in the oral medicine clinic or in the dental surgery. The aetiology of this condition is thought to be vascular changes at the base of the skull. Whilst many features of the pain may be similar to those of classical migraine, there are differences (Table 15.7). The patients are much more commonly young males and they may experience 1–8 attacks per day. Alcohol and vasodilators may precipitate attacks, but they also occur spontaneously. Cluster headache is less common than migraine. During an attack there are repeated episodes of pain, usually of about 30 minutes in duration, with a variable interval between. The pain is usually located behind and around the eye, with extensions to the maxilla and to the temporal area. The pain lasts for 30–120 minutes and is usually accompanied by vascular changes. Autonomic symptoms are often present, such as weeping of the eye on the affected side and congestion of the nasal mucous membranes. The attacks often occur at regular times at night and disturb sleep—hence the pseudonym 'alarm clock pain'. Spontaneous remission can occur after several months of attacks. The characteristic group-

Table 15.7 Comparative features of migraine and cluster headaches

Migraine	Cluster headaches
Age and gender	
Slightly more common in females, can occur at any age, mainly 2nd–3rd decades	Mainly young males, > 20 years
Site	
Usually unilateral temporal, occipital, or frontal muscles	Unilateral, orbital region
Nature of pain and intensity duration	
Severe throbbing, pulsating continuous, hours–days (4–72 h) usually day time. Up to 12 attacks per month	Severe boring episodic 30–180 min, often at night. Can be several attacks per day.
Precipitating factors	
Stress, foodstuffs for some patients	Alcohol for some patients
Prodromal symptoms	
Aura-phase. Common neurological symptoms (e.g. visual disturbances, speech problems, numbness)	Aura phase is uncommon
Associated features	
Family history common. May be sensitive to light, smells, noise. vomiting is common	Family history uncommon. Vascular changes on affected side (lacrimation/nasal congestion)
Treatment	
Avoidance of precipitating factors NSAIDs, 5HT_1 agonists.	Avoidance of precipitating factors. Sumatriptan, NSAIDs

ing of attacks of pain over a short period followed by long periods of remission has led to the term 'cluster headache'. Some patients do not have these episodic occurrences and they are then diagnosed as having chronic cluster headaches.

The pain often responds to antimigraine drugs in the same way as migraine itself but subcutaneous injection of sumatriptan is thought to be the treatment of choice during an attack. There are very clear diagnostic criteria for this condition, which has led to high-quality multicentre randomized controlled trials of therapy.

Characteristics of cluster headaches

- Male to female ratio, 9:1
- Predilection for young males
- Episodic severe pain of 30 min to 3 hour duration that can wake a patient from sleep
- Centred over orbital region
- Accompanied by lacrimation and nasal congestion
- Alcohol may provoke pain

Tension-type headache

Tension-type headache is now the term recommended to describe a variety of poorly defined conditions, such as 'tension headache', 'stress headache', and 'muscle contraction headache', that are very common. Tension-type headaches are characterized by pain that is mild to moderate in severity, and the distribution is bilateral. The complaint is one of a feeling of tightness, constriction, or pressure. The pain may affect the frontal, occipital, and temporal muscles. The headache may be episodic or chronic and is not accompanied by systemic disturbance or neurological signs.

The causes of tension-type headache are poorly understood, but muscular tension and stress are thought to be important. Overwork, fatigue, an emotional crisis, and menstruation are common precipitating factors. It is worth noting that tension-type headaches do not usually wake the patient from sleep. Similar symptoms may be experienced by patients who have drug-related headaches, hypertension, or hyperthyroidism. A minority of patients may suffer from both tension-type headache and migraine.

Treatment of tension-type headaches involves avoidance of trigger factors such as alcohol, improving sleep patterns, taking more exercise, or using relaxation techniques or other stress-coping strategies. Drug treatments consist of the intermittent use of simple analgesics such as aspirin, paracetamol, or NSAIDs. Caffeine-containing drugs should be avoided. Most patients with episodic tension-type headaches have short-lasting attacks and respond well to simple analgesics. However, around 2–3 per cent of sufferers have chronic tension-type headaches with intractable symptoms that are resistant to simple analgesics. Some of these

are potentiated by overuse of analgesics. The use of tricyclic antidepressants may be helpful but, ideally, should be used in conjunction with cognitive and behavioural approaches.

Facial pain: miscellaneous conditions

Two conditions that should be mentioned because they may very occasionally cause facial pain are temporal arteritis and auriculotemporal syndrome (Frey's syndrome). It is important that the dentist is aware of the former lesion because early diagnosis can prevent serious complications.

Giant cell arteritis (temporal arteritis/cranial arteritis)

Giant cell arteritis is an inflammatory condition that typically affects the walls of medium-sized arteries. The lumen of the vessel becomes compromised and, as a consequence, ischaemia of the tissues supplied by the artery may occur. Giant cell arteritis can affect many parts of the body (polymyalgia rheumatica), but the head is often involved. When the temporal artery is involved it is called temporal or cranial arteritis.

Temporal arteritis

In temporal arteritis the pain is localized to the temporal and frontal regions—this corresponds to the area supplied by the superficial temporal artery. The pain is described as a severe throbbing ache, but paroxysmal pain is also occasionally described. In between attacks of pain the affected area may be very tender to the touch and the temporal artery may be tortuous, pronounced. The pain may be initiated by eating and, as a consequence, weight loss may ensue. The masticatory pain is due to ischaemia of the muscles and should be differentiated from temporomandibular pain disorders. The patients, most of whom are in older age groups and predominantly female, also complain of general malaise and diffuse muscular and joint pains. There may also be degeneration of vision because of involvement of the retinal artery and subsequent ischaemia of the optic nerve. The essential pathology of this condition is generalized inflammation with an infiltrate of giant cells. This condition can affect other vessels in the head and neck (for example, lingual arteritis).

It is important that this condition is recognized and treated as early as possible, because it may otherwise progress to cause irreversible damage to the optic nerve. Patients should therefore be assessed on an emergency basis. Diagnosis is made on clinical grounds, largely dependent on the evidently enlarged and painful artery and on elevated erythrocyte sedimentation rate (ESR). The ESR is markedly raised (over 100 mm in 1 hour) and C-reactive protein (CRP) levels may also be elevated. A normal ESR virtually rules out temporal arteritis. Absolute diagnosis depends on the finding of a typical giant-cell inflammatory process in a biopsy of the affected vessel, which should only be done in patients who have a raised ESR. Treatment is with high doses of systemic steroids, of the order of 60 mg of prednisolone daily, until symptoms disappear. Patients are maintained on a lower dose of steroids for up to 2 years.

Characteristics of temporal (giant cell) arteritis

- A vascular disease primarily affecting elderly people—mean age 70 years
- Sudden-onset pain or headache that may be initiated or exacerbated by eating
- Blindness is a recognized complication—it is therefore important to promptly diagnose and treat this condition
- The ESR is abnormally high; arterial biopsy may demonstrate granulomatous arteritis
- Differential diagnoses: temporomandibular joint disorders: trigeminal neuralgia
- Treat with high-dose systemic steroids

Auriculotemporal syndrome (Frey's syndrome)

The auriculotemporal syndrome is caused by damage to the auriculotemporal nerve as it passes through the substance of the parotid gland in the early part of its course. It is a rare condition that may be the result of a wide range of pathological processes within the gland, both inflammatory and neoplastic, or of surgical trauma (postgustatory neuralgia). The symptoms are of erythema and sweating in the cutaneous distribution of the auriculotemporal nerve. The symptoms are usually in response to gustatory stimuli. In approximately 10 per cent of cases the condition is accompanied by pain in the distribution of the auriculotemporal nerve. The pain is often described as 'burning' in nature. Between attacks of pain there may be anaesthesia or paraesthesia of the skin in the affected area. The term 'gustatory neuralgia' has been proposed for this pain. No effective treatment has been identified for this condition.

Frey's syndrome is a recognized complication of surgical trauma (for example, parotid gland surgery and temporomandibular joint surgery), but it can also be due to accidental trauma, local infection, sympathetic dysfunction, and parotid pathology. It is evident, therefore, that, once the condition is recognized, confirmation of the diagnosis and subsequent treatment depend on a full investigation of the involved parotid gland. The topical application of an antiperspirant may be helpful in controlling the sweating.

Neurological disturbances

Facial nerve deficits

Deficits of the seventh cranial nerve (facial nerve) may result from a central or peripheral cause and it is essential to distinguish between these two types of neurological lesion.

Characteristics of Frey's syndrome

- Flushing and sweating in the cutaneous distribution of the auriculotemporal nerve following a gustatory stimulus
- Pain is uncommon (less than 10 per cent of cases)
- Trauma, local infection, local surgery, sympathetic dysfunction, and central nervous system disorders are possible aetiological factors

1. *Upper motor neurone lesions* are central lesions that affect the nerve fibres responsible for movement in the lower facial muscles. In such a lesion, the muscles over the maxilla and mandible are weakened, but those of the forehead are unaffected. This is because the motor nerves to the muscles of the forehead are regulated by both cerebral hemispheres, with free crossing of nerve fibres. In contrast, the muscles of the lower part of the face are innervated only by nerves controlled in the opposite hemisphere. In these lesions the emotional movements of the whole of the face may be unaffected since these are initiated by upper motor neurones separated from the pyramidal motor fibres that serve the facial muscles for normal function.

2. *Lower motor neurone lesions* affect both the upper and lower facial muscles. The forehead and face are equally affected. In these cases the pathological process is peripheral to the facial motor nucleus in the pons. The most common cause of such a paralysis is Bell's palsy (discussed below) but a wide variety of lesions affecting the facial nerve below the base of the skull (including some in the parotid gland) may be responsible for symptoms. Emotional movements are also lost in the area since the lesion responsible affects the common path of all the peripheral fibres.

Peripheral paralysis is subdivided into intrapetrosal and extrapetrosal lesions. When the lesion affects the facial nerve in the intrapetrosal tract, the chorda tympani and stapedius nerve are also involved. There may, therefore, be a hearing deficit (hyperacusia) and loss of taste on the anterior two-thirds of the tongue on the affected side. Since the chorda tympani is given off within the facial canal at the base of the skull, lesions occurring below this will not affect the sense of taste.

The nerves responsible for motor function to the face are shown in Table 15.8.

Anaesthesia and paraesthesia

The onset of anaesthesia or paraesthesia, either slowly or suddenly, in the distribution of a nerve may have localized or generalized significance; Table 15.9 lists possible conditions that may cause orofacial anaesthesia or paraesthesia.

Local causes of anaesthesia in branches of the trigeminal nerve include direct trauma to the nerve (as in fractures, traumatic

Table 15.8 The nerves responsible for motor control of the head and neck

Number	Cranial nerve	Muscles
V	Trigeminal	Masticatory muscles
VII	Facial	Muscles of facial expression
IX	Glossopharyngeal	Uvula, soft palate, base of tongue, pharynx
XI	Accessory	Trapezius
XII	Hypoglossal	Tongue

Characteristics of upper motor neurone disease

- A central lesion that causes partial paralysis of the facial muscles
- The lower facial muscles, contralateral to the lesion, are paralysed
- The orbicularis oculi and frontalis muscles, which receive bilateral cortical fibres, have limited function
- The blink reflex and movement of forehead muscles unaffected

Characteristics of lower motor neurone disease

- A lesion affecting the facial nerve along its intra- or extrapetrosal course
- There is paralysis of the facial muscles around the eye, forehead, and mouth, the blink reflex is lost, and drooling is common
- There may be taste and hearing deficits if the lesion is situated within the intrapetrosal tract

Causes of facial palsy

Intracranial causes	Extracranial causes (including intrapetrosal lesions)
Cerebrovascular accidents	Incorrect placement of local anaesthetic
Cerebral tumours	Iatrogenic (following resection of tumour)
Neurological diseases	Parotid tumour
Multiple sclerosis	Heerfordt's syndrome
Head injuries	Melkersson–Rosenthal syndrome (Chapter 12)
Ramsey Hunt syndrome (Chapter 4)	

Table 15.9 Conditions that may cause orofacial anaesthesia or paraesthesia

Local	Systemic
Local anaesthetic	Multiple sclerosis
Trauma	Intracranial lesions
Resorption of the alveolar ridge exposing mental foramen	Hyperventilation/tetany Medication Psychogenic
Infection (osteomyelitis, herpes zoster)	
Malignancies	

extractions, sagital split osteotomies), pressure on the nerve by a foreign body (such as a tooth root or root canal medicament), inflammatory changes in relation to the nerve (especially osteomyelitis), and neoplasms encroaching on the nerve. More generalized neurological conditions that may affect the trigeminal nerve in this way include multiple sclerosis and the neuropathy of mixed connective tissue disease (Chapter 11). Similar changes may occur as the result of a variety of intracranial space-filling lesions such as an acoustic neuroma (Fig. 15.2).

Following a cerebrovascular accident there may be a range of neurological abnormalities affecting the face and mouth. Among the more difficult to deal with are the changes in sensation, proprioception, and muscular control, which may make denture-wearing very difficult for the affected patient.

> Following a cerebrovascular accident there may be a range of neurological abnormalities affecting the face and mouth.

Bell's palsy

Bell's palsy is the name given to an acute paralysis of the facial nerve. It is practically always unilateral and no obvious cause is found in the vast majority of cases. It is thought that some cases

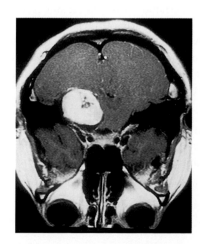

Fig. 15.2 Magnetic resonance scan showing a mass in the cerebellopontine angle. (Patient presented with 'facial numbness')

may have a viral aetiology; possibly herpes simplex virus. Bell's palsy is the most common lower motor neurone lesion and, depending upon the severity of the condition, some or all of the muscles of expression on the affected side may be weakened or paralysed. The extent of the paralysis is easily seen if the patient is asked to smile, to close the eyes, and to furrow the brow. There may or may not be loss of taste sensation on the anterior lateral part of the tongue on the affected side, depending on whether or not the chorda tympani nerve is involved. Approximately half the patients complain of severe pain in the area of the parotid gland or the ear—spreading down the mandible—although this generally precedes the paralysis or occurs in the early stages of the condition. The facial appearance is characteristic. The impaired function of the seventh cranial nerve can be demonstrated by asking the patient to smile, close their eyes, and attempt to purse their lips. The affected side will be unable to perform these actions.

> Prompt diagnosis and treatment of Bell's palsy may prevent functional and aesthetic impairment.

One currently recommended treatment regime for Bell's palsy is a combination of systemic steroids and aciclovir. The antiviral is advocated because of the possible involvement of the herpes simplex virus. Aciclovir is given at a dose of 400 mg, four times daily. Steroids are administered in high dosage—60 mg prednisolone daily for 5 days, then reducing the dose over the same period of time, is a reasonable regime. The rationale behind this approach is unproven, but it is thought that steroids may be advantageous by reducing oedema around the facial nerve. Some workers have suggested that it needs to be instituted within the first 24–72 hours of onset of the Bell's palsy. Others suggest that it should be adopted only if spontaneous resolution does not take place. There is no conclusive evidence from randomized controlled trials that steroids or antiviral agents, given alone or in combination, provide any long-term benefit for patients with Bell's palsy. Nonetheless, it is the authors' view that, unless there are significant contraindications to steroid therapy, it should be started with a systemic antiviral agent at the earliest opportunity after diagnosis. This is in an attempt to avoid the possibility of long-term cosmetic deformity that accompanies an unresolved facial palsy. It is important to protect an eye that remains partially open, either by an eye pad or shade.

Management of Bell's palsy

- Initial high-dose prednisolone, reducing after 5–7 days
- Systemic antiviral therapy
- Ensure adequate eye protection

Most patients with Bell's palsy recover within a few weeks, but for the chronic cases supportive or corrective treatment may

be necessary. A simple splint or a modification to an existing denture may help support the soft tissues and improve the facial profile of the affected side. Referral to physiotherapy departments for electrical stimulation of the paralysed facial muscles may also be helpful. Galvanic stimulation is considered to be worthwhile because it stimulates muscle contraction, possibly promotes motor end-plate function, and is of psychological benefit. Hand-held, patient-operated small nerve stimulators are now available for this purpose. Surgical treatment may be considered in some patients for cosmetic reasons, but there is little evidence that this approach is successful. Facial palsy as a manifestation of the Melkersson–Rosenthal syndrome is fully discussed in Chapter 12.

Multiple sclerosis

Multiple sclerosis (disseminated sclerosis) is a disease featuring progressive demyelination of nervous tissue with episodes of relapse and remission. This results in permanent and increasing disability. The condition affects mainly young adults, it is slightly more prevalent in females, and the usual age of onset is 20–40 years. The disease can present with a wide range of symptoms (Table 15.10) depending upon the sites of lesions in the brain. Diagnosis of the condition depends upon clinical features, magnetic resonance imaging (to demonstrate the central areas of demyelination), and exclusion of other neurological deficits.

Patients with multiple sclerosis (MS) may present with pain resembling trigeminal neuralgia. This can occur at any stage of the disease and it can be a presenting feature. If trigeminal neuralgia is the first manifestation of MS, the patients are often younger than the trigeminal neuralgia population as a whole and their neuralgia is often bilateral.

The clinician should, however, consider the possibility of multiple sclerosis when a patient younger than 50 years old presents with symptoms suggestive of trigeminal neuralgia. It is important, however, that this suspicion is not voiced to the patient until they have been fully assessed by a neurologist. Multiple sclerosis does not necessarily give rise to symptoms that mimic classical trigeminal neuralgia—it may give rise to persistent pain, with no identifiable trigger areas. Paraesthesia and allodynia may also be features of the condition. Multiple neurological deficits are usually present such as muscle weakness, visual disturbances,

Table 15.10 Common symptoms of multiple sclerosis

Type of symptom	Description
Visual	Loss of visual acuity and colour vision and eye pain (due to optic neuritis); diplopia
Weakness of the limbs	Tingling or paraesthesia may be present
Vertigo	
Ataxia	

and sensory loss. The management for the facial pain is similar to that for trigeminal neuralgia.

Multiple sclerosis (MS) is diagnosed in 2–4 per cent of patients with trigeminal neuralgia.

Extrapyramidal syndromes

Extrapyramidal syndromes are neurological disorders that affect pathways other than the principal ones concerned with voluntary movement. They are characterized by abnormality of muscular action with tremors. Parkinsonism is the best known condition of this kind.

It has recently become evident, however, that symptoms of a similar kind may occur following the use of certain drugs, especially in elderly patients. In particular, sedatives and tranquillizers of the phenothiazine group have been implicated. These patients may occasionally come to the dental surgeon for diagnosis since the dyskinetic symptoms are often most evident in the muscles of the masticatory apparatus. This can make dental treatment difficult. Repetitive movements or tremor of the tongue or mandible, which may be of a bizarre nature, should be suspected as having a drug-induced origin in patients of this older age group. Treatment is by withdrawal of the offending drug, although resolution may take some time.

> Extrapyramidal syndromes are neurological disorders that affect pathways other than the principal ones concerned with voluntary movement.

Discussion of problem cases

Case 15.1

Q1 What is the usual drug of choice for this patient and what starting dose would you prescribe?

Carbamazepine is the first drug of choice. A reasonable regime would be to commence the patient on 100 mg twice daily, increasing by 100 mg every two to three days until the paroxysms of pain are controlled. Caution is required in elderly patients as they may be very susceptible to the side-effects. A pain diary is useful to monitor the effects of the drug.

Q2 What warnings and information would you give to the patient?

The patient should be warned about the following possible side-effects: tiredness; dizziness; ataxia; double vision; and inability to concentrate—patients report that they feel 'spaced out' or like a 'zombie'.

They should be instructed:

- not to drive whilst experiencing the side-effects listed;
- to be cautious when drinking alcohol;
- to contact the hospital or medical practitioner if a rash develops.

The patient should be told that the drug is an anticonvulsant and not a conventional analgesic. It should, therefore, be taken regularly, not 'on demand' like other analgesics and, preferably, 30 minutes before a meal. The patient should be told that they need to be reviewed regularly, that the dose of anticonvulsant may need to be increased, and that blood tests will be required. Pain relief should occur, for the majority of patients, within 24 hours, although the full therapeutic benefit may not be attained for 2–3 weeks.

Q3 What investigations do you need to carry out before starting on this drug?

The patient should have blood taken so that some baseline indicators can be obtained (full blood count, liver function tests, and electrolytes; see text).

Q4 If your patient had presented taking warfarin, would you envisage any management problems?

Carbamazepine is a hepatic microsomal enzyme inducer. Therefore, if taken concurrently with any other drug that is metabolized by the liver, a pharmacokinetic drug interaction will occur. In this case warfarin will be metabolized more quickly and, consequently, the serum warfarin levels will fall. This will invariably reduce the efficacy of warfarin and the patient's prothrombin time will be altered—the international normalized ratio (INR) will drop. This could increase a patient's susceptibility to thromboembolic sequelae. The dose of warfarin will, therefore, probably need to be increased and monitored whilst the patient is taking carbamazepine and for a short time after cessation of the anticonvulsant. Patients on warfarin carry a warning card and this will give information about their dose, INR, and a contact number for their anticoagulation clinic. This clinic will adjust the patient's warfarin dose if necessary.

Case 15.2

Q1 How would you manage this situation?

The patient is exhibiting symptoms of a lower motor neurone palsy. You need to check that the signs are unilateral and that the patient has not recently been experiencing facial weakness or symptoms of a neurological deficit, such as paraesthesia. The left-sided facial musculature should be checked for function to ensure that this is a lower motor neurone problem and that the patient is not suffering from an upper motor neurone lesion such as a cerebrovascular accident; although this would be unlikely in this particular case. The most likely diagnosis is a transient facial nerve palsy resulting from the deposition of local anaesthetic around the seventh cranial nerve (usually into or near the parotid gland). Facial nerve paralysis is evident within minutes of the injection and the duration of facial weakness is usually less than 12 hours. If a longer-acting local anaesthetic solution such as bupivacaine has been used then resolution will be delayed. It is, however, unlikely that bupivacaine would be routinely used for restorative procedures.

The following actions are advised.

- Reassure the patient; explain that it is an uncommon but well recognized complication of the anaesthetic technique that was used.

- Use an eye patch over the affected eye to prevent corneal damage (the patient should be wearing protective glasses during the treatment).

- Assess the general condition of the patient and continue treatment if she is happy to do so. If the patient appears distressed, the tooth should be temporized (further preparation may be required for this) to ensure that the patient will not experience any postoperative discomfort or pain from the molar tooth.

- Review next day to ensure that the paralysis has resolved. A telephone call, if possible, later that day is good practice.

- Write the details of the incident clearly in the case notes stating what information was given to the patient and the details for patient follow up.

Projects

1. Describe how you would assess the function of the cranial nerves.

2. Describe the intracranial course of the trigeminal and facial nerves.

3. What information is available for patients with trigeminal neuralgia: (a) in the form of leaflets; (b) on the internet?

4. Acute sinusitis can be mistaken for pain of dental origin; what is the evidence for the efficacy of antimicrobial therapy in this condition?

16

Temporomandibular disorders

Investigation of the stomatognathic system
- History
- Examination
- Imaging
- Arthroscopy

Temporomandibular pain dysfunction syndrome (TMPDS)
- Management

Internal derangement
- Disc displacement with reduction
- Disc displacement without reduction

Rheumatoid arthritis

Osteoarthrosis (osteoarthritis)

Masseteric hypertrophy

Tumours

site, and radiation of any pain. Exacerbating, relieving, and associated factors should also be identified. In disorders of the TMJ the following four features are very important in helping the clinician arrive at a diagnosis.

1. *Pain history.* Pain may originate primarily within the TMJ or from the muscles of mastication—both arthralgic and myogenic pain may be present. Pain may be felt as a dull ache over the area of the joint, the ear, over the temporal fossa, or over the maxilla. The pain may be bilateral or unilateral and is usually described as being constant, but with acute exacerbations. It is during these acute exacerbations that the radiation of the pain from the joint often occurs. In some instances associated pain in the neck, upper arm, occipital area, or along the lingual nerve may be reported. The severe attacks of pain occur predominantly in the early morning in some patients, whereas in other patients they are more common at the end of the day. Acute episodes may also be precipitated after a meal, at the wide opening of the mouth, or during the night when lying heavily on one side of the face.

   Muscular pain associated with temporomandibular pain may cause a headache. It is possible that some practitioners may confuse the diagnosis with migraine. Similarly, pain arising within the joints themselves may be attributed to earache. Many patients found to have painful joints will have had an ear examination with negative results

2. *Joint sounds.* The patient most commonly complains of a click. This click represents the movement of one component of the joint over the others, and can mean that the disc is slipping out of place, sticking, or malfunctioning. Joint sounds are quite common and are not always significant. The presence of a click does not, on its own, indicate that treatment is required. Clicks may be quite loud and readily audible, and this may cause social embarrassment when eating. In other cases, however, a stethoscope is required to hear the sound. Although an acute episode of pain and clicking may be precipitated by movement of the TMJ, patients may find that pain is associated with periods in which clicking is minimal. There may be a click on both opening and closing—this is referred to as a reciprocal click. Apart from the single loud click, other sounds may be heard in the joint on stethoscopic examination (auscultation). Crepitus (a grating or gravel-like sound) is most commonly heard in osteoarthrosis. Care must be taken in the use of the stethoscope to eliminate the crackling sound produced by laying the bell of the instrument over hair. The resulting crackling sound can easily be mistaken for joint crepitation.

3. *Restriction of opening.* The patient may report difficulty on wide opening, often associated with the imminent onset of a loud click. In other instances the difficulty may be in applying pressure on closing the mouth. The inability to open the mouth wide, due to reflex muscular spasm (contraction) of the masticatory muscles, is called trismus and is usually a temporary rather than permanent condition. Patients with TMJ problems often complain that their jaw locks. This may mean that the jaw cannot open normally. It sticks or 'locks' and this restricts opening. This is thought to be due to the disc being 'squashed and bunched up' anteriorly, preventing further opening. This is usually termed a 'closed lock' situation and is mainly due to anterior disc displacement without reduction and may follow disc laxity and stretching or possibly tearing or perforation in the posterior bilaminar zone area of the disc. Alternatively, the term 'locking' refers to the mandible temporarily becoming 'stuck' in an open position—the patient is not able to close or open the jaw further. This complaint is not the same as dislocation. Dislocation refers to the displacement of the head of the condyle out of the glenoid fossa to a position anterior to the articular eminence.

   - Trismus is the inability to open the mouth wide due to reflex muscular spasm (contraction) of the masticatory muscles and is usually a temporary rather than permanent condition.
   - Dislocation of the TMJ refers to the displacement of the head of the condyle out of the glenoid fossa to a position anterior to the articular eminence.

4. *Swelling.* Patients with TMJ disturbances occasionally complain of swelling over the maxilla, but there is no clear reason for this. A slight degree of soft-tissue swelling may be occasionally noted on examination. In a few other instances patients may complain of tenderness and swelling in the area of the parotid, presumably an effect brought about by the close proximity of part of this gland to the TMJ. In these cases it may be a matter of some difficulty to distinguish between parotid involvement in joint disturbance or joint involvement in a parotid pathology.

Thorough dental, medical, and social histories are required. Any history of trauma to the TMJ should be explored and the outcomes of any previous treatments, if any, should be ascertained. It is also important to identify if the patient suffers from other pain syndromes, and if they have high levels of emotional stress. (Chapter 17 describes the assessment of psychological factors in some detail.)

Examination

The clinician should have a sound knowledge of the functional anatomy of the TMJ and associated structures prior to undertaking an examination of the patient. Examination of the TMJ and masticatory muscles should begin by observing the degree of symmetry of the mandible and face, and by observing the path of excursion of the mandible on opening and closing. It is helpful to focus on a specific landmark (such as the mesial incisal edge of a mandibular central incisor) whilst asking the patient to open and close their mouth—in this way any lateral deviation will be noted. The amount of mandibular opening should be recorded. An inter-incisal opening of approximately 35–45 mm is within the normal range. Loud joint sounds may be heard during mandibular function. In order to examine the joint by palpation the examiner should be in front of the patient so that movement of the mandible may be related to those palpated in the condylar heads. A single finger is placed over each condylar head while the mandibular movements are carried out. Abnormal tenderness associated with the lateral aspect of the joints is detected by light pressure over the condyle and the immediate pre-auricular region. Examination of the posterior joint can be undertaken by intra-auricular (intra-meatal) palpation—the little fingers are positioned in the external auditory meatus followed by the gentle application of forward pressure. Faint joint sounds may be heard by using a stethoscope placed over the condyle head while mandibular movements are performed.

> The clinician should record the amount of mandibular opening. An inter-incisal opening of approximately 35–45 mm is within the normal range.

Muscular tenderness associated with joint disturbance may be detected by palpation of the masseter and temporalis muscles. The reader must be cognizant of the origin and insertions of the masticatory muscles. Clinical examination of the masseters is carried out by asking the patient to clench the teeth firmly together and palpating a muscle manually. When the masseters are contracted, the examining finger is run up the anterior muscle border intraorally, counterpressure being exerted from the external surface. When the examining finger reaches the zygomatic origin of the masseter, tenderness becomes evident and is shown by the patient's reaction. A similar test should be carried out on the opposite side. The temporal origin of the temporalis can be assessed extraorally when the patient is clenching, but the insertion of the tendon is felt intraorally by running the little finger up the anterior border of the mandibular ascending ramus. It is not practical to directly palpate the medial and lateral pterygoid muscles. The lateral pterygoid muscles can, however, be assessed by applying lateral pressure to the mandible and asking the patient to resist the force applied. Spasm of this muscle will elicit pain or tenderness in the pre-auricular region.

> Muscular tenderness associated with joint disturbance may be detected by palpation of the masseter and temporalis muscles.

Dentition

Following the examination of the TMJ and associated muscles, a careful dental examination should be undertaken. The clinician should identify and treat orodental pathology that may be a source of pain. The occlusal relationship of the teeth, both static and dynamic, is recorded. Centric occlusion (CO) and centric relation (CR) should be identified and their relationship noted. In the majority of patients these positions are not coincident. There should be a small (1 mm) anterior slide from CR to CO. Large slides should be noted, particularly if the slide is in a lateral direction. Occlusal interferences should be identified during mandibular excursions and the presence of faceting, fractured restorations, and tooth wear noted. Soft-tissue evidence suggestive of bruxism is ridging of the buccal mucosa and lateral borders of the tongue. Study casts should be taken as a baseline record.

Features suggestive of bruxism

- Tooth-wear facets that match in mandibular border (para-functional) movements
- Crenated (pie-crust) lateral border of the tongue
- Ridging of the buccal mucosa
- Masseteric hypertrophy
- History of repeated fracture of restorations

Imaging

The complex anatomy of the TMJ has led to the development of many radiographic views. The main value of plain film radiography is to identify gross anatomical or functional changes that would indicate an underlying organic cause. Early bone pathology is not usually detected and erosions must be quite advanced to be seen on plain films. A standard panoramic radiograph may be helpful to exclude dental disease but this is not a good view for showing the articular surfaces of the TMJ. An 'open mouth' dental pantomograph will show the condylar necks and lateral view of the condylar heads (Fig. 16.1). The relation of the condyle heads to the disc and fossae are not, however, well displayed. Transpharyngeal views also give the bony outline of the condyle and the lateral aspect of the articular surface. Transcranial views, with the mouth open and closed, demonstrate condylar anatomy and the range of movement in the joint, including the size of the joint space (Fig. 16.2).

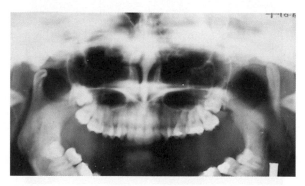

Fig. 16.1 Panoramic view with mouth open showing condyle heads and necks.

Left side

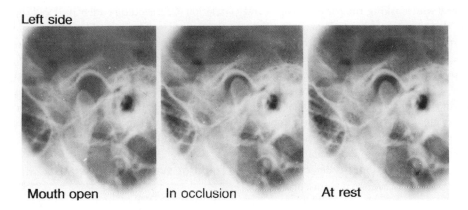

Mouth open   In occlusion   At rest

Fig. 16.2 Transcranial views of temporomandibular joint with mouth open, teeth in occlusion, and at rest.

Computerized tomography (CT) is useful for imaging the hard-tissue detail. Magnetic resonance imaging (MRI) visualizes both soft-tissue detail and bony outline (Fig. 16.3) as well as being useful in determining the position, function, and form of the disc when the mouth is open and closed. This is required in the preoperative assessment prior to disc surgery.

Arthrography involves the injection of a radio-opaque contrast agent into the joint space (usually the lower one) to delineate articular surfaces and the disc. This technique remains the only truly dynamic study of the joint and the most sensitive examination for identifying disc perforations. Arthrography is indicated in chronic temporomandibular pain dysfunction syndrome that has not responded to initial treatment modalities and also for persistent locking and limited mouth opening of unknown aetiology. The technique is not, however, always well tolerated by patients and carries a relatively high radiation dose. It has now largely been replaced by MRI.

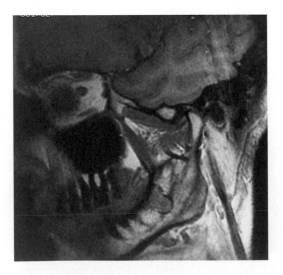

Fig. 16.3 Sagital magnetic resonance scan showing dento-alveolar complex, including the temporomandibular joint.

- An 'open mouth' dental pantomograph will show the condylar necks and lateral view of the condylar heads, but the relation of the condyle heads to the disc and fossae are not well displayed.
- Transpharyngeal views give the bony outline of the condyle and the lateral aspect of the articular surface.
- Transcranial views, with the mouth open and closed, demonstrate condylar anatomy and the range of movement in the joint, including the size of the joint space.

Arthroscopy

Mini-arthroscopy may be an investigative or therapeutic procedure. This minimally invasive technique allows for the direct examination of the upper joint space. Lower joint space arthroscopy is not usually performed due to the small size of the space between the disc and the condylar head in comparison to the size of the instruments used for mini-arthroscopy. Lysis of the upper joint space, lavage, capsular distension, removal of intraarticular adhesions and loose bodies, disc release, and the placement of corticosteroid preparations may be performed with arthroscopical surgery. On rare occasions more extensive intraarticular surgery may be undertaken, such as biopsy and disc repositioning. TMJ arthrocentesis maybe carried out as an isolated procedure, to provide articular lysis and lavage, but without the necessity of using expensive arthroscopical equipment.

Temporomandibular pain dysfunction syndrome (TMPDS)

There are many synonyms used to describe this condition—myofacial pain dysfunction, facial arthromyalgia, facial pain dysfunction, masticatory muscle disorder. The term temporomandibular pain dysfunction syndrome (TMPDS) will be used in this text. This condition is the most prevalent disorder of the TMJ and affects predominantly female patients. Epidemiological data suggests that 40–80 per cent of patients with disorders of the TMJ are female. In TMPDS the predominant complaint is of pain, which may take any of the forms previously described. This pain may be associated with limitation of opening or with joint sounds, also as previously outlined. The patients quite often admit to a history of psychological stress, although overt psychiatric abnormality is unusual.

There may be a history of previous joint clicking, limitation of opening, trauma, or recurrent dislocation. Questioning may elicit the presence of a habit that alters mandibular positioning or action. Some patients may hold the mandible in a particular position, usually a protrusion or lateral position, when engaged in some mental activity. There may be a history of biting on some foreign body, such as a pen or pencil. The patient may be aware of grinding their teeth, but a history of bruxism is often supplied by some other member of the patient's family or a partner. Examination may reveal one or several of the following: limitation of opening of the mouth; deviation of the mandible on opening; clicking heard or felt in the joint; gross malocclusion leading to abnormal joint movements, or minor degrees of malocclusion with abnormal cuspal guidance of closure; gross occlusal attrition; occlusal interferences; unsatisfactory dentures; tenderness of the muscles of mastication.

Signs and symptoms associated with TMPDS

- Pre-auricular pain that may radiate to other sites
- Tenderness of the joint on palpation
- Limited jaw movement or deviation of mandible on opening and closing
- Tenderness of masticatory muscles on palpation
- Joint sounds (clicks, crepitus)
- Headache

Clinically, there is tenderness or pain of the TMJ and muscles of mastication—this may be bi- or unilateral. Limitation of mandibular opening and joint sounds are often present. In most patients with chronic symptoms, radiographs of the joints reveal no abnormality of structure, although limitation or increase in joint movement may be seen.

The aetiology of TMPDS is unclear. Many theories have been postulated, including skeletal jaw relationships, occlusal disharmonies, lack of posterior teeth, and unilateral tooth loss, but there is no clear evidence to support these. Interestingly, relatively few patients with complete dentures appear to present with TMPDS. Parafunctional clenching and grinding and abnormal posturing of the jaw have been implicated as initiating or perpetuating factors in some patients—it is hypothesized that repetitious adverse loading causes microtrauma of the masticatory system. Psychosocial factors such as anxiety and depression may predispose certain patients to temporomandibular disorders and

may also serve to perpetuate the symptoms. In some patients there is a history of trauma. Both yawning and dental treatment have also been implicated. Care must be taken in differentiating the pain due to temporomandibular disturbances from that arising from dental causes or from facial pain of the types described in Chapters 15 and 17. In particular, the differential diagnosis between facial pain of psychogenic origin and that caused by chronic temporomandibular dysfunction in patients undergoing emotional stress is difficult. In fact, the two conditions occasionally seem to merge in a patient with physical signs of TMJ dysfunction, but with the demonstrative, anxious, obsessive outlook typical of the patient converting hidden anxieties into facial pain symptoms. Some patients with TMPDS have a history of general pain disorders. Needless to say, in such cases, the initial presumptive diagnosis should be of joint dysfunction. Only when all physical signs of TMPDS have been addressed by treatment, should the diagnosis of psychogenic pain be more firmly entertained. It is in observing the reaction to treatment that the differential diagnosis is perhaps best made. Irrespective of the aetiology of chronic temporomandibular pain, the psychological response to pain cannot be ignored in the management of this condition—Chapter 17 explores this further.

Disc displacement has been implicated as being important in the aetiology of TMPDS. However, abnormalities in the location of the disc have been noted in many patients with and without TMPDS.

Management

A full discussion of the management of temporomandibular disorders is outside the scope of this book and this is only a brief overview. In view of the fact that the aetiology is poorly understood, it is not surprising that the management of this condition is contentious. The range of management options used for TMPDS is listed in Table 16.1. Many patients with TMPDS are successfully managed in practice by offering an explanation for the symptoms and reassurance, together with occlusal appliances if indicated. Initial management should always be conservative, and preferably it should be non-invasive and reversible. These requirements are important for the management of TMJ disorders because a successful outcome cannot be ensured. The value of reassurance and counselling cannot be underestimated. Patients should be told about the nature and prognosis of this condition. An information leaflet is helpful to reinforce this. A minority of patients will be worried that they have a serious, even life-threatening, condition and information can allay such fears. There may also be a strong placebo response to the different treatment modalities advocated for TMPDS.

The successful management of TMPDS cannot be guaranteed. Therefore the initial treatment of TMPDS should be:
- non-invasive
- reversible

Many patients respond to reassurance (± a removable occlusal appliance)

Table 16.1 Spectrum of management strategies for temporomandibular disorders

Initial (conservative) management	Further (specialist) management
Reassurance	Psychological intervention
Education	Occlusal adjustment
Habit management (e.g. jaw exercises, awareness of daytime jaw clenching)	Occlusal rehabilitation (e.g. restorative, orthodontic, orthognathic surgery)
Modification of function (e.g. chewing, yawning, singing)	Antidepressants Psychotherapy
Rest	Intraarticular steroids
Anti-inflammatory agents and analgesics (local and systemic)	Manipulation under general anaesthesia
Muscle relaxants (e.g. diazepam)	Surgery (e.g. arthrocentesis, arthroscopy, or open articular surgery at arthrotomy)
Occlusal splints (removable)	Psychiatric liaison clinic/pain clinic
Physiotherapy	

The use of occlusal appliances, or splints as they are commonly called, is frequently helpful for some patients, and studies have demonstrated that there is a significant placebo effect. Occlusal appliances should be removable and give full occlusal coverage. There is no place for the routine use of splints that only give partial occlusal coverage—such splints may cause unwanted tooth movement. Table 16.2 highlights some important points concerning the provision of occlusal appliances, whilst Table 16.3 gives details of the three splints most commonly used for TMJ disorders.

Jaw exercises and various forms of physiotherapy may all play a part in treatment. Exercises to correct faulty patterns of activity—such as deviation on opening and closure—may be helpful. Therapy with analgesic or relaxant drugs may have a limited use,

Table 16.2 Points to remember when providing removable occlusal appliances in the management of temporomandibular disorders

Prior to construction of occlusal splints:
Undertake a pretreatment analysis of the stomatognathic system
Make comprehensive written records
Archive study models with an occlusal record prior to splint therapy
All occlusal appliances:
have a placebo effect
alter occlusal contacts
decrease occlusal forces transmitted to teeth
Do *not* use partial coverage splints (risk of uncontrolled tooth movement)
Reinforce the need for good oral and appliance hygiene

but only over a restricted period of time. Nonsteroidal anti-inflammatory drugs (NSAIDs) are the analgesics of choice, provided that there are no contraindications to their use. The use of benzodiazepines for their muscle relaxant properties may be helpful in acute cases where there is trismus. In addition, their hypnotic action can be beneficial in ensuring sleep. It is imperative that only short courses of benzodiazepines are used, ideally 2 weeks or less, because of the potential risk of dependence. Benzodiazepines are, therefore, only of value during the acute phase of TMPDS.

There is no evidence that permanent occlusal rehabilitation is of value for TMJ disorders and such treatment should only be undertaken with specialist advice. In a small number of cases orthodontic treatment or a combined approach using orthognathic surgery is indicated. Most maxillofacial surgeons would only perform orthognathic surgery for a patient with a temporomandibular disorder if, in addition to the articular signs and symptoms, the patient was having problems from the malocclusion and underlying skeletal relationships due to inadequate function or for aesthetic reasons. In a few cases of chronic TMJ disorders, antidepressant drugs, with or without psychotherapy, may help. TMJ surgery should be reserved for patients with a clearly identifiable joint abnormality, such as a displaced or damaged disc. There are other prerequisites for surgery. As a general rule the condition tends to be self-limiting and is not thought to progress to a degenerative joint condition in the majority of cases. TMJ surgery should not be carried out until the following criteria have been met.

1. A mechanical intraarticular joint problem should have been proven by the use of specialized imaging, such as MRI.

2. All exhaustive nonsurgical reversible treatment measures have failed to control the presenting signs and symptoms.

3. The patients' symptoms deleteriously affect their day to day activity to the extent that they have a poor quality of life.

Chronic TMPDS that is resistant to conservative management may require the modalities used to treat chronic pain of psychogenic origin.

Internal derangement

Internal derangement is a common disorder and is due to the permanent displacement of the articular disc, which has an abnormal relationship to both the glenoid fossa and articular eminence.

Internal derangement is a common disorder and is due to an abnormal relationship of the disc to the condyle, glenoid fossa, and articular eminence. This condition is different from TMPDS because the articular disc is permanently, not intermittently displaced, as in TMPDS. The click in true articular derangement is continuous—not intermittent. Pain is not always a feature, espe-

Table 16.3 Characteristics of commonly used occlusal appliances in disorders of the TMJ

Soft vacuum-formed splints

Useful mainly for muscular (myofacial) signs and symptoms

Soft full coverage splints, better tolerated in the lower arch

Quick to make—impression required of only one arch

Do not conform to a specific occlusal prescription, but can be made in different thicknesses

Not amenable to occlusal adjustment

Worn at night time

Good for acute TMPDS; can make bruxism worse in some patients

Last approximately 6 months

Stabilization splint

Hard acrylic, full coverage splint

Technically demanding and time-consuming to make. Requires impressions of both arches and a record of centric relation. A face bow is required in difficult occlusal cases.

Maxillary or mandibular appliance but maxillary is often easier to adjust

Worn at night time, for long-term use

Designed to provide an ideal occlusion at rest and in function (i.e. centric occlusion—maximum simultaneous occlusal contacts—ideally this should equate to centric relation. There should be incisal and canine guidance with no posterior interferences)

Anterior repositioning splint

Mandibular or maxillary hard acrylic, full occlusal coverage

Require impressions of both arches and an occlusal record with the mandible protruded

Indicated for disc displacement with reduction (i.e. click disappears when patient is asked to open and close from a protrusive mandibular position)

For functional use, as much as possible; ideally worn 24 h/day for about 12 weeks

Avoid in adolescents to prevent it acting as a functional orthodontic appliance

Objective is to allow the disc to reposition

---

cially in the early stages of this condition. Disc displacement may be divided into two presentations—each has a different treatment modality.

Disc displacement with reduction

- Reproducible reciprocal clicking
- Disc displacement shown by imaging and absence of degenerative bone disease

In addition, there may be pain, deviation of jaw movements, no limitation of opening.

Disc displacement without reduction

- Persistent limitation of mouth opening (≤ 35 mm) with history of sudden onset
- Disc displacement shown by imaging and absence of degenerative bone disease

In addition there may be pain and clicking.

Disc displacement with reduction

In this condition the disc is displaced during opening and closing. During function the malaligned disc 'reduces' or improves its structural relationship with the condylar head. In disc displacement with reduction there is a reciprocal click, noted during opening and closing, that is not always painful, and jaw deviation on opening and closing is common. The reciprocal click is usually eliminated when the patient opens and closes from a protruded mandibular position, often with the incisors in an edge to edge position confirming the presence of anterior disc displacement with reduction. This condition does not always merit treatment, especially if the only presenting problem is that of a clicking joint. The management of this condition may range from counselling to the provision of a stabilization splint and physiotherapy. Muscle relaxants are occasionally used and, in a minority of cases, surgery may be considered. The condition may deteriorate with the disc becoming progressively more displaced and possibly interfering with opening of the mandible, leading to disc displacement without reduction and a closed lock situation.

Disc displacement without reduction

In this condition the disc is displaced during opening and closing. The malaligned disc does not improve its structural relationship with the condylar head during function—the disc is permanently displaced, usually in an anterior or anteromedial direction. There is a history of the jaw locking, because the misaligned disc mechanically obstructs the condyle during jaw opening. There is usually no evidence of any articular clicking of a reciprocal nature, although a previous history of such clicking—followed by locking—may be given. The disc displacement may, on occasion, be reduced from a protruded mandibular position, although this is not always the case. The implication is that the protruded mandible has placed the condyle in a position where it is in a normal functional relationship with the disc—as opposed to compressing the posterior part of the disc (bilaminar zone). In other cases, the closed lock is not reducible with anterior mandibular repositioning (protrusion) and, consequently, the disc displacement is permanent. Counselling, physiotherapy, and muscle relaxants can be of value in these cases and an anterior repositioning splint may also be indicated. Surgery may be suitable for a minority of patients.

> Disc displacement can sometimes be reduced from a protruded mandibular position.

Rheumatoid arthritis

Rheumatoid arthritis is a common multisystem, autoimmune, inflammatory disease. It is now accepted that the TMJ is involved to some extent in a large proportion of patients with generalized rheumatoid disease. It is, however, unusual for the patient to present, undiagnosed, with primary symptoms for the TMJ. When patients with rheumatoid arthritis do seek treatment for TMJ problems the major complaint is of limitation of opening and crepitus, stiffness, and pain followed by aching. Significant pain as a symptom is rare. Crepitus is the most common clinical sign on examination—joint tenderness and functional abnormalities may also be seen. Symptoms are usually bilateral. Radiographic evidence of changes has been found in a high proportion of these patients, manifesting as erosions, proliferations, and flattening of the condylar head. As in other joints, the disease process may occur in a phasic manner, acute exacerbations being followed by either a healing phase or a secondary chronic phase. Ankylosis of the TMJ can occur. Rarely, it is possible for the patient to develop an anterior open bite deformity caused by destruction of the condyles and the loss of condylar and posterior and occlusal face height.

Immunological tests for rheumatoid arthritis were outlined in Chapter 2. A raised erythrocyte sedimentation rate (ESR) and hypergammaglobulinaemia are usually present, together with an elevated titre of rheumatoid factor and antinuclear and other antibodies. These tests may prove positive before systemic changes have been noticed. It is also worth remembering that a significant proportion of patients with rheumatoid arthritis have Sjögren's syndrome. These individuals may develop salivary gland pathology that presents as facial pain. Sjögren's syndrome is described in full in Chapter 8.

Nonsteroidal anti-inflammatory analgesics are the mainstay of treatment for rheumatoid arthritis. However, more severe cases are treated by disease-modifying drugs such as methotrexate or azathioprine. Surgery of the TMJ may be indicated for ankylosis and cases of severe condylar destruction. In some patients prosthetic joint replacement or autogenous (costochondral) grafting may be required to decrease pain, improve appearance, or restore function.

Osteoarthrosis (osteoarthritis)

Changes may take place in the TMJ as part of a generalized, degenerative arthritic condition. Osteoarthrosis is a metabolic defect of articular cartilage and is usually asymptomatic in the TMJs and is seen as a chance finding on radiographs. Radiographic changes may not always be evident but, when present, they are variable and include a reduction in joint space and erosions of the articulating surfaces of the condyle and of the fossa. Osteophytes may occasionally be seen at the anterior edge of the condyle.

Most patients with osteoarthrosis are female and over the age of 50 years. Pain is rare and the history is usually of joint sounds and gradually increasing stiffness. The joint may be tender to pressure and crepitations are often heard and felt when the joint is moved. Movement may also be restricted. When pain is present it tends to be localized to the pre-auricular region—in contrast to the myofacial pain distribution of TMPDS. The rheumatoid factor is negative and the ESR normal in these patients. Symptomatic anti-inflammatory analgesics are usually effective for osteoarthrosis and muscle relaxants are occasionally indicated. Surgery is rarely appropriate.

Masseteric hypertrophy

Unilateral enlargement of the muscles of mastication, and of the masseter in particular, occasionally occurs as a response to serious derangement of the occlusion leading to unilateral mastication. It may also, however, occur with little or no occlusal disharmony and, in fact, may be bilateral rather than unilateral. In the affected patients the complaint is usually only of increasing facial asymmetry. On examination the masseter (or masseters) is found to be enlarged as a whole, often with a marked increase overlying the mandibular insertion. When the masseter is defined for examination by asking the patient to clench the teeth, the muscle is easily palpated, the lower part often standing out and resembling a soft-tissue mass. Plain radiography (posterior–anterior mandible) or a dental panoramic view may show a marked concavity at the insertion of the masseter, at the periphery of which there is lipping of the bone. If electromyographic facilities are available, it is may be possible to demonstrate atypical muscle activity in all the muscles of mastication. Magnetic resonance imaging is useful in defining normal anatomy and hypertrophy of the muscle and in identifying any other pathology (Fig. 16.4).

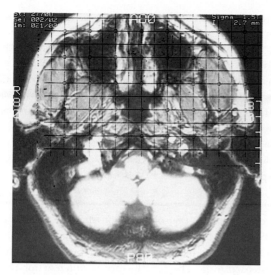

Fig. 16.4 Axial magnetic resonance scan showing pterygoid and masseter muscles.

Management of masseteric hypertrophy with injection of botulinum toxin has been reported, but there is no convincing evidence of its long-term benefit.

Tumours

Pseudotumours, such as synovial chondromatosis, and true tumours of the TMJ are rare. Osteomas (Fig. 16.5) and chondromas form the majority of these and are benign and restrict mandibular opening. They may also result in occlusal problems with occasional skeletal and jaw deformities. Malignant osteosarcomas are exceptionally rare in the TMJ, although malignant tumours of nearby structures, such as the parotid gland, may involve the TMJ area by secondary invasion.

Discussion of problem cases

Case 16.1 Discussion

Q1   What are the likely causes for this patient's trismus?

Trismus is the reduced ability to open the mandible due to reflex muscular spasm (contraction) of the masticatory muscles. The

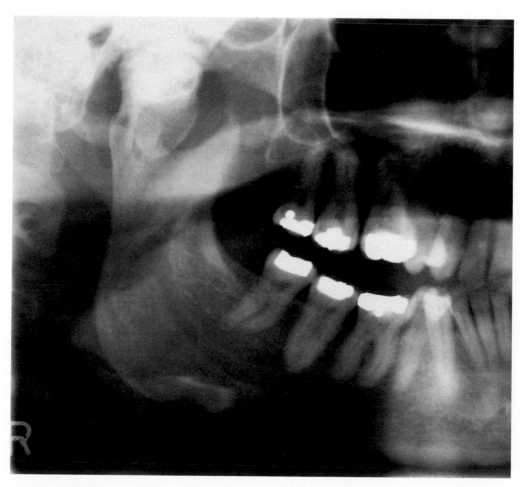

Fig. 16.5 An osteoma of the neck of the condyle.

term is, however, often used more broadly to refer to an inability to open the mouth fully, for example, due to ankylosis of the TMJ following trauma or fibrosis of the masticatory muscles following exposure to external beam therapeutic radiation.

The most likely cause of this 20 year old's recent history of pain and trismus is a dental infection. At her age this may be associated with an impacted mandibular third molar due to pericoronitis. Questioning the patient about her dental history will be helpful. If the condition is pericoronitis, it is possible that the patient is aware that she has an erupting tooth and may have experienced similar symptoms in the past. A radiograph is essential to confirm the position of a partially erupted tooth. The patient may have had an inferior dental nerve block for recent treatment and this occasionally results in damage to the muscles due to inflammation or haematoma formation.

Q2   List the possible aetiologies for acute and chronic limitation of mouth opening.

The most common causes of trismus are infection (for example, pericoronitis, sialadenitis), acute TMPDS, and trauma. The trauma may be iatrogenic (following removal of mandibular third molars or inferior dental nerve blocks) or a result of violence or an accident (facial and condylar fractures, damage to the muscles of mastication). The causes of trismus are listed in Table 16.4.

Case 16.2 Discussion

Q1   What conditions may be responsible for this patient's pain and what could you do, in the first instance, to help you reach a definitive diagnosis?

Table 16.4 Causes of trismus

Extra-articular	Intra-articular
• Infection/inflammation in related structures (e.g. pericoronitis, sialadenitis)	• Infective arthritis
	• Osteoarthrosis
	• Rheumatoid arthritis
• Haematoma, inflammation, or infection following mandibular fracture block injections	• Ankylosis of TMJ
	• Intra-capsular condylar frac-
	• Dislocation
• Trauma (post-operative oedema, facial trauma)	
• TMPDS	
• Tetany	
• Tetanus	
• Fibrosis due to burns or radiation	
• Systemic sclerosis and submucous fibrosis	
• Neoplasm	

Table 16.5 Causes of pain in or adjacent to the temporomandibular joints

• TMPDS	• Iatrogenic—inflammation following mandibular block injection or removal of mandibular third molars
• Internal derangement (disc displacement)	
• Arthritis	• Salivary gland disease (e.g. mumps, autoimmune sialadenitis, malignancies)
• Osteoarthrosis	
• Odontogenic infection	
• Trauma—fractures	• Giant cell arteritis (ischaemic pain)
• Atypical facial pain	• Malignancies
	• Ear problems

This edentulous 70-year-old patient may be suffering from TMPDS, despite the fact that it is less common in edentulous and elderly patients. An older patient with crepitus may be suffering from osteoarthrosis. The pain history is different for these two conditions. A plain film of the TMJs, such as an open jaw dental pantomograph may show irregularities of the condylar surface such as erosions or osteophytes in osteoarthrosis.

This patient has two problems, pain and overclosure with his dentures—these may or may not be related. In the first instance, one of the dentures could be fitted with a soft occlusal splint and the patient reviewed over a 6-week period to see if the pain has reduced. The splint will increase the occlusal vertical dimension and this may be beneficial in reducing the pain. This is a reversible procedure and a helpful one prior to constructing new dentures for this patient. NSAIDs may be prescribed (providing there are no contraindications). If symptoms do not resolve after the construction of new dentures, physiotherapy may be considered. This patient may need referral to a specialist clinic if a radiographic assessment has not been undertaken or if the pain fails to respond to the management outlined above.

Q2   There are several causes of pain that may present in or adjacent to the temporomandibular joints. Make a list of the possible differential diagnoses.

Table 16.5 lists causes of pain in or adjacent to the temporomandibular joints.

Projects

1. Describe the features of the different anatomical zones of the articular disc and list the origin and insertion of all the muscles of mastication. Explain with the aid of diagrams the differences between disc displacement with reduction and disc displacement without reduction.

2. What are the surgical treatments available for TMPDS?

3. What role does the physiotherapist play in the management of TMPDS?

17

Psychogenic orofacial problems

Chronic orofacial pain
- Atypical facial pain
- Atypical odontalgia
- Oral dysaesthesia (Burning mouth syndrome)
- Management of chronic orofacial pain

Disturbances in taste and salivation

Delusional symptoms

Dysmorphophobia

Self injurious behaviour

Eating disorders

Drugs and alcohol

Psychogenic orofacial problems

Problem cases

Case 17.1

A 55-year-old female patient presents with a 3-month history of a 'burning and tingling sensation on the tip of the tongue'. The patient relates the onset of symptoms to the provision of new replacement complete dentures.

Q1 How would you investigate this lady's symptoms and what are the possible causes?

Case 17.2

A new patient presents to your practice and gives a 3-year history of toothache. On examination the patient has a heavily restored dentition.

Q1 Discuss how you might differentiate between pain of dental origin and atypical odontalgia in this patient.

Case 17.3

A 60-year-old edentulous female is seen by a colleague in your dental practice. This lady has a 3-month history of facial pain, which is increasing in intensity. The examining dentist thinks that the patient has either atypical facial pain or trigeminal neuralgia. Radiographs do not show any significant abnormality and the dentures are satisfactory. You are asked to give your opinion.

Q1 What information from the pain history and clinical examination would you use to differentiate between these two conditions? (You will also need to read Chapter 15 to answer this question.)

Introduction

A substantial number of orofacial problems may occur as a manifestation of psychosomatic disease. These include atypical facial pain, tension headaches (see Chapter 15), oral dysaesthesia (including burning mouth syndrome), and disturbances in taste and salivation. Psychological symptoms may aggravate or initiate disease. Many conditions that have organic causes can have significant psychosomatic components, such as asthma and migraine. It has been estimated that approximately one-third of all consultations between patients and their medical practitioner are essentially about psychological problems. Diagnosis of a psychosomatic symptom does not necessarily imply that the patient has an underlying psychiatric illness. A transient emotional disorder, such as an anxiety state or stressful life events, can frequently give rise to orofacial symptoms. Patients who are emotionally disturbed may present with physical symptoms and there is an unfortunate tendency to dismiss these as being 'imaginary'. It is important to appreciate that emotional disturbances can have an effect on the hormonal, vascular, and muscular systems, and may produce physical symptoms such as xerostomia or facial pain. The dentist, however, must always be very careful to eliminate any organic cause for patients' symptoms before diagnosing them as being due to an underlying emotional or psychological problem.

> Emotional disturbances (anxiety, depression, and stress) can exacerbate or cause physical symptoms.

It is also important to bear in mind that patients with orofacial pain of psychogenic origin may still develop pain of dental origin. It can be all too easy for a clinician to be less discriminatory in assessing 'new pains'. A thorough pain history and dental examination are always required when the pain history alters. Patients with a history of psychological problems frequently feel that they have been 'labelled' and are prejudged by the medical and dental profession. The clinician needs to keep an 'open mind'. The patient should be able to recognize that his or her complaint is being taken seriously. It is always worth remembering that a patient may have an undiagnosed, life-threatening condition.

Examples of psychosomatic diseases

Oral dysaesthesia	Atypical facial pain
Temporomandibular dysfunction	Tension headaches
Disruptive gagging	Chronic fatigue syndrome
Dry mouth	Panic attacks
Anorexia nervosa	

The busy dental surgery is not the ideal place to elicit a social history and patients may be reluctant to discuss personal problems in such an environment. However, many patients build up a relationship of trust with their dentist, particularly if they have been under his or her care for a while. Taking a social and psychological history is often time-consuming but can be invaluable if it provides an insight into orofacial symptoms with no demonstrable organic cause. A patient may appear to be coping bravely with a condition until questioned about lifestyle and emotional well-being. Table 17.1 suggests several questions that may be useful in assessing how a patient is coping with a chronic condition such as atypical facial pain or burning mouth syndrome. The use of psychometric questionnaires can be helpful. However, many require skillful interpretation. The Hospital Anxiety and Depression (HAD) scale is a relatively straightforward indicator of a patient's anxiety and depression. It can assist the clinician in identifying emotional problems in patients. The scale was devised for use in non-psychiatric hospital departments and can be filled in by the patient over a few minutes, and quickly scored by the clinician.

Patient confidentiality is of the utmost importance and must be maintained in all aspects of clinical dentistry. This point must be stressed to all members of the dental team.

> The successful management of chronic pain conditions requires that psychological issues are addressed.

Terminology can sometimes be confusing to the uninitiated. Somatization is a term used to describe the process whereby an individual's psychological and social distress are manifested as bodily symptoms that cannot be wholly attributed to organic pathology. Somatoform disorders are therefore psychogenic conditions. However, there are strict criteria that should be fulfilled before a diagnosis of somatoform disorder is made.

> Somatization is a term used to describe the process whereby an individual's psychological and social distress are manifested as bodily symptoms that cannot be wholly attributed to organic pathology.

Table 17.1 Useful questions when taking a history of pain with suspected psychogenic origin

How are you sleeping?
Has your appetite been affected by this condition?
Does the complaint stop you enjoying yourself (e.g. socializing with friends)?
How do your family/partner/friends react to your condition?
What do you think (or do you have any idea what) has caused the pain?
Do you do anything to help you cope with your pain /discomfort?
Does anything take your mind off the pain (e.g. exercise, relaxation, drinking alcohol)?

Chronic orofacial pain

Atypical facial pain

Clinical features

This is a relatively common cause of non-odontogenic facial pain, which is encountered particularly in middle-aged women. Atypical facial pain is characterized by a continuous dull ache. If the pain is not continuous, it is present for most of the time. The descriptors of the pain can be variable and are often emotive. The pain frequently affects the maxilla and can be bilateral or unilateral. However, it is not unusual for it to be poorly localized. The pain is not usually provoked by facial movements, and generally fails to respond to simple analgesics. Characteristically, it affects the non-muscular sites of the face and an episode may last for hours or days, although it can be intermittent. The pain is frequently aggravated by fatigue, worry, or emotional upset.

> Atypical facial pain is characterized by a continuous dull ache that can be bilateral or unilateral but frequently affects the maxilla.

Several specialist opinions may have been sought and numerous investigations undertaken prior to the patient presenting to the oral medicine clinic. Typically, patients have been seen by (or already have appointments for) ENT specialists, physicians, maxillofacial surgeons, and neurologists. Many have sought treatment from practitioners of alternative medicine. Table 17.2 summarizes the features of atypical facial pain.

A number of studies have suggested that atypical facial pain is often provoked by some form of dental treatment, such as extractions or restorative procedures, but it may also be initiated or exacerbated by stressful life events such as bereavement, divorce, or illness in the family. The patients frequently complain of pain elsewhere in the body, which may have been diagnosed as irritable bowel syndrome, tension headaches, or dysmenorrhoea

Table 17.2 Features of atypical facial pain

Dull, nagging nature but pain descriptors may not be consistent
Emotive adjectives may be used to describe the pain
Pain intensity may vary
Unilateral or bilateral distribution of pain but location may change with time
Pain is not usually related to anatomical distribution of a nerve
Simple analgesics are usually ineffective
Pain exacerbated by stress and/or dental treatment
History of other chronic pain disorders is common
No obvious underlying organic signs
History of extensive restorative and/or surgical treatment to resolve the pain is common
Frequently patient has been seen by several specialists for this condition

Table 17.3 Chronic medical conditions frequently associated with atypical facial pain

Irritable bowel syndrome
Dyspepsia
Headaches
Dysmenorrhoea
Neck and/or back pain
Fibromyalgia
Chronic fatigue syndrome

(among many other possibilities), so that there is frequently a complex (and perhaps inaccurate) history of chronic ill health. It has been estimated that up to 80 per cent of patients with psychogenic facial pain have other chronic pain conditions (see Table 17.3). There is also considerable overlap of symptoms between atypical facial pain and chronic temporomandibular pain dysfunction. Some authorities believe that the two groups are indistinguishable. It is certainly the case that some patients with atypical facial pain may give a history of intermittent temporomandibular joint (TMJ) dysfunction, and others report symptoms of oral dysaesthesia.

Atypical odontalgia

Atypical odontolagia (idiopathic odontalgia) is a variant in which the pain is localized to one tooth (or a number of teeth) that appears to be clinically and radiologically sound. This situation is very difficult to diagnose. The symptoms can resemble those of pulpitis and periodontitis and repeated replacement restorations fail to resolve the pain. Operative intervention can often aggravate the condition. Classically, the offending tooth is root-filled in an attempt to eliminate pain of pulpal origin. Periradicular surgery may then be carried out. Ultimately, the tooth is extracted. The pain is then frequently transferred to an adjacent tooth or teeth. On occasion, this can result in an aggrieved patient blaming the dentist for taking the wrong tooth out. In the absence of teeth the pain may then persist in the alveolus. Exploratory surgery and ridge-smoothing procedures may be tried before a diagnosis of atypical facial pain is made.

A provisional diagnosis of atypical facial pain can often be made after listening to the patient's history, but it is essential to eliminate all other demonstrable causes of facial pain, particularly those due to dental conditions. Patients who give a history suggestive of sensory disturbance, or have evidence of a cranial nerve deficit, must be referred for specialist evaluation and imaging, to eliminate the possibility of a latent neoplasm or generalized neurological disorder.

> Patients with unexplained sensory deficits of cranial nerves should be referred for further investigation to exclude space-occupying lesions and undiagnosed neurological conditions.

The results of one study have shown that about half the patients presenting with symptoms of atypical facial pain were suffering from an underlying psychiatric disturbance, most commonly a depressive illness or neurosis. Adverse life events are frequently revealed on closer questioning of patients with atypical facial pain, and include marital difficulties and chronic ill health in the family. Chronic anxiety and bouts of depression are also important factors in this type of facial pain. Unfortunately, some patients with atypical facial pain do not readily accept the importance of underlying psychological factors and such individuals are frequently difficult to manage. They often prefer to pursue numerous further investigations or exploratory surgery, which, as mentioned previously, may exacerbate the situation. It is essential not to imply to the patient that there is anything 'imaginary' involved in their pain as this may be met with disbelief and, in some cases, anger. Despite going to great lengths to avoid patients misinterpreting your diagnosis, they are frequently of the opinion that you think their pain or condition is 'all in their mind'. This belief may be so firmly held that the patient will refute your diagnosis and decline your advice. The authors find it helpful, while discussing the situation with the patient, to compare the pain to that of a 'stress-induced' headache, which may occur as a result of cramped muscles or blood vessels. The concept of a parallel with a 'stress headache' is generally well accepted by patients, who are able to appreciate that this is not generally due to any underlying pathology.

> Patients with atypical facial pain often want a physical solution to their condition.

There are several options available to the clinician in the management of facial pain. Counselling and reassurance may be all that is required by some patients, but others may require psychotropic medication, with or without psychotherapy. These options are outlined at the end of this section.

Oral dysaesthesia

Oral dysaesthesia is a term used to denote disturbances of oral sensation. It includes conditions such as burning mouth syndrome, but also encompasses symptoms of abnormal taste (dysguesia) or xerostomia in cases where there are no clinical signs or discernible cause. A number of differing features of oral dysaesthesia may occur in the same patient.

Burning mouth syndrome

Burning mouth syndrome (BMS) (stomatodynia in an older terminology) is a condition in which the patient presents with a complaint of a generalized soreness or burning sensation in the mouth. The tongue is frequently affected (glossopyrosis or glossodynia) but the burning sensation can affect all parts of the oral mucosa and in some instances is localized to a small discrete area. Some patients with these symptoms may have, on examination, some readily recognizable abnormality, such as geographic tongue that is responsible for the symptoms. Others have a completely normal appearance of the oral mucosa and it is this group who are included in the diagnostic category of BMS. A full assessment of these patients is essential to eliminate any identifiable cause, such as systemic disease or clinically undiagnosed oral candidosis. Screening tests should be undertaken routinely to exclude haematinic deficiencies or endocrine problems such as diabetes (see Tables 17.4 and 17.5). A number of patients who complain of a burning mouth also have a dry mouth and should be investigated to eliminate conditions such as Sjögren's syndrome (Chapter 8).

Denture-induced problems should be eliminated as far as possible, but it must be appreciated that some individuals cannot tolerate dentures, however well constructed. A very small proportion of patients with BMS will have had their problem ascribed

Features of burning mouth syndrome

- Predominantly middle-aged females (7 females:1 male)
- Generalized or localized burning of the oral mucosa
- Oral mucosa looks normal

Table 17.4 Burning mouth syndrome: underlying conditions

Diabetes
Haematinic deficiencies—vitamin B_{12}, iron, folate*
Salivary gland hypofunction.
Candidosis
Parafunctional habits (chronic trauma)
Gastro-oesophageal reflux disease (GORD)
Depression
Allergy to restorative or denture materials

* Vitamin B_1, B_2, B_6 deficiencies have also been implicated but there is little scientific evidence to support this association.

Table 17.5 Burning mouth syndrome: investigations

Detailed clinical history
Full clinical examination
Blood tests
Full blood count
Serum B_{12} + folate
Red blood cell folate
Serum ferritin
Blood glucose
Microbiology—quantitative assessment of carriage of oral *Candida**
Assessment of salivary gland function

* Isolation of *Candida* species is not indicative of a candidal infection. Therefore, a routine swab is of limited use if there are no clinical signs. Quantitative assessments are only undertaken in specialist centres.

to an allergy to denture materials, and it may be extremely difficult to dissuade patients from this attractive, but unlikely cause. Allergy to denture materials can occur but is very uncommon. Irritation due to leaching out of excess acrylic monomer has also been reported, but should not occur if the dentures have been processed correctly. In one survey of patients presenting with a burning mouth, the patients were predominantly (but not exclusively) female with a mean age of around 60 years and wearing complete dentures. The majority complained of a burning sensation in the tongue and upper denture-bearing area. The next most common site was the mucosa of the lips and, then, other sites of the oral mucosa. From the results of this survey it would appear that three groups of patients emerged: those with a demonstrable source of local irritation (50 per cent); those with an identifiable systemic abnormality (30 per cent); and those with a psychogenic background (20 per cent). Systemic factors included haematological deficiencies and undiagnosed diabetes, but other female endocrine abnormalities were not prominent.

The result of one study has suggested that single or combined deficiencies of vitamins B_1, B_2, or B_6 may be present in a number of patients with BMS, and that vitamin therapy may benefit such individuals. However, other studies have failed to show any response to these vitamin B supplements. Serum levels of zinc have been investigated in patients with BMS, but there is no convincing evidence that zinc deficiency is involved in the pathogenesis of this condition.

A number of patients diagnosed as suffering from BMS have no identifiable underlying cause for their complaint. These idiopathic cases frequently have an underlying psychogenic cause, such as chronic anxiety or depression. Many have a cancer phobia and know of someone who has suffered from oral cancer. It is therefore helpful to explore the patients' beliefs about their condition. This may involve asking them directly if they think they might have cancer. Some patients with this condition respond well to reassurance, supplemented by an information leaflet about BMS. However, others may require psychiatric intervention, in the form of antidepressant medication with or without psychotherapy (see next section). An overview of management options for BMS is given in Table 17.6.

Management of chronic orofacial pain

The management of chronic orofacial pain is usually undertaken in a hospital environment where the patient can be fully investi-

Table 17.6 Management of burning mouth syndrome

Eliminate
Systemic disease
Local causes (e.g. candidosis)
Counselling
Cognitive behavioural therapy—refer to clinical psychologist for assessment
Antidepressant therapy

gated and the response to medication and psychotherapy monitored. On receipt of referral from a dentist it is often advisable to write to the patient's medical practitioner to enquire if there is any relevant medical, psychological, and psychiatric history. This allows invaluable information concerning previous therapies and treatment to be collated and assessed. Similarly, it is important for the oral physician to keep the medical practitioner informed about patient management.

A number of dental schools in the UK and elsewhere now have psychiatric liaison clinics that can provide an ideal environment for the patient to be introduced to psychiatric advice.

Patients can find the diagnostic labelling of a condition very reassuring. A small proportion of patients are extremely anxious or agitated because they believe that they have a serious or life-threatening condition such as cancer. Reassurance may be all that is needed for some patients. Some patients can demonstrate remarkable insight into their condition, and counselling or a psychological approach to therapy may be helpful.

Antidepressant medication

Tricyclic antidepressants, such as dosulepin hydrochloride (dothiepin) or nortriptyline, have been used successfully in other forms of chronic pain, such as back pain, and their analgesic action appears to be independent of the antidepressant action. These drugs have been shown to be effective in atypical facial pain and BMS but they do have some side-effects, such as drowsiness and dry mouth. It is helpful to make it clear to the patient that the antidepressant is being given for its pain control properties and that it is not likely to lead to any form of addiction. Patients will often appreciate the pain-relieving properties of antidepressants if they are made aware of their use in other chronic pain conditions such as arthritis, chronic back pain, and postherpetic neuralgia. It is also helpful to inform patients that chronic pain often causes a reactionary depression. Drowsiness has already been mentioned as a side-effect of tricyclic antidepressants and this may be problematical. An alternative would be to use one of the nonsedating selective serotonin reuptake inhibitors (SSRIs) such as sertraline. However, if a patient with chronic orofacial pain is having difficulty sleeping, the sedating properties of tricyclics may be helpful. Xerogenic side-effects limit their use in oral dysaesthesia.

Benefits from therapy with tricyclic antidepressants

- Analgesic effects
- Improved sleep
- Mood elevation

Cognitive behavioural therapy

There are several types of psychological approach to the management of psychogenic problems including chronic pain. Cognitive behavioural therapy (CBT) is one technique that may be used by clinical psychologists. In essence, CBT explores an individual's emotions, thoughts, attitudes, and beliefs. The

Side-effects of antidepressants

Tricyclic antidepressants

These commonly have the following side-effects:
- sedation;
- dry mouth;
- constipation;
- blurred vision;
- urinary retention.

These effects are due to the anticholinergic (more specifically, antimuscarinic) activity of tricyclic antidepressants. The individual drugs within the tricyclics do vary in their propensity to cause side-effects (for example, there are tricyclics that have increased sedative properties). Some members have additional side-effects. Tolerance to side-effects does occur in many patients. The side-effects are reduced by commencing therapy on low doses and then increasing the dose gradually. Therapy for elderly patients should always be initiated at low doses because the hypotensive properties of tricyclics predispose to dizziness and possible syncope.

Selective serotonin re-uptake inhibitors (SSRIs)

These have fewer antimuscarinic side-effects than tricyclics. The typical side-effects are:
- gastrointestinal disturbances such as nausea, dyspepsia, vomiting, abdominal pain, diarrhoea, and constipation;
- headache;
- sexual dysfunction.

   Abrupt cessation of therapy with SSRIs is not recommended as it can be associated with headaches, paraesthesia, dizziness, and anxiety.

   Hyponatraemia is a possible side-effect of all antidepressants in the elderly and may be manifest as drowsiness, confusion, or convulsions.

consequences that these have on behaviour are also assessed. Frequently the therapist will discover that a person's assumptions and beliefs may be unhelpful and irrational. This is often the case in patients who have 'cancer phobia'. Their beliefs aggravate their anxiety. The goal of CBT is to replace dysfunctional cognitive structures with more realistic functional ones—cognitive restructuring. Table 17.7 shows the stages involved in CBT. A case history of one patient with BMS is given in the text box.

   Complete pain relief is not always feasible and patients should be made aware that CBT can help the patient understand their condition and symptoms and hopefully 'turn down' the

Table 17.7 Major components of cognitive behaviour therapy with chronic pain patients*

Step 1 Assessment
Pain levels
Intensity
Frequency
Duration
Quality
Signal of impending pain episode or attenuation
Emotional reactions to pain
Worry
Anxiety
Depression
Anger and hostility
Cognitions and beliefs
Self-efficacy (i.e. 'Can I cope with the pain?' or 'Can I do what the clinician is expecting me to do?')
Locus of control
Expectations of pain (over a time course, or in certain situations)
Behaviour
Medication (prescribed and non-prescribed)
Activity levels
Avoidance of painful area (when eating, positioning tongue)
Encouraging sympathy and support from others
Step 2 Derive formulation (see Fig. 17.1)
Step 3 Cognitive restructuring
Relaxation
Distraction: used intermittently during critical moments (e.g. peak levels of pain intensity)
Beliefs: change negative and catastrophic thinking (e.g. 'This continuous pain means I must have cancer')
Step 4 Behavioural changes
Activity: increase physical and social behaviour
Attention: decrease attention from others in response to pain behaviour
Avoidance: reduce the degree of avoiding areas of mouth with increased sensitivity
Medication: review the use of excessive medication and rationalize to effective levels

* Adapted, with permission, from Humphris, G.M., Longman, L.P., and Field, E.A. (1996). Cognitive-behavioural therapy for idiopathic burning mouth syndrome: a report of two cases. *British Dental Journal* 181, 204–8.

Cognitive behavioural therapy: a case history

An example of this behavioural approach is illustrated in Fig. 17.1. This flow diagram represents a hypothesis or 'formulation' for a patient with BMS who presented to the authors' clinic. It summarizes the important features of his symptoms and the factors that may influence the condition. This 38-year-old male noticed his oral dysaesthesia shortly after major life events—redundancy, marital breakdown, restricted access to his children, and moving back to reside in his parents' home. The patient had no identifiable physical cause for his BMS and was referred for psychological assessment. The patient attended three 50-minute sessions, which allowed the clinical psychologist to construct the formulation in Fig. 17.1. The psychologist hypothesized that the major life events produced anxiety. The patient presented with symptoms of severe pain, anxiety, panic attacks, and depression. His anxiety was exacerbated by the belief that his condition was due to cancer. The patient was socially isolated and had no formal structure to his day. The patient was amenable to psychological intervention and attended three further sessions for therapy. The patient was encouraged to develop a more structured lifestyle (regular sleep, eating properly), social activities were increased, and the belief that he had oral cancer was refuted. Relaxation techniques were demonstrated to the patient and methods to help the patient cope with the pain—coping strategies— were suggested. The patient was pain-free at a 6-month review appointment.

This case history is adapted, with permission, from Humphris, G.M., Longman, L.P., and Field, E.A. (1996). Cognitive-behavioural therapy for idiopathic burning mouth syndrome: a report of two cases. *British Dental Journal* 181, 204–8.

pain volume. Pain diaries have proved to be a useful tool in helping patients understand that their environment can influence pain.

Disturbances in taste and salivation

Patients who complain of an unpleasant taste in whom no abnormality of any kind is detected are very difficult to manage.

Patients commonly report a sour, metallic, or bitter taste and are typically middle-aged females. These individuals often become quite obsessional about their condition and are frequently concerned that they have halitosis as well as a bad taste. Others complain of a dry mouth, despite the fact that the oral mucosa appears moist and salivary flow is normal. Symptoms of BMS sometimes coexist and some describe delusional symptoms such as sand or grit in the mouth or an excessive discharge of mucus. The complaint can be associated with significant detrimental changes in diet and lifestyle.

There are several conditions that may cause an alteration in taste and halitosis (see Chapter 6) and these should be excluded or treated in the first instance. Many patients have a combination of symptoms described above, which can be manifestations of an underlying cognitive disorder. Financial worries, bereavement, and cancer phobia are frequently revealed. Patients may respond to reassurance but a number will require psychological management.

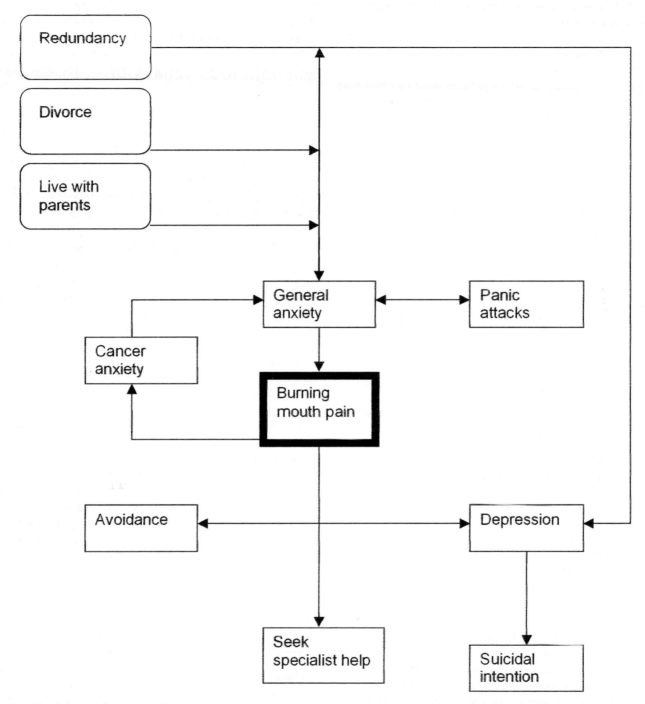

Fig. 17.1 Psychological formulation for a patient with burning mouth syndrome. The major factors are shown with hypothesized associations (arrowheads indicate the direction of influence). (This case history is adapted, with permission, from Humphris, G.M., Longman, L.P., and Field, E.A. (1996). Cognitive-behavioural therapy for idiopathic burning mouth syndrome: a report of two cases. *British Dental Journal* 181, 204–8.)

Delusional symptoms

A small number of patients have delusional symptoms involving the oral cavity. A delusion is an abnormal belief, from which the individual cannot be dissuaded and which is not in keeping with his or her cultural background. These patients may have a history of psychiatric illness so it is prudent to liaise with the medical practitioner. One group of patients that may be encountered by the dental surgeon are those who suffer from delusional halitosis. Despite intensive oral hygiene regimens and numerous investigations, these patients insist that their breath smells when it does not. Such patients are very difficult to manage and frequently have no other manifestation of a psychiatric disorder. Delusional halitosis is a form of a monosymptomatic hypochondriacal psychosis. Another presentation of this condition is the 'phantom bite syndrome' in which patients insist that they have an abnormal bite, while others have a false belief that there are lumps or seeds under the oral mucosa. It is important that the dentist identifies the patient who is deluded about their occlusion. Irreversible occlusal rehabilitation in these patients is to be avoided. Patients with delusional symptoms do not readily accept psychiatric assistance or a psychologically based explanation of their symptoms. It is advisable for the clinician to inform the general medical practitioner about his or her concerns. Organic causes of dental and facial pain should be excluded before diagnosing a delusional state. Early recognition of delusional symptoms may protect the patient from undergoing protracted investigations and unnecessary treatment.

> A delusion is an abnormal belief, from which the individual cannot be dissuaded and which is not in keeping with his or her cultural background.

Dysmorphophobia

The term dysmorphophobia is rather misleading because it is not a phobia. The patient with dysmorphophobia has a serious preoccupation with an aspect of their physical appearance that they feel is defective. The physical abnormality may be a minor physical problem or it may be imaginary. The sufferer has a feeling of 'ugliness' and a desire for corrective treatment. Whilst any part of the body may be targeted, a facial feature is most commonly involved, for example, the teeth or facial profile. The effects of this disorder on the sufferer are variable but the patient may become dysfunctional and require hospitalization. Suicide attempts can be a feature. Patients with dysmorphophobia may be relentless in their pursuit for dental or surgical treatment to rectify their perceived deformity. Such therapies may serve to enhance the patient's morbid preoccupation. Dissatisfaction, anger, and litigation may ensue. Clinicians should carefully explore a patient's requests and expectations before embarking upon cosmetic procedures and be wary of patients who thinks that treatment is a magical cure for their problems. The patient with dysmorphophobia is not always easy to diagnose. The borders between an acceptable and abnormal appearance are open to subjective interpretation. When an underlying psychological problem is suspected as the main reason for the patient's dissatisfaction with their appearance, it may be advisable to seek a specialist opinion before commencing treatment.

Changes in the classification of psychiatric disease have redefined dysmorphophobia into non-delusional and delusional variants. The delusional type is a psychotic disorder and the non-

delusional has been named 'body dysmorphic syndrome', but for the purposes of this chapter no distinction has been made between these two variants.

Self-injurious behaviour

There are some patients who cause self-harm to their orofacial tissues—this may or may not be intentional. Self-injurious behaviour is well recognized in several groups of patients with developmental, physical, or learning disabilities. Examples of these conditions are epilepsy, profound neurodisability, cerebral palsy, autism, Lesch–Nyhan syndrome, and Riley–Day syndrome (congenital indifference to pain). Trauma to the lip, cheek, and tongue are commonly seen in these groups of patients. Table 17.8 suggests some management options that may be used, but treatment is rarely simple and not always successful.

> A factitious disorder is a psychological or psychiatric disorder characterized by the compulsive, voluntary production of signs and symptoms of a disease for the sole purpose of assuming a 'patient's role' and in the absence of other secondary gain.

Patients who deliberately cause self-mutilation present a difficult assessment and management problem. Self-harm is commonly associated with depressive disorders. The orofacial lesions can be variable in presentation and site. Gingivitis artefacta, which consists of destructive lesions to the gingivae, is well recognized in the literature. Often such lesions are caused with a finger nail. Similar traumatic injuries, such as traumatic ulceration, may occur on the oral mucosa ('factitious stomatitis') and on the skin ('dermatitis artefacta'). The diagnosis can be difficult but the lesion is nearly always in an area accessible to the patient and the clinical features are often inconsistent with the history and other orofacial conditions. Patients rarely admit to causing such lesions and it can be difficult to persuade the

Table 17.8 Management of self-injurious behaviour in patients with disabilities

Local
Topical anaesthetics
Topical antiseptics
Sutures to close wound
Bite-raising appliances
Occlusal guards and lip bumpers to displace soft tissues
Restoration of broken teeth
Dental extractions
Occlusal adjustment to teeth
Systemic
Analgesics
Antibiotics for spreading infections

patient that they are in need of specialist help. Behavioural therapy can be beneficial. However, some patients may require psychotropic medication.

Eating disorders

Anorexia nervosa and bulimia nervosa are common conditions in the Western world. Eating disorders present an enormous challenge to society and the health-care professions. Eating disorders occur in both females and males, but are more common in females with a ratio of 10:1. Broadly speaking, anorexics avoid food and consequently lose weight, in contrast to bulimics who have episodes of binge eating and purging. Purging may involve the abuse of laxatives, enemas, diuretics, and exercise; self-induced vomiting is also common. This may be considered an oversimplification as the differences between the two conditions are sometimes not so clear-cut. Anorexics can also suffer from self-induced vomiting.

Eating disorders

- Anorexia nervosa: food avoidance; underweight; distorted body image
- Bulimia nervosa: binge eating and purging; usually normal body weight

Anorexia nervosa is less common than bulimia and the median age of onset is 17 years, but it has been reported in patients as young as 8 years old. Comorbidity with other psychiatric and personality disorders is well recognized—depression, social phobia, and obsessive compulsive disorder are common. Medical conditions associated with malnutrition occur, such as renal failure, liver dysfunction, amenorrhoea, and dehydration.

Bulimia nervosa is more common than anorexia and is thought to affect approximately 2 per cent of young adult women. Unlike anorexics, bulimics are usually of normal body weight, but many have a history of anorexia or obesity. As with anorexia there are high levels of associated psychiatric or psychological problems. Systemic disease can also accompany bulimia. Oesophageal erosions are common and frequent vomiting and misuse of laxatives can cause potassium depletion. The resultant hypokalaemia predisposes the patient to myocardial instability and fatal arrhythmias can occur.

Anorexia and bulimia can both have a significant impact on dental hard tissues. Acid erosion of dental hard tissues is described in Chapter 18. Self-induced vomiting and a high intake of acidic drinks and foods are the prime causes of tooth wear in patients with eating disorders.

Parotid gland enlargement can also be a feature of eating disorders, and mucosal lesions have been reported in patients with bulimia. This is because the fingers or objects used to induce vomiting can traumatize the mucosa, in particular the soft palate. Stomatitis may also occur due to nutritional or haematinic

deficiencies. The dentist therefore not only has a role in the prevention and management of oral disease in these patients, but also in the identification of eating disorders. The dental practitioner may be able to encourage the patient to acknowledge the need for professional help and liaise with the patient's general medical practitioner.

Drugs and alcohol

Drug dependency, including alcoholism, may present problems in the oral medicine context, as in many others. Perhaps the most significant drug-related problem affecting dentistry is the intravenous drug–HIV–hepatitis relationship. It is quite clear that many drug-dependent patients may have problems of nutritional and immune abnormality, resulting in oral changes such as those discussed in earlier chapters.

The term 'alcoholism' is used as a generic term, approved by the World Health Organisation, to describe all types of alcohol-related problems. It has been estimated that 1 in 10 members of the population has a serious alcohol problem. Physical problems that may result from excessive alcohol intake are widespread and affect all systems. A summary is given in Table 17.9. Many of the effects of alcohol abuse can impact upon the management of the dental patient, but of particular relevance to oral medicine are nutritional deficiencies—often folate deficiency—that may result in stomatitis and other problems, as detailed in Chapter 13. Psychological problems may include depression and may manifest themselves as orofacial problems, such as the burning mouth syndrome or atypical facial pain. Occasionally, patients with chronic pain conditions may resort to alcohol or other drugs in the hope that

Table 17.9 Effects of alcohol abuse on general health

System affected	Effect
Cardiovascular system	Hypertension
	Cardiomyopathies
	Dysarrythmias
Immune system	Increased susceptibility to infection
	Increased susceptibility to malignancies
Haematology	Deficiency of haematinics and clotting agents
Metabolism	Hypoglycaemia, electrolyte deficiencies, malnutrition
Gastrointestinal system	Gastritis, ulceration, malabsorption, hepatitis, cirrhosis, pancreatitis
Neuromuscular system	Myopathies, neuropathies, dementia
Psychiatric	Depression, anxieties, suicidal ideation, psychoses
Orodental tissues	Tooth wear, salivary gland swelling, apthous stomatitis
Fetus	Fetal alcohol syndrome

they will help control their pain. The role of a high intake of alcohol together with tobacco use in the aetiology of oral malignancy was discussed in Chapter 10.

Haematological screening in an alcohol-dependent patient may show a macrocytosis in the presence of normal folate levels. The reason for this is not clear. Liver function tests may very well be normal as these tests show great individual variation.

It should be appreciated that alcohol and drug addictions are well recognized in the medical or dental professional and this includes the student population (see Project 1 at the end of this chapter).

Discussion of problem cases

Case 17.1 Discussion

Q1   How would you investigate this lady's symptoms and what are the possible causes?

A full history should be taken. It is important to know if the symptoms were attenuated or absent when the dentures were left out. An intraoral examination is required to identify if there is any mucosal abnormality present. The patient relates the onset of symptoms to the provision of new replacement complete dentures. The dentures, therefore, should be assessed for lack of freeway space. The new dentures may have been made with an unacceptable increase in the occlusal vertical dimension. Alternatively, the denture teeth may not have been placed in the neutral zone. It is always helpful to examine the patient's old dentures (if she still has them) to compare the denture designs in relation to a patient's complaints.

It is possible that the patient has developed parafunctional habits, such as rubbing the tongue against the denture, since the dentures were fitted. Patients are often unaware of this. If the denture tooth position is thought to be satisfactory, a soft occlusal splint may be helpful in 'breaking' the habit.

Allergy to denture-base materials is exceptionally rare, and a mucosal problem is more likely to be a result of an excess of uncured free monomer. If this is the case, the symptoms should resolve if the dentures are not worn. In addition, the monomer should cease to leach out of the denture with time. Some patients seem unable to tolerate dentures and a full denture history is essential. It is necessary to enquire if the patient has successfully worn dentures before (including partial dentures).

If the patient's dentures are found to be adequate and the oral mucosa appears normal, then the patient should be fully investigated for BMS as outlined in Table 17.5. Table 17.4 lists the underlying conditions that can cause BMS.

Case 17.2 Discussion

Q1   Discuss how you might differentiate between pain of dental origin and atypical odontalgia in this patient.

When a tooth has had many dental interventions or has a large restoration present, it is often all too easy to find an imperfection present that may be thought to be responsible for the symptoms. When a large filling or a crown is present, it is reasonable to consider that a pulp could be inflamed or infected or that a painful root-filled tooth could require re-treatment or periradicular surgery. In clinical practice, therefore, it can often be difficult to exclude a dental cause in a tooth with chronic

Table 17.10 Characteristics of pain in dental conditions

Pulpitis
Variable presentation from mild to severe pain. Reversible pulpitis may present as sharp pain with hot, cold, and sweet stimuli (osmotic or thermal changes in pressure). Pain may be localized to affected tooth or adjacent teeth, but can be referred to affected side of face (unlikely to cross midline). Defective restorations, caries, or occlusal trauma are possible causes. Analgesics can be helpful but not antibiotics. Chronic pulpitis can also present as a poorly localized dull ache
Cracked tooth
Vague or inconsistent history of pain during eating; may be sensitive (sharp pain) to thermal stimuli. There may be an intermittent dull ache. Pain is not always elicited by the same stimuli, and it may be difficult to elicit pain clinically.
Pain usually localized but can be referred (similar manner to pulpitis). Affected tooth is usually restored, crack(s) may be visible but are not necessarily pathological. Relief is obtained when occlusal forces no longer stress the fracture line (e.g. piece of cusp fractures off)
Periradicular periodontitis
Throbbing pain, mild to severe. Pain should be well localized. The following may be present: a sinus, a localized alveolar swelling, a periodontal pocket.
Antibiotics and analgesics may have been effective in reducing or eliminating the pain. The affected tooth is usually restored or carious; alternatively, there is a history of trauma. Relief should be obtained when the source of infection is removed (e.g. a necrotic pulp)
Pericoronitis
Dull ache with acute exacerbations. Pain tends to be well localized. Most commonly, the mandibular third molar is involved. Pain can radiate across the affected side of the jaw. Pain worse on eating. Very rarely is sleep disturbed.
The painful tooth is usually partly erupted or has an operculum with an associated periodontal stagnation area. Antibiotics and analgesics may have been helpful. Relief is obtained when: (1) the tooth is taken out of occlusion (preventing trauma to the operculum); (2) the operculum is removed; (3) the tooth is extracted; or (4) the tooth erupts fully

Table 17.11 Trigeminal neuralgia and atypical facial pain: differential diagnosis

Trigeminal neuralgia	Atypical facial pain
Age (years)	
50+	30–60
Pain intensity	
Remarkably severe	Intensity may vary from mild to severe, but usually a 'background', low-intensity pain is present
Pain descriptors	
Stabbing, sharp, lancinating pain of a few seconds duration. Paroxysms may follow in quick succession	Dull, throbbing, gnawing, nagging, pulling, occasionally sharp
	Florid and emotive adjectives are used
	Descriptors may be inconsistent
Location/distribution/radiation of pain	
Mandible or maxilla	Maxilla is the most common site
Well localized	Not always well localized and site may change
Unilateral	Uni- or bilateral
Follows anatomical distribution of one sensory division of the trigeminal nerve (occasionally more than one division is involved)	Does not usually follow anatomical distribution of nerves
	Can be bilateral and can cross midline
	Can radiate over whole of face
Duration of pain	
Brief—usually only seconds	Continuous
Trigger zones for pain	
Yes, well defined	Not usually present
Periodicity of pain	
Intermittent	Continuous or intermittent
Precipitating factors	
Moving or touching a trigger zone. Mild stimuli may provoke an attack	Stress, life events
Relieving factors	
Carbamazepine—response to treatment usually good	Antidepressants—response variable
Peripheral nerve block with local anaesthetic injection temporarily relieves pain	Local anaesthetic injection into area often fails to relieve pain
Commonly used analgesics are not beneficial	Analgesics are occasionally some help, but not always
	Pain may not be problematic during sleep
Pain behaviour	
A 'frozen face' appearance	Variable presentation
Speech and facial appearance are altered if the associated facial movements cause pain	Patient may have developed habits, e.g. touching or picking the affected site
Avoids touching trigger zone	
History	
Other chronic pain syndromes not usually present	Frequently a longstanding history of pain
	Frequent restorative and surgical intervention is common
	High prevalence of chronic ill health, especially other chronic pain syndromes

symptoms. It is always easier to make a diagnosis of atypical odontalgia (a variant of atypical facial pain) when a succession of interventions have been carried out without success. It is therefore essential that detailed dental and pain histories are taken. A patient with atypical odontalgia may have a history of repeated restorations, followed by root treatment, crown placement, and an apicectomy. It is not unusual to find out that adjacent teeth have had similar treatments for chronic pain. Teeth may also have been extracted. The clinician needs to establish if any treatment was beneficial. The effect of any medications that have been used for the pain should be assessed. In atypical odontalgia it is unlikely that simple analgesics and antibiotics will have relieved the pain. Despite this, patients may still have a high daily intake of analgesics.

The nature of the pain is also important. Patients with atypical odontalgia/facial pain may also give a history of pain and altered sensations that are variable. It is not unusual for a patient with atypical odontalgia to have a definite view of what started the pain. Dental causes for consideration in the differential diagnosis are given in Table 17.10—compare these with the features of atypical facial pain listed in Table 17.2.

Case 17.3 Discussion

Q1 What information from the pain history and clinical examination would you use to differentiate between these two conditions?

To distinguish between trigeminal neuralgia and atypical facial pain the clinician will need to listen carefully to the pain history and notice the patient's demeanour and mannerisms. The descriptors that the patient uses to describe the pain are often very important. A simple pain questionnaire such as the McGill pain questionnaire can be very helpful. Table 17.11, whilst not exhaustive, is of value in differentiating between trigeminal neuralgia and atypical facial pain.

Projects

1 The British Dental Association have produced a publication entitled *Drugs and alcohol: addiction in the dental profession, problems and solutions*. What is the role of the 'dentists' health support programme' in relation to dentists with alcohol and addiction problems?

2 The Hospital Anxiety and Depression (HAD) scale can be useful when assessing a patient with chronic pain. Obtain a copy of this psychometric questionnaire and find out how to evaluate a completed form.

18

Disorders of the teeth and bone

Disorders of the teeth
- Hypodontia
- Variation in eruption
- Variation in the size of teeth
- Non-carious tooth surface loss
- Discoloration of the teeth
- Disturbances of the structure and enamel and dentine

Disorders of bone
- Inherited and developmental disturbances
- Metabolic and endocrine disorders
- Disorders of unknown aetiology: Paget's disease

Disorders of the teeth and bone

Problem cases

Case 18.1

A 14-year-old boy is unhappy with the appearance of his front teeth. He does not like their 'blotchy appearance'. Clinical examination reveals the presence of small white flecks on the enamel surfaces of most of the teeth. The enamel surfaces are not pitted. The teeth have no restorations present and are caries-free. The discoloration is intrinsic.

Q1   What are the differential diagnoses for this boy's dental condition?

Q2   What additional information do you need to help you make a definitive diagnosis?

Case 18.2

An 18-year-old girl presents to your surgery because she is unhappy about the appearance of her front teeth and complains that her front teeth are getting thinner. She reports that her teeth are sometimes sensitive to hot and cold. Examination reveals exposed dentine on the palatal surfaces of the maxillary incisors and canines. There is also exposed dentine on the occlusal surfaces of the maxillary first permanent molar teeth.

Q1   What are the possible causes of tooth wear in this case?

Q2   What condition would you suspect if the patient also presented with swollen parotid glands and appeared to have generalized skeletal muscle wastage?

Disorders of the teeth

The teeth are poor indicators of generalized disease. Following their calcification, metabolic processes have little effect on the structure of the teeth. Structural abnormalities almost invariably reflect changes occurring in the period during which the teeth were being formed. Apart from structural variation, abnormalities in the numbers, size, and shape of the teeth occasionally occur, in conjunction with abnormalities of the bones or of the skin and other epidermally derived structures. When numbers of missing teeth, supernumerary teeth, or abnormally shaped teeth are observed, it is as well to consider the possibility of some such complex association. It must always be remembered that teeth

Table 18.1 Dental anomalies and associated diseases

Dental anomaly	Associated systemic/ genetic disease
Disorders of tooth development	
Anodontia, oligodontia	Hypohidrotic ectodermal dysplasia, Down's syndrome
Supernumerary teeth	Cleidocranial dysplasia, Gardner's syndrome
Macrodontia, microdontia, taurodontism, dilaceration, gemination	Down's syndrome, Klinefelter's syndrome
Dentinogenesis imperfecta, amelogenesis imperfecta, enamel hypoplasia, dentine dysplasia, fluorosis	Osteogenesis imperfecta, congenital syphilis, rickets, hypophosphatasia
Disorders of eruption and shedding	
Premature eruption	Hyperthyroidism
Delayed eruption	Cretinism, rickets, cleidocranial dysplasia, hereditary gingival fibromatosis, Down's syndrome
Impaction of teeth	Cleidocranial dysplasia

missing from the arch may either be congenitally absent, have been extracted, or may be unerupted. The major post-eruption changes that occur are the losses of tooth substance caused by caries, attrition, erosion, and abrasion. This chapter will discuss some of the disorders mentioned. The list is not, however, exhaustive and the reader is referred to a textbook of oral pathology. Table 18.1 highlights some dental anomalies that are associated with genetic or systemic disease.

Hypodontia

Hypodontia (oligodontia), the congenital absence of teeth, represented by the loss of one or two teeth with no apparent associated abnormalities is not uncommon. The most common teeth to be missing are the last in each series. Most surveys, however, show that one or more third molars are missing in approximately one-quarter of the population. A study carried out in an English population and excluding the third molars has shown that the teeth most likely to be missing are the lower second premolars

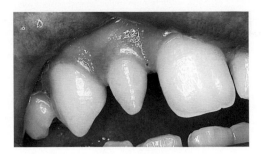

Fig. 18.1 A conically shaped tooth in the position of an upper lateral incisor.

(40.9 per cent) followed by the upper lateral incisors (23.5 per cent) and by the upper second premolars (20.9 per cent). The pattern of missing teeth does, however, vary from population to population. A common finding in hypodontia is the presence of small and conically shaped teeth replacing normal units of the dentition (Fig. 18.1). Hypodontia in the primary dentition is a relatively rare occurrence.

The congenital absence of teeth associated with abnormalities of the bone or ectodermal appendages is relatively rare. The dysplasia involved may be attributed to ectodermally derived structures or to more complex syndromes in which there are both dermal and bony abnormalities.

Variation in eruption

The wide normal range makes it difficult to specify accurately the dates of eruption of either the deciduous or the permanent teeth. Several factors have been found to affect the date of eruption, including racial origin and such unlikely influences as the socioeconomic environment. In general, earlier bodily development is reflected in early eruption of the teeth.

Markedly premature eruption of the permanent teeth is very rare. It has been suggested that it may occur in cases of hypersecretion of those hormones that influence development. It is somewhat more common to note premature eruption of the deciduous teeth. Frequently, no systemic factor is found to account for this. It should perhaps be mentioned that teeth present at birth in a few children (the neonatal teeth) do not represent premature eruption. These are supernumerary teeth and part of a separate predeciduous dentition.

Delayed eruption of the deciduous teeth may occur in endocrine deficiency states and it has been shown that, in Down's syndrome, not only are the eruption dates somewhat retarded in general, but also there is often an unusual sequence of eruption. It is very difficult to ascribe a characteristic dental picture to many of the endocrine abnormalities since, in a number of cases, varying and contradictory effects have been described. In many such patients the most obvious abnormality is disproportion in the sizes of the teeth and the jaws, this in turn leading to gross irregularity of the occlusion. The presence of supernumerary or unerupted teeth may delay or prevent eruption. Cleidocranial

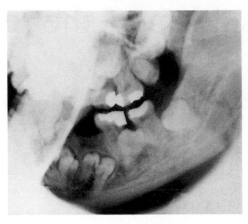

Fig. 18.2 Multiple unerupted teeth in cleidocranial dysplasia.

dysplasia, although rare, is a well known syndrome in which there are multiple additional teeth associated with unerupted teeth (Fig. 18.2).

Variation in the size of teeth

The size of the teeth of any individual is determined largely by inherited factors. Extreme variation in size, either in the direction of small teeth (microdontism) or in the direction of large teeth (macrodontism) may be accompanied by no other growth abnormality. Conversely, endocrine growth disorders leading to gigantism or dwarfism may be accompanied by no corresponding variation in tooth size. The size of the teeth alone bears no relationship to metabolic factors in the vast majority of instances.

Non-carious tooth surface loss

Attrition, erosion, and abrasion are commonly seen in dental patients. The clinical appearance of the teeth may be suggestive of a specific cause for tooth wear but caution should be exercised in the identification of a single aetiological agent. Tooth wear is usually a multifactorial process. The presence of attrition or erosion may be of interest to the oral physician. Wear facets in opposing arches that match in parafunctional positions of the mandible are indicative of bruxism. This may be significant in the aetiology of a headache that is present on waking or in myofacial pain.

> In any individual, tooth wear usually has a multifactorial aetiology.

Erosion is the loss of dental hard tissue by a chemical process that does not involve bacteria (Fig. 18.3). The causes of erosion are listed in Table 18.2. The active substances may be endogenous or exogenous. Acidic foodstuffs and beverages are commonly implicated. These include citrus fruit and juice, and many soft drinks including fruit squashes and cordials, mixer-type drinks, and many others. A highly significant cause of erosion is the self-induced vomiting of bulimia nervosa, which may result in widespread loss of enamel, particularly from the palatal surfaces of the

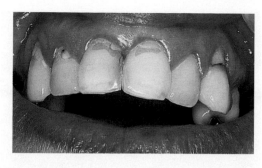

Fig. 18.3 Acid erosion with cervical lesions and loss of normal enamel contour.

Table 18.2 Causes of dental erosion

Extrinsic acids
Beverages (e.g. fresh fruit juices, cordials, carbonated drinks, wine, fruit teas)
Foods (e.g. citrus fruit, pickled foods)
Industrial processes (e.g. wine tasting, battery manufacture, metal plating)
Intrinsic acids
Gastro-oesophageal reflux disease (GORD)*
Eating disorder—bulimia nervosa
Morning sickness in pregnancy
Rumination (voluntary regurgitation)

* This may be secondary to other conditions, e.g. alcoholism.

upper anterior teeth and the cusps of permanent molars. Parotid enlargement and a non-specific mucositis may also be seen in the bulimic patient. Patients with gastric conditions that result in chronic acid regurgitation will present with this type of tooth wear.

- Anorexia nervosa can be associated with dental erosion because of a high intake of acid drinks and fruit
- Bulimia nervosa is associated with dental erosion because teeth are exposed to intrinsic (gastric) acid

Discoloration of the teeth

Widespread coloration of the teeth occurs in a few diseases in which abnormal blood pigments circulate. Of these, infantile jaundice is the most common. In this condition the deciduous teeth may be coloured blue-green due to the laying down of a pigment in the immediate postnatal dentine zone. A less common, and now virtually eliminated, cause of tooth discoloration is haemolytic anaemia of the newborn caused by rhesus incompatibility. Following the haemolysis, pigments may be deposited in the skin and in the teeth, which may take on coloration that varies from grey to green-grey and to brown. Coloration of the teeth also occurs in some other considerably rarer situations in

which abnormal pigments circulate, for example, in porphyria. However, a far more common cause of tooth discoloration is tetracycline staining. It need hardly be said, however, that the number of young patients with tetracycline staining is rapidly reducing with the almost total withdrawal of this group of antibiotics from 'at-risk' groups.

Disturbances of the structure of enamel and dentine

When the normal sequence of enamel matrix formation and calcification is disturbed, a series of abnormalities may be produced. These may be distinguished as hypoplasia, when the quantity of enamel is reduced, or as hypocalcification, in which the degree of calcification is unsatisfactory. The two conditions may be combined and various clinical conditions may be differentiated. A parallel range of disturbances in the formation of dentine may also occur, but these are not so well differentiated as in enamel. The use of the term 'hypoplasia' can be confusing and requires explanation, since it is used both in the strictly scientific sense as mentioned above and also in a clinical sense to describe a generalized disturbance of enamel structure caused by some form of systemic disturbance.

This group of conditions can be conveniently divided as follows:

(1) enamel or dentine developmental defects resulting from localized disturbances;

(2) enamel or dentine developmental defects resulting from generalized disturbances;

(3) genetically determined defects of enamel formation or genetically determined defects of dentine formation.

Defects due to local causes

When an infection occurs in association with a deciduous tooth the permanent successional tooth developing below it may undergo a disturbance of development. In such cases the enamel is usually distorted and pitted. This condition is easily recognized by its restriction to a single successional tooth.

Defects due to generalized causes

Widespread infections or nutritional disturbances during the tooth enamel development period may adversely affect the laying down of enamel. Such conditions affect all the teeth developing at the time and it is often possible to time accurately the onset of the disturbance by the position of the defect on the teeth. In general, the deficient enamel forms a band around the tooth corresponding to the period of disturbance (Fig. 18.4). The band may be wide or narrow and, in some circumstances, the banding may be incomplete. It has been suggested that the enamel opacities seen in some patients may represent a minor form of this condition. Unless the disturbance of tooth formation is unusually severe, the teeth do not seem to be unduly susceptible to attack by caries. Histologically, the dentine that developed at the same

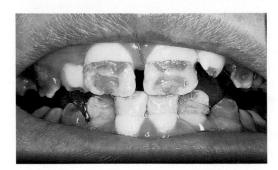

Fig. 18.4 Enamel hypoplasia as a result of a general disturbance during development.

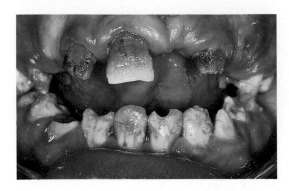

Fig. 18.6 Hypoplasia in a patient with disturbed calcium metabolism.

time as the affected enamel may show slight deficiencies, but this does not result in clinical abnormality.

Prenatal syphilis may produce defects in tooth development. The spirochaete may lodge in the enamel organ and interfere directly with the formation of the enamel. The effects are generally confined to the anterior permanent teeth and to the first permanent molar. The typical molar form of the syphilitic tooth is the mulberry molar in which the shape of the tooth is well expressed by its name; these teeth are also termed Moon's molars. The typical variation in the anterior teeth takes the form of a conical, screw-driver shape with a notched incisal edge called a Hutchinson's incisor (see Chapter 4).

If the development of the teeth occurs when large amounts of fluorides are ingested, mottling of the enamel may occur. The effect of fluorosis may be recognized by the presence of opaque white patches in the enamel, often arranged in a band-like formation. Unlike the teeth in other forms of hypoplasia, the teeth affected by fluorosis are susceptible to a brown discoloration (Fig. 18.5) that may resemble amelogenesis imperfecta. Similar idiopathic mottling may occur in teeth of patients from non-fluoride areas, but this is rare.

Hypoplasia or hypocalcification of the enamel may occur in patients suffering from generalized ectodermal disease (such as epidermolysis bullosa) or from disturbances of calcium metabolism such as hypoparathyroidism. These conditions clearly represent the final result of abnormal tooth germ formation and

abnormal calcification, respectively. Many other diseases may produce dental abnormalities of a similar type. These changes are, however, rare. It is unlikely that the generalized disease process will have gone unrecognized by the time that the tooth abnormality has become evident in the majority of these patients (Fig. 18.6).

It will be evident that the diagnosis of the abnormalities of tooth structure described above depends largely on the recognition of the clinical appearance of the teeth. Radiography apart, there is very little in the way of supplementary tests or investigations that will add to a carefully carried out clinical examination of the patient, an examination that should evidently include a careful medical and family history. In virtually all cases laboratory tests prove unproductive.

Defects due to genetic causes

AMELOGENESIS IMPERFECTA

Amelogenesis imperfecta is a hereditary developmental defect of enamel. The condition may show as either a hypoplasia of the enamel or as a hypocalcification. If an early phase of enamel formation is disturbed, the amount of matrix laid down is reduced, but the calcification is complete. We thus have a thin and irregular layer of hard enamel. This is the hypoplastic type (Fig. 18.7). Severe attrition may occur early in life. In the hypocalcified type

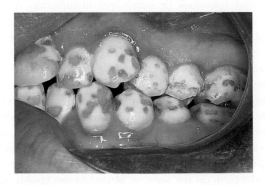

Fig. 18.5 Fluorosis.

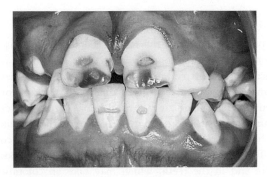

Fig. 18.7 Hypoplastic enamel. The enamel is imperfect, but is hard.

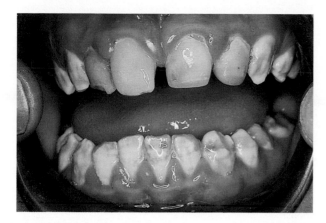

Fig. 18.8 Hypocalcified enamel. The enamel is soft and eroded.

a later stage of enamel formation is disturbed and we have a normally thick layer of poorly calcified enamel. In this case, the whole of the enamel is soft and eroded with loss of much enamel by attrition and exposure of the dentine (Fig. 18.8). In both forms the deciduous and permanent dentitions may be affected. The dentine retains its normal structure in both cases.

DENTINOGENESIS IMPERFECTA

In this condition there is failure of development of the dentine with normal enamel development. It is a hereditary condition and affects both the deciduous and permanent dentitions. The teeth erupt usually with normal morphology, but have a grey or brown colour. They show a rather iridescent coloration, which leads to the term 'hereditary opalescent dentine'. The pulp chambers are often reduced in size and may be obliterated. Although the enamel is of normal structure, it readily breaks away, leaving the dentine exposed.

Occasionally, this condition occurs as part of a generalized condition of osteogenesis imperfecta in which the imperfect calcification of the bones leads to frequent fractures. Often in such cases there is a deficiency in the sclera of the eye leading to a blue coloration.

Disorders of bone

Diseases of bone have traditionally been divided into three groups: genetic, inflammatory, and metabolic. In reality, this classification is rather simplistic. For example, the classification of Paget's disease is problematic because the aetiology of this condition is uncertain. Nonetheless, the classification remains a useful one for many conditions. Relatively few disorders of bone present with any frequency for investigation in the oral medicine clinic. Fibrous dysplasia and Paget's disease are seen only occasionally. However, some genetically determined diseases have an impact on dentistry in general, because they are part of generalized syndromes involving bone and epidermal appendages (including teeth). In these complex syndromes the predominant oral condition is variation in the size, number, morphology, and, some-

Table 18.3 Blood chemistry in diseases of bone

	Levels in blood of		
	Calcium	Phosphate	Alkaline phosphatase
Normal	2.2–2.7 mmol/l	0.8–1.4 mmol/l	Variable†
Paget's disease	N	N	++
Monostotic fibrous dysplasia	N	N	N
Polyostotic fibrous dysplasia	+	N	+
Primary hyperparathyroidism with bone lesions	+	N/–	+

* N, Normal; +, a moderate rise' ++, a marked rise; –, a moderate fall.

† Alkaline phosphatase values: normal levels for the age group should be determined from the specific laboratory. Usual adult values up to 125 IU/l.

times, structure of the teeth. Cleidocranial dysplasia and osteogenesis imperfecta are examples of such syndromes.

Inflammatory bone disease is marginally within the field of oral medicine, although the classic presentation of osteomyelitis of the jaws is now very rare. In this chapter, cleidocranial dysplasia and fibrous dysplasia are respectively classified as 'inherited' and 'developmental' conditions. The metabolic bone diseases discussed in this chapter are gigantism, acromegaly, osteoporosis, and osteomalacia. Hyperparathyroidism is essentially an endocrine disease but has bony manifestations in the jaws that are of obvious importance.

The screening procedure that is likely to provide the first evidence of a metabolic bone abnormality is an estimation of serum calcium, phosphorus, and alkaline phosphatase. Table 18.3 gives details of the levels in the conditions mentioned in this chapter. When interpreting the results for alkaline phosphatase it is important to be aware that there can be wide variations depending upon the age of the patient and the activity of the disease.

Inherited and developmental disturbances

Cleidocranial dysplasia

In cleidocranial dysplasia (dysostosis) there is an abnormality of membrane bone formation. The changes observed are lack of calcification of the clavicle, flattening of the frontal bone, and the presence of a number of supernumerary teeth. These teeth are often of complex form, resembling units of the normal dentition, and frequently remain unerupted (Fig. 18.2). It may appear that the patient is suffering from hypodontia because of the failure to erupt of large numbers of teeth within the jaws. Radiographs of the skull (showing wormian bones) and clavicles (demonstrating clavicular aplasia or hypoplasia) should confirm the diagnosis. The absence of clavicles enables patients to bring their shoulders forward to approximate in the midline. A flattened nasal bridge and a high-arched narrow palate may also be present.

Fibrous dysplasia

Fibrous dysplasia is a fibro-osseous lesion of the bone and may involve one (monostotic) or several (polyostotic) bones in the body. The cause of the condition is unknown and it is generally regarded as a developmental disorder. Diagnosis is based upon clinical symptoms, radiological appearance, biochemical investigations, and possibly histopathology.

Fibrous dysplasia

- Monostotic fibrous dysplasia is essentially a single lesion affecting the jaws without any other skeletal or other generalized abnormality.

- Polyostotic fibrous dysplasia is a generalized condition that may affect the jaw bones.

MONOSTOTIC FIBROUS DYSPLASIA

This is a condition that may arise in either male or female patients and is associated with very little other disturbance of bone or any other tissue. It is more common than the polyostotic form. The lesions occur more often in the maxilla than in the mandible. The essential change in this condition is the replacement of the normal bone architecture by a partially calcified fibrous mass with a histology suggesting an acceleration of the normal bone metabolism of osteoclasis and osteogenesis. The degree of ossification of the lesion is widely variable. Tissue removed from a lesion may vary from a very soft and haemorrhagic specimen to a relatively hard and well ossified tissue. This process is not associated with any generalized change. In particular, the accepted blood chemistry determinants (calcium, phosphorus, and alkaline phosphatase) remain unchanged. In the case of well-demarcated lesions of fibrous dysplasia, there is a great deal of discussion as to whether these represent benign, neoplastic changes. This question has been, to some extent, sidestepped by the adoption of the term 'fibro-osseous lesion'.

The characteristic feature of fibrous dysplasia is of an otherwise symptomless swelling of the mandible or maxilla (Fig. 18.9). In the case of the maxilla, the swelling may encroach on the antral cavity (Fig. 18.10). There is virtually no other complaint and all investigations of a biochemical nature prove to be unproductive. The only useful investigation is radiography, although the appearance of fibrous dysplasia may be very variable. In general, the basic pathological process of decalcification and recalcification is reflected in a mottled appearance of the bone on radiography. This, however, depends on the stage and the rapidity of the process. In those patients in whom the process is slow and includes a significant element of calcification, the mottling will be minimal and the expanded bone will have an almost normal appearance. If the decalcification of bone is predominant at the

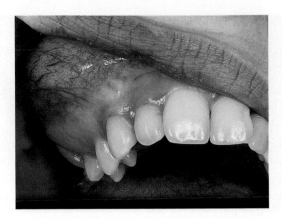

Fig. 18.9 Fibrous dysplasia. A monostotic lesion of the right maxilla.

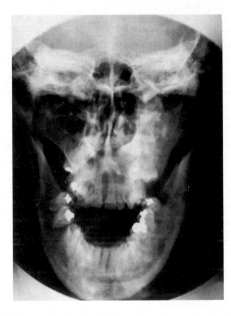

Fig. 18.10 Fibrous dysplasia. Radiograph of lesion in the left maxilla.

time of radiography, then the radiographic appearance will reflect this fact.

Management of monostotic fibrous dysplasia should be highly conservative. There is no medical treatment available and, since the lesions progress to a self-limiting static phase over a few years, it is almost always better to await events before carrying out surgery. The extent of this surgery should be determined entirely by cosmetic factors. Since neoplastic change is virtually unknown in this condition, there is no need to attempt to remove the whole of the lesion and, in fact, this is often an almost impossible task. It is generally accepted, therefore, that simple cosmetic contouring of the facial skeleton is best carried out after growth is complete.

POLYOSTOTIC FIBROUS DYSPLASIA

This condition is very much less common than monostotic fibrous dysplasia. It is virtually always associated with widespread changes throughout the skeleton and in other systems of the body that are collectively known as Albright's syndrome. In this condition areas of bone throughout the body are replaced by fibrous tissue with widely differing amounts of new ossification included within them. This often leads to multiple fractures and to gross distortion of the skeleton. In Albright's syndrome, the bony lesions are associated with patchy melanotic skin pigmentation (café-au-lait spots) and, in the case of females, sexual precocity. This condition is a far more active one than that of monostotic fibrous dysplasia and this is reflected in the blood chemistry changes. In polyostotic fibrous dysplasia the serum alkaline phosphatase is often greatly elevated, as in the serum calcium. This is in contrast to monostotic fibrous dysplasia when no such changes can be shown.

Albright's syndrome

- Polyostotic fibrous dysplasia
- Melanotic skin pigmentation
- Precocious puberty in females

Metabolic and endocrine disorders

Gigantism and acromegaly

Hypersecretion of growth hormone is usually associated with an adenoma of the anterior pituitary gland. The clinical manifestations of the condition are dependent upon the time of onset of the hypersecretion. In children with open epiphyses, gigantism occurs, leading to generalized overgrowth of the skeleton, organs, and soft tissues. When the epiphyses have fused, overproduction of growth hormone causes acromegaly—only bones with the potential for growth will enlarge. Acromegaly is accompanied by renewed growth of the mandibular condyle, hands, and feet with overgrowth of some soft tissues. Condylar growth results in mandibular prognathism. As a consequence of this, teeth, when present, become spaced. Changes occur in the facial tissues—the

Table 18.4 Acromegaly: orofacial features

Macroglossia
Facial palsy
Mandibular growth
Facial pain
Temporomandibular joint pain
Malocclusion
Proclination of anterior teeth
Increased interdental spaces
Posterior and anterior cross-bites
Hypercementosis
Coarsening of facial features
Skin hyperhidrosis, acne

lips and nose become thickened, resulting in a coarsening of the face. The tongue may also enlarge (macroglossia). Acromegaly is also accompanied by serious systemic complications such as, raised intracranial pressure, headaches, blindness, hypertension, cardiomyopathy, and diabetes mellitus. The orofacial features of acromegaly are summarized in Table 18.4. An enlarged tongue is a commonly reported feature of acromegaly. The dentist may therefore have an important role to play in the diagnosis of the disease (see Chapter 6). Rarely, patients with acromegaly may present with facial pain.

Treatment of acromegaly depends upon the cause of the condition. Ideally, growth hormone levels need to revert to normal. Treatments include surgery (usually transphenoidal resection of the tumour) and radiotherapy to the tumour. Drug therapies (for example, bromocriptine or somatostatin analogues such as octreotide) may also be used. Surgery may also be required to correct some of the skeletal and dental consequences of the disease.

Hyperparathyroidism

Hyperparathyroidism is caused by oversecretion of parathormone (PTH). Parathormone mobilizes calcium from bone to increase the serum calcium levels. This is achieved by increased intestinal absorption of calcium and increased reabsorption of calcium by the renal tubules, but mostly by increased osteoclastic bone resorption.

Primary hyperparathyroidism is usually due to an adenoma of the parathyroid glands. Secondary hyperparathyroidism is increasing in prevalence and is a consequence of chronic depressed plasma calcium levels. This is most frequently due to chronic renal failure (Chapter 13) or longstanding malabsorption (for example, coeliac disease; see Chapter 12). The management of primary hyperparathyroidism is usually surgical. The treatment of secondary hyperparathyroidism is dependent upon treating the cause.

PRIMARY HYPERPARATHYROIDISM

Primary hyperparathyroidism may be mild and asymptomatic but in severe cases may be life-threatening due to uncontrolled hypercalcaemia and renal failure. The condition is frequently diagnosed incidentally when calcium is measured as part of a biochemistry profile—this is generally before there is extensive destruction of the bone. Cyst-like, osteolytic swellings (brown tumours) of the jaws can develop; these are histologically indistinguishable from giant cell granulomas of the jaws. Radiographically, they are well defined radiolucencies and may be multilocular. They occur more frequently in the mandible and the maxilla. In hyperparathyroidism there may be loss of the lamina dura and generalized rarefaction of the jaw bones.

The diagnosis should be confirmed with investigation of blood chemistry, which reveals raised plasma calcium and raised PTH. The plasma phosphate level is often low but may be normal, particularly if there is an element of renal failure. Plasma alkaline phosphatase is only raised when there is bone involvement.

Hypoparathyroidism

This condition is usually iatrogenic, following removal of the parathyroid glands. Early-onset hypoparathyroidism can affect calcified tissues and result in hypoplastic enamel, short roots, and incomplete hypomineralization of dentine (see earlier section on teeth). All of these changes are due to hypocalcaemia.

Osteoporosis

Osteoporosis is a condition in which the skeletal bone structure undergoes degradation both of bone matrix and calcium, that is, a reduction in bone mass per unit volume. Serum biochemistry indices are normal. There is skeletal rarefaction and low trauma fractures often occur, including vertebral fractures. Osteoporosis is probably the most common disease of bone. Women are more likely to be affected than men. In the edentulous patient with osteoporosis the residual alveolar ridges may resorb more rapidly. Osteoporosis may limit the sites available for implant placement and adversely affect the prognosis of endosseous implants. Conversely, the presence of functioning implants may reduce the rate of progression of osteoporosis.

There are many risk factors that have been identified: increasing age, postmenopause (especially early menopause); steroid therapy (Chapter 3); hyperthyroidism and primary hyperparathyroidism; and immobilization. The disease occurs most commonly in postmenopausal females, and hormone replacement therapy can be helpful in prevention and treatment. Biphosphonate therapy is widely used and has been shown to increase bone density and reduce fracture risk.

A well documented iatrogenic cause of osteoporosis is systemic steroid therapy and 50 per cent of patients on prednisolone (5 mg/day or more) for more than 3 months of each year are likely to develop osteoporosis. The prophylaxis of osteoporosis for patients on long-term steroid therapy is fully discussed in Chapter 3.

Rickets and osteomalacia

Rickets is a condition that occurs in children as a result of deficient calcification of the bones and (unusually) the teeth. It is essentially due to lack of vitamin D, because of either nutritional deficiency, malabsorption, or impaired metabolic processes. In this condition the bones are poorly formed and, as a result, badly shaped. It is said that the teeth are not affected in this condition, but in fact, some patients with a history of rickets have signs of hypoplasia of the teeth (Fig. 18.11). Osteomalacia is the adult equivalent of this condition, that is, defective bone mineralization in bone that has stopped growing. Osteomalacia may occur in pregnancy (particularly in those of Asian origin), in malabsorption (such as in coeliac disease), or in renal disease. There is a failure of mineralization during normal bone turnover. Calcium plasma levels tend to be low, phosphate levels can be normal or low, and alkaline phosphatase levels are raised. Osteomalacia is rarely diagnosed in the oral medicine clinic.

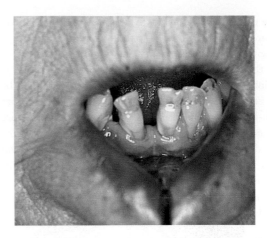

Fig. 18.11 Dental hypoplasia in a patient with a history of rickets.

Disorders of unknown aetiology: Paget's disease

Paget's disease (osteitis deformans) is a widespread condition of old age and is found in a large proportion of older patients at autopsy. Radiographic signs of Paget's disease may be seen in about 3 per cent of the population aged over 40 years—most will be asymptomatic. Paget's disease is similar to fibrous dysplasia, in that both represent an imbalance of the osteogenic and osteolytic processes occurring in bone formation. Activity is not related to physiological requirements and the final result is bone growth. Paget's disease can affect any bone in the body—those most commonly affected are the pelvis, spine, sacrum, femur, tibia, and skull. It often occurs initially in the skull and facial bones. The classic complaint of a patient is that his or her hat has become too tight, but an equally common complaint is of dentures that are becoming 'too small'. The bone growth in Paget's disease particularly affects the vault of the skull and maxilla, although the mandible may also be involved (Fig. 18.12). The expansion of the bone of the base of the skull leads to closure of the foramina and resultant neurological changes such as deafness. Nerve compression may also lead to 'neuralgia-like' symptoms in the trigeminal nerve. This should always be considered as a possible diagnosis in older patients, particularly when there are other symptoms such as deafness. Apart from neuralgia-like symptoms the patient may complain of pain within the bone itself. This is a common symptom known as bone pain. Radiographically, the bone is reputed to have the appearance of cotton wool. There is loss of normal bone trabeculation and, in later stages, areas of sclerosis can be seen—giving rise to the cotton wool appearance. Since cementum is essentially bone, this is also affected by the changes of Paget's disease, and hypercementosis is a common finding in these patients. Malignant change in the affected bone is a reputed complication, although the incidence of osteosarcoma is low and usually occurs in patients with polyostotic Paget's disease. Cardiac failure because of high output into the expanded blood spaces of the bone is a well-recorded, but rare complication.

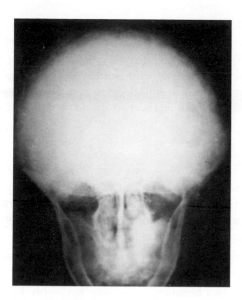

Fig. 18.12 Paget's disease. Radiograph showing expansion of the skull and 'cotton wool' appearance of the bone.

The cause of Paget's disease is unknown. Viral and genetic factors have been implicated. Diagnosis of Paget's disease in the first instance is clinical, confirmed by imaging (radiography and a radioisotope bone scan) and by blood chemistry, the characteristic finding being an increased (sometimes greatly increased) serum alkaline phosphatase level. Other bone markers are often abnormal in Paget's disease. For example, urinary deoxypyridinoline is elevated in active Paget's disease and falls in response to treatment. Patients with suspected Paget's disease are usually referred to a specialist in metabolic bone disease. Bisphosphonates (for example, pamidronate or risedronate) are very effective in the treatment of Paget's disease because of the inhibitory effects this class of drug has on osteoclasts. The net result is a reduction in bone turnover and, consequently, in progression of the disease.

There are a number of important dental considerations when treating patients with Paget's disease. Extraction of teeth may be difficult because of hypercementosis and there may be profuse postoperative haemorrhage because of the irregular and increased blood supply to the new bone. Paget's disease should, if possible, also be rendered biochemically inactive by bisphosphonates prior to surgery, as this will reduce the vascularity of the affected bone. Patients with this condition are also more susceptible to infection following any form of intervention and any extraction or oral surgery procedure should be covered by antibiotic prophylaxis. These problems of haemorrhage and infection lead to great caution in taking biopsies in Paget's disease. Since this is a condition that can be diagnosed by non-interventive means, the question of confirmatory biopsy should be approached with great reserve. A summary of the salient clinical features of Paget's disease is given in Table 18.5.

> Prior to exodontia Paget's disease should be rendered chemically inactive by bisphosphonates—this will reduce the vascularity of the affected bone.

Table 18.5 Summary of clinical features in Paget's disease

Predominantly a disease of later life, rare under 40 years, often asymptomatic
Results in erratic increased bone growth, bone density, and deformation
Skull frequently affected
Hat size becomes too small
Cranial nerve deficits possible
Serum alkaline phosphatase may be elevated
Radiographic features
'Cotton wool appearance'
'Hypercementosis, possible root resorption'
Further dental considerations
Appearance of diastemas between teeth, occlusal derangement, lip incompetence
Dentures become too tight
Possibility of difficult extractions
Risk of postextraction bleeding and/or infection
Can cause facial pain or paralysis

Discussion of problem cases

Case 18.1 Discussion

Q1   What are the differential diagnoses for this boy's dental condition?

The opacities are present on most teeth—therefore it is unlikely that this is chronological hypoplasia. The most likely diagnosis of this 14-year-old's condition is dental fluorosis, but the dentist needs to consider genetic causes such as amelogenesis imperfecta.

Q2   What additional information do you need to help you make a definitive diagnosis?

On rare occasions, it may not be possible to differentiate between fluorosis and amelogenesis imperfecta. However, the information gained by asking the questions below usually allows a definitive diagnosis to be made.

1. Was the primary dentition affected?

2. Do any other members of the family have a similarly affected dentition?

3. Has the patient lived in an area where the water supply was fluoridated or had a naturally high fluoride level?

4. Were fluoride supplements used during the period of calcification of the crowns of the teeth?

The presence of discoloration in the primary dentition would support genetic influences, although the primary dentition is not invariably affected. A hereditary condition is also supported by the occurrence of the condition in a family member who belongs to a different generation or lives in a different geographical area. The presence of enamel opacities in siblings is not a helpful discriminator.

Dental fluorosis is a common enamel defect, resulting from an increase in concentration of fluoride in the microenvironment of ameloblasts during enamel formation. Fluorosis therefore results from systemic intake of fluoride during enamel formation. Investigation of the fluoride history is essential. Levels of fluoride in the water supply can be obtained from the appropriate water supplier. It is also possible that fluorosis could be due to fluoride supplements (toothpaste; fluoride drops, tablets, or mouthwashes).

Case 18.2 Discussion

Q1   What are the possible causes of tooth wear in this case?

Tooth wear usually has a multifactorial aetiology. The clinical signs decribed in case 18.2, however, are highly suggestive of dental erosion. This does not negate the possibility of nutrition and abrasion being important co-destructive aetiologies. A full medical and dental history, including a dietary analysis will be required to try to identify if the acid is dietary or gastric in origin. The intake of food and beverages with erosive potential needs to be assessed. A history of acid reflux and vomiting should also be explored. It should be remembered that gastric reflux may be silent (asymptomatic) and that patients may not admit to self-induced vomiting.

Q2   What condition would you suspect if the patient also presented with swollen parotid glands and appeared to have generalized skeletal muscle wastage?

A patient who presents with dental erosion, enlarged parotid glands, and generalized muscle wastage is likely to have an eating disorder, and bulimia nervosa should be suspected.

Projects

1   List the disorders of teeth that you are likely to see in patients. Divide these disorders into: (a) those with a prenatal and postnatal aetiology; (b) those that are congenital or acquired conditions.

2   Identify the different causes and clinical presentations of tooth discoloration.

3   Undertake a literature search using key words 'Paget's disease' and 'dentistry'. What are the different ways in which patients present with undiagnosed symptomatic Paget's disease to dental, oral medicine, or maxillofacial clinics? What are the problems in managing a dental patient who has a diagnosis of Paget's disease?

19

Medical emergencies in dentistry

The prevention of medical emergencies

Administration of drugs
- Routes of administration of drugs

Emergency drugs and equipment

Management of emergencies

Medical emergencies in dentistry

Life-threatening emergencies are rare but can occur at any time in dental practice. Dentists must be able to provide acutely ill patients with life-saving measures prior to the arrival of specialist help. It is essential, therefore, that they are trained in the management of medical emergencies that they might precipitate or encounter.

Medical emergencies that may be encountered in dental practice and that require prompt management

- Vasovagal attack
- Seizures
- Angina
- Asthma attack
- Hypoglycaemia
- Myocardial infarction
- Anaphylaxis
- Cardiac arrest

The prevention of medical emergencies

Medical emergencies are usually unexpected but rarely occur without warning. The decline in a patient's health whilst in the dental chair is likely to be preceded by signs and symptoms and early recognition of an unwell or deteriorating patient can sometimes abort an acute problem.

Dentists examine and treat a population of patients with variable health status. Advances in medical care and a trend for longevity means that an increasing number of medically compromised patients present for dental care. It is important that the risks associated with the management of these patients are assessed. A detailed medical history is of paramount importance. When assessing the significance of a patient's medical problems, it is helpful to consider the following questions.

- What are the effects, if any, of the medical condition(s) on the proposed treatment?

- What effect will the proposed treatment have on the disease?

- Are adverse drug reactions or interactions anticipated?

It is not possible to be familiar with all significant drug interactions and the clinician should have immediate access to a regularly updated reference text, such as the *British National Formulary*. Another invaluable source of advice, in the UK, is the Drug Information Service, which has a unit dedicated to the management of drug-related problems associated with dental treatment.

Dental patients may become severely anxious and experience acute somatic symptoms prior to, or during dental treatment. A panic attack is an extreme acute manifestation of this. Physiological and psychological stressors may present a serious risk to a medically compromised patient. Methods of pain and anxiety control are of paramount importance in the management of medically compromised patients. For example, in a dental phobic who suffers from hypertension and angina, it is important to ameliorate a patient's physiological response to anxiety-provoking procedures—the use of sedation can be beneficial in this situation.

An awareness of potential problems or complications associated with medical conditions can sometimes prevent a critical incident. For example, hypoglycaemia is an acute complication of both type 1 and 2 diabetes mellitus. The timing of dental appointments should be discussed with the patient so that they are compatible with the patient's diabetic management, allowing adherence to usual eating schedules. If a dental procedure (for example, multiple extractions) is likely to result in dietary restrictions, consultation with the patient's physician or dietitian may, on occasions, be advisable. However, in many diabetics, it is the patient who has the required expert knowledge.

Dentists use local anaesthetics on a daily basis and these agents have an excellent safety record. It is, however, important that clinicians do not become complacent about their side-effects and toxicity. The maximum recommended dosage of a local anaesthetic must not be exceeded and caution should be exercised when using more than one preparation. It should also be remembered that topical anaesthetics such as lidocaine gels or mouthwashes will be absorbed and will, therefore, contribute to drug levels in the systemic circulation. The maximum safe dose of local anaesthetics should be significantly reduced in patients who have concurrent disease, are on certain medications, or are very young or elderly.

When considering the maximum dose of local anaesthetic consider the following.

Patient factors
Age
Weight
Vascularity of the tissues being anaesthetized
Concurrent disease
The local anaesthetic
Anaesthetic agent
Concentration
Manufacturer's instructions
Vasoconstrictor

Circulatory collapse has been reported in patients undergoing surgical procedures and this has rarely been attributed to adrenal insufficiency that has resulted from steroid therapy. Some authors advocate that patients who are taking steroids regularly or have done so within the past 6 months should receive a pretreatment dose of steroid or double their daily dose perioperatively. The use of steroid cover is a contentious issue and pretreatment protocols are not universally accepted. It is the authors' opinion that the role of steroid prophylaxis for dental procedures has, in the past, been overstated. Evidence-based research is required to settle this debate.

The recognition of the unwell patient and the assessment of his or her suitability for treatment are important skills for a clinician to develop. Dentists will only encounter a limited number of emergencies and all of these can result in the collapse of the cardiovascular system. Therefore, it is essential that dentists regularly update their knowledge on the prevention and management of relevant medical emergencies. The best way of addressing this is by having regular scenario training with all of the dental team. Whilst rehearsal of basic life support using manikins is mandatory for any clinician, respiratory and cardiac arrest should not be the only emergencies that are the subject of scenario training. It should also be remembered that collapse may occur anywhere on the premises and may affect a member of staff or a companion of a patient. It is not always possible, therefore, to have immediate access to the medical history of the casualty.

> Dentists have an ethical and professional duty to be cognizant of appropriate guidelines for the management of acute medical problems that might occur—they also need to have the skills and resources to follow this guidance.

When assessing the risks that are associated with treating a patient it can be helpful to grade the level of systemic disease that a patient has in terms of how that condition limits the daily activities of a patient. The American Society of Anesthesiologists (ASA) classification for fitness for anaesthesia can be helpful in assessing the significance of a patient's medical condition (Table 19.1). This

Clinical risk management

Clinical risk management is a systematic process for the identification, analysis, and control of adverse events or potential risks. Clinicians should always:

- take a full documented medical history;
- be aware of possible adverse reactions (if unsure seek expert advice);
- know the principles in the prevention and management of medical emergencies;
- regularly rehearse and develop the management of emergencies with the dental team and record all training sessions;
- be familiar with their working environment;
- ensure that regular checks are carried out on emergency equipment and the expiry dates of emergency drugs; these checks should be recorded.

Table 19.1 Classifications of the American Society of Anesthesiologists (ASA)

Classification	Description
I	Fit and well
II	Mild systemic disease that does not interfere with day to day activity (e.g. well controlled asthma)
III	Moderate to severe systemic disease that is limiting but not incapacitating. Day to day activity may be altered (e.g. well-controlled insulin-dependent diabetes mellitus, angina pectoris, chronic bronchitis). The medical status may be upset by treatment
IV	Severe systemic disease that is a constant threat to life; the disease is severely limiting and incapacitating (e.g. unstable angina, severe haemophilia). The medical condition is unstable and unpredictable
V	Moribund, not expected to survive 24 hours

system is also used by dental sedationists for patient assessment. It is unlikely that a patient who is ASA I or II will require any modifications to dental treatment whilst a patient who is ASA III may have a significant drug history and may be susceptible to potential drug interactions.

Administration of drugs

There are several routes available for the administration of emergency drugs and these are expanded upon in Table 19.2. It is worth noting that some routes are more useful than others and it is the first four techniques that have most relevance to dental practice. Drugs can be administered via an enteral or parenteral route. Enteral routes require that a drug is absorbed from the gastrointestinal tract. This includes drugs that are delivered by buccal, oral, or rectal administration.

Table 19.2 Routes of drug administration

Route	Onset of action	Example
Oral	30–120 min	Aspirin, glucose
Inhalation	1–5 min	Oxygen, nitrous oxide, salbutamol
Sublingual/buccal	1–2min	GTN, glucose gel
Intramuscular	5–15 min	Adrenaline (epinephrine; for anaphylaxis) Glucagon
Subcutaneous	15–20 min	Hydrocortisone
Intravenous	20–30 s	Adrenaline (epinephrine ; for cardiac arrest) Diazepam
Rectal	6–20 min	Diazepam suppositories
Intratracheal	1–5 min	Adrenaline (epinephrine)
Intraosseous	Up to 5 min	Adrenaline (epinephrine)

Routes of drug administration

Oral administration

The onset of action of a drug is usually slow following oral administration and can be adversely affected by the presence of food and the low pH. Oral administration is only suitable for the conscious patient and is not appropriate for the majority of drugs used in medical emergencies. There are, however, two acute situations when the use of an orally administered drug may prevent serious sequelae. Aspirin should be used as soon as possible in the post-myocardial infarction patient and glucose should be given in the conscious hypoglycaemic patient.

Inhalation administration

The onset of action following the administration of an inhaled drug is very rapid. Oxygen and bronchodilators such as salbutamol are used successfully by this method. Whereas in a conscious patient supplementary oxygen is usually given at a flow rate of 2–6 l/min, in resuscitation procedures a minimum flow rate of 8–12 l/min is used.

Sublingual and buccal administration

Drugs given by the buccal or sublingual routes are absorbed rapidly across the mucosa which is highly vascularized. These routes are particularly useful when a significant proportion of the drug is metabolized by the liver when it initially enters the hepatic circulation. This is referred to as the 'first-pass' effect. Glyceryl trinitrate (GTN) has a significant 'first-pass' effect and is ineffective when swallowed—nearly 100 per cent of it is immediately metabolized by the liver after absorption from the alimentary tract. It is essential, therefore, that patients do not swallow tablets that are intended for absorption across the oral mucosa.

Intramuscular (IM) administration

The intramuscular route has a slower rate of onset of action than intravenous (IV) administration and is greatly influenced by the local tissue perfusion. The mid-deltoid region of the upper arm is a good site for an IM injection because it is easily accessible and is well perfused. The tongue is often cited as a convenient place for the intramuscular administration of emergency drugs. However, local bleeding and possible swelling could exacerbate airway problems and, as a consequence, this technique is not advocated by the authors.

Intramuscular administration is the route of choice for adrenaline (epinephrine) in anaphylaxis. Hydrocortisone, glucagon, and chlorpheniramine may be given by the IM route if IV access is not possible. The maximum volume that can be given at any one injection site is usually 5 ml. However, this is unlikely to be relevant to dentists in an emergency situation.

Subcutaneous (SC) administration

The subcutaneous route involves placing a drug in the adipose tissue beneath the dermis. The onset of action of drugs given subcutaneously is much slower than for drugs given by the IM route, because adipose tissue is usually poorly perfused.

Intravenous (IV) administration

Intravenous access allows a drug to be administered quickly and reliably. It is the preferred route of drug administration in advanced life support. The most frequently used method of achieving secure venous access is with a plastic cannula mounted over a needle. The needle is removed once the cannula is correctly located. The size of cannula depends upon whether it is to be used for rapid fluid administration (when a large diameter is indicated) or for drug administration alone (in which case smaller-gauge cannulae can be used). In an emergency situation the largest vein and cannula available should be used. A metal butterfly needle is not recommended, as venous access is not secure.

The superficial veins in the arm are most frequently used to site an IV cannula. Intravenous drug administration requires specialist skills and regular practice. Many dentists do not undertake IV cannulation on a routine basis and would be unlikely to gain vascular access in an emergency situation when the venous circulation may be compromised.

Rectal administration

The absorption of drugs from the rectum is similar to that obtained following the intramuscular administration of a drug. This route can be beneficial when a drug is broken down by gastric and intestinal enzymes or is pH-sensitive, and also when a patient cannot take medication orally. In poorly controlled epileptics, especially patients with learning disabilities, diazepam administered rectally may be used to control seizures.

Tracheal administration

It is not always possible to obtain intravenous access in a collapsed patient. This can be particularly problematic in intra-

Table 19.3 Emergency drugs: indications for use and mechanisms of action*

Drug	Indications (dose)	Mechanism of action	Comments
Oxygen	Any medical emergency	To supplement oxygen intake and prevent cerebral hypoxia	Oxygen can be used in most emergencies
Adrenaline[†] (IM) 1:1000 (1mg/ml)	Anaphylactic shock (0.5mg, repeated at 5 min intervals if required)	This directly acting sympathomimetic amine has α- and β-adrenergic activity. The α-agonist activity reverses peripheral vasodilatation and preserves blood flow to essential organs. The β-activity relaxes bronchial smooth muscle (dilates the airways), increases coronary blood flow and the force of myocardial contraction, and suppresses histamine and leukotriene release	IM route is much more effective than the SC route
Adrenaline[†] (IV) 1:10 000 (1mg/10ml)	Cardiac arrest (1 mg repeated every 3 min)	This directly acting sympathomimetic amine has α- and β-adrenergic activity. The objective is to increase cerebral and coronary perfusion	IV route preferred
Glucagon (IM)	Diabetic hypoglycaemia (unconscious) (1mg)	This polypeptide hormone increases serum glucose by mobilizing glycogen stores	IV or SC routes can be used, but very few dentists are skilled in IV access and absorption is delayed with the SC route
Salbutamol (inhaler)	Asthma (100 μg)	β$_2$-adrenergic agonist activity relaxes bronchial smooth muscle	
Glyceryl trinitrate spray (sublingual)	Cardiac/chest pain (400 μg metered dose)	Vasodilatation of the coronary arteries occurs	
Glucose (oral)	The conscious hypoglycaemic patient	Rapid absorption elevates serum glucose levels	Glucose gels for rapid buccal absorption are available
Diazepam (IV)	Status epilepticus (10 mg)	Benzodiazepine that facilitates the action of γ-aminobutyric acid (an inhibitory neurotransmitter)	Caution: slow IV injection, risk of respiratory depression. Other anticonvulsants may be required
Chlorphenamine (IV)	Adjunctive treatment for anaphylaxis (10–20 mg)	Helps reverse histamine-mediated vasodilatation	Slow IV injection, can give IM. This is a second-line drug
Hydrocortisone (IV)	Adjunctive treatment for anaphylaxis Adrenal shock (200 mg)	Helps reduce late sequelae of anaphylaxis by reducing capillary permeability, reducing leukocyte and macrophage migration and inhibiting the mediators of inflammation	Can give IM
Aspirin (oral)	Myocardial infarction (150–300 mg)	Anti-platelet action decreases platelet aggregation; antithrombotic effect reduces mortality after cardiac infarction	If given, inform paramedics/hospital staff
Solvents (e.g. water)		Solvents may be required to dissolve drugs that are presented as powder (e.g. glucagon, hydrocortisone)	

* Drug protocols are constantly being updated and modified as new scientific information becomes available. It is the duty of the clinician to keep up to date with current guidance. Only adult doses are given in this table.

† Adrenaline is also known as epinephrine.

venous drug abusers and patients who have severe hypovolaemia. Adrenaline (epinephrine), atropine, and lidocaine can be successfully administered by the intratracheal route. It is implicit in this technique that the patient has been intubated with an endotracheal tube. A laryngeal mask airway will not facilitate the intratracheal administration of drugs.

Intraosseous administration

This route is often used in paediatric resuscitation. It can be useful in adults when no other method of access is possible. A special cannula is usually inserted into the medullary cavity of the tibia—aspiration of bone marrow indicates correct positioning. Administration of drugs must be followed by a flush of fluid.

Emergency drugs and equipment

There are often local, regional, and national variations in the guidance issued relating to which emergency drugs should be kept in a dental surgery. Clinicians should exercise their professional judgement in the light of current practice and the relevant contemporaneous guidelines and recommendations from authoritative bodies. Practitioners need to assess the drugs most appropriate to their needs and this will be influenced by the type of practice they have. For example, additional drugs will be required if intravenous sedation or general anaesthesia is undertaken on the premises.

The clinician needs to be familiar with the preparation and administration of drugs in an emergency situation. A single drug is often available in several presentations—for example, hydrocortisone is available as a powder for reconstitution with water or as a liquid in a glass ampoule or a preloaded syringe. Some emergency drugs are available in preloaded syringes and these have several advantages. They require the minimum of preparation (this can save valuable time), can reduce the possibility of operator error, and simplify training protocols. It is prudent to ensure that all emergency drugs are capable of a natural rubber latex-free delivery. The frequently recommended drugs for use in the dental surgery in an emergency are given in Table 19.3. The mechanisms of action of the drugs are also briefly summarized. There is merit in dentists only carrying drugs that are essential for the first-line management of acute medical problems. It is the authors' opinion that the following drugs are the most useful, first-line drugs for the immediate management of an emergency: oxygen, adrenaline (1mg/ml), salbutamol inhaler, GTN, glucose for oral administration, and glucagon. Table 19.4 lists emergency equipment that should be present in a dental surgery. This list is a guide and is not intended to be exhaustive.

This chapter has not taken into account drugs that are used in sedation. If sedation with benzodiazepines is carried out, then flumazenil should be readily available in case the patient has been oversedated. It should also be remembered that a combination of 50 per cent nitrous oxide with 50 per cent oxygen may be a useful analgesic and anxiolytic in a patient, post myocardial infarction.

Table 19.4 Emergency equipment required in the dental surgery*

Pocket mask†
Self-inflating bag, valve, and mask with reservoir†
Oropharyngeal airways‡
Nasopharyngeal airways‡
Oxygen therapy masks
Tubing and appropriate connectors to attach oxygen cylinders to oxygen masks
Syringes and needles to deliver drugs by a parenteral route in an emergency
IV cannulae and adhesive tape
Independently powered portable suction apparatus with wide-bore aspiration tips.
Blood pressure monitor§

* Equipment should be free from natural rubber latex.
† These will allow the provision of intermittent positive pressure ventilation to the lungs.
‡ A range of sizes should be available.
§ This has not usually been recommended as an essential item. However, it may be helpful in the assessment of the unwell patient.

It is the responsibility of the dentist to ensure that regular checks are undertaken on all emergency equipment and emergency drugs. These checks should be recorded.

Management of emergencies

Table 19.5 details the management of medical emergencies that may occur in dental practice. Fainting (vasovagal attack, syncope) is the most frequently encountered cause of collapse in dental practice. The brief loss of consciousness that occurs in fainting is due to an abrupt fall in cardiac output that leads to a reduction in cerebral blood flow. The dental team should recognize the characteristic signs that precede collapse and take appropriate action—sometimes this may prevent loss of consciousness. It should be remembered that, occasionally, syncope may not have a benign cause and can be associated with serious cardiac dysrhythmias or a transient ischaemic attack (mini-stroke).

Algorithms for cardiopulmonary resuscitation are constantly being revised and the clinician needs to be aware of current protocols. Table 19.6 outlines the basic procedure for the assessment and management of the collapsed patient. When a patient has lost consciousness the clinician needs to constantly assess and monitor the patient's airway, breathing, and circulation. This sequence of actions is often abbreviated to 'ABC', and this acts as an *aide-mémoire*. This enables the clinician to quickly ascertain if the patient is breathing and still has a cardiac output. If the patient has suffered a respiratory or cardiac arrest, then specialist help is urgently required. In the meantime the dental team must perform cardiopulmonary resuscitation to ensure some cerebral blood flow. This will hopefully prevent irreversible hypoxic brain

Table 19.5 Medical emergencies and their management

Causes	Signs	Management
Faint		
Transient hypotension and cerebral ischaemia	Weakness, dizziness, pallor, sweating, nausea, confusion, tachycardia followed by a bradycardia, loss of consciousness.	Place patient in a supine position with the legs elevated above the level of the heart to improve cerebral flow
Predisposing factors include hypoglycaemia, anxiety, fear, pain, and fatigue	Minor convulsions or incontinence can occur.	A patient who is sitting may lower their head by placing it between their knees, this is not as effective as lying a patient down. Lay a pregnant patient on her side. Administer oxygen. Reassure the recovering patient, a glucose-rich drink may be helpful. When a member of the dental team recognizes that a patient is likely to faint the patient should be placed in a supine position—this may prevent loss of consciousness. If the patient fails to regain consciousness promptly other causes of loss of consciousness must be considered.
Hypoglycaemia		
Anxiety, infection	Cold and clammy skin, trembling. Irritability, confused, aggression, and uncooperative behaviour. Drowsiness and disorientation.	*Conscious*: glucose drink, tablets or gel *Unconscious*: intramuscular glucagon (1 mg/ml) or an IV glucose infusion (25 ml of 50% solution). Administer oxygen Always monitor patient and maintain airway. Transfer to hospital.
Epileptic seizure		
Known epileptic Poorly controlled or non-compliance with drug regime Stress, hypoglycaemia; may accompany a faint. Overdose of local anaesthetic may cause seizures.	Loss of consciousness Muscle rigidity followed by jerking movements; incontinence may occur. Confusion may be present during recovery	Protect from injury (remove potentially harmful objects, use pillows around patient if these aid their protection). Administer oxygen and maintain airway if possible. If the patient can be discharged home, ensure that they are accompanied—they might have post-ictal confusion. Status epilepticus is probable if seizure continues in excess of 7 minutes; therefore emergency services should be called. If status epilepticus is diagnosed diazepam (up to 10 mg) by slow IV injection may be given; it is not always efficacious
Asthma		
Pre-existing disease that is poorly controlled, anxiety, infection, exercise, exposure to an antigen	Breathlessness with wheezing on expiration. If untreated, breathing may become increasingly difficult	Salbutamol inhaler or nebulizer and oxygen. Place the patient in a comfortable position. If there is no improvement summon emergency services Hydrocortisone IV or IM may be given Status asthmaticus is a life-threatening condition
Chest pain		
Angina, myocardial infarction	Usually a crushing retrosternal pain, irregular pulse, may experience breathlessness, nausea, or vomiting	Sublingual GTN, oxygen, Place patient in a comfortable position—consult with the patient. In a patient with a known history of angina ask if the symptoms are typical. Call emergency services if pain does not subside in 3 minutes (possibility of a myocardial infarction (MI)). Possible administration of oral aspirin (300 mg) if MI suspected; nitrous oxide and oxygen, if available, can be helpful to reduce pain and anxiety. Monitor. If loss of consciousness follow the protocol for cardiopulmonary resuscitation.
Hyperventilation		
Stress, pain, or expectation of pain. This is often a response to unfocused fears. Can be associated with chronic generalized anxiety disorder	Rapid breathing, tachycardia, trembling, dizzy, faint, sweating Paraesthesia, muscle pain/stiffness Can lead to tetany. Patients can complain of chest pain	Reassure Ensure comfortable position Stop treatment Rebreathe expired air

Table 19.5 Medical emergencies and their management *continued*

Causes	Signs	Management
Anaphylaxis		
Exposure to an antigen to which the patient has been sensitized, commonly drugs (most notably penicillins) or natural rubber latex. Anaphylaxis to local anaesthetic is extremely rare	Initial flushing of the skin may occur followed by oedema of the head and neck. Altered sensations such as paraesthesia around mouth and fingers. Pallor, cyanosis will accompany acute breathing difficulties with bronchospasm and/or severe hypotension. Loss of consciousness and cardiac arrest can occur	Lay flat, elevate legs Maintain airway and administer oxygen Call expert assistance Immediate adrenaline (0.5 ml of 1:1000) IM; repeat if necessary Hydrocortisone and chlorphenamine are 2nd-line drugs
Cerebrovascular accident		
Ischaemia, haemorrhage, or embolism in a cerebral artery	A stroke (partial or total weakness on one side of the body), dysarthria, aphasia, hemiplegia, and possible loss of consciousness	Lay flat and administer oxygen, maintain airway, monitor Summon expert help.
Local anaesthetic toxicity		
Overdose	Lightheadedness; visual or hearing disturbances. Agitation, confusion, seizures, respiratory distress. Loss of consciousness, respiratory and cardiac arrest.	Administer oxygen, maintain a comfortable position Call emergency services Monitor patient
Adrenal shock (Addisonian crisis)		
Stress in a patient who has adrenal suppression (e.g. induced by disease or long term steroid therapy)	Pallor, rapid weak pulse, rapidly falling blood pressure, loss of consciousness	Lay patient flat. Administer oxygen, 200 mg hydrocortisone (IV is the preferred route but IM can be used) Summon expert help. This is rare—consider other causes
Respiratory arrest		
Status asthmaticus, airway obstruction	No breathing; central pulse present (initially)	Follow basic life support algorithm for rescue breathing. If untreated, will become a cardiac arrest
Cardiac arrest		
Myocardial infarction Circulatory collapse Anaphylaxis Hypoxia Respiratory arrest	Unconscious; no central pulse	Follow basic life support algorithm; this will involve assessment of responsiveness, airway, breathing, and circulation (ABC). Expert assistance should be summoned as soon as possible to ensure early defibrillation (if indicated) and administration of emergency drug (advanced life support algorithms)

Some authorities suggest that an IV benzodiazepine should be given to the patient who has seizures following overdose of local anaesthetic. This is not advised because it carries the risk of respiratory depression

Table 19.6 Assessment and management of the collapsed adult patient.

Assess	Action	Comments
Is the patient conscious?	If yes, is expert help required? If no, call for help from staff	Ensure that it is safe to approach before assessing the patient
Airway	Establish and maintain airway*	Is there debris to remove from the mouth?
Breathing (look, listen, and feel)	If breathing, is expert help required? If not breathing, call emergency services† and start artificial ventilation‡	
Circulation	If yes, continue with ventilation If no, start external cardiac compressions	Palpate a major pulse (e.g. carotid pulse)

* An endotracheal tube or laryngeal mask airway should only be used if the operator is skilled in their use.

† If a person is available send them to meet the emergency team at the entrance to the building or clinic.

‡ Positive pressure ventilations should ideally be undertaken with a self-inflating bag connected to oxygen. A single rescuer may prefer to use expired air with a pocket mask attached to an oxygen supply.

damage. In the event of a cardiac arrest, a successful outcome is greatly influenced by the early application of advanced life support skills. The majority of primary adult cardiac arrests present in ventricular fibrillation and patient survival is dependent upon early defibrillation.

Projects

1. Patients who require specialist care following their medical emergency will need to be transferred to an appropriate unit. In the UK paramedics will transfer the patients. Specify what information you would need to give in the 'hand-over' of the patient to the emergency/specialist care team.

2. Identify the expert committees/panels that issue advice on the emergency drugs and equipment that should be held at your dental practice. Ascertain how frequently the drugs and equipment are checked in the clinical environment in which you work.

Appendix

These mouthwashes should be kept in the refrigerator. The shelf-life of mouthwashes is approximately 2 weeks.

Chlortetracycline mouthwash

Formulary. To make 200 ml (10 ml tds), use:

- chlortetracycline, 4 g
- mucilage of tragacanth, 50 ml
- distilled water to 200 ml

  Monitor patient for oral candidosis.

Triamcinolone (plain) mouthwash

Formulary. To make 200 ml (10 ml tds) use:

- triamcinolone for the concentration required (see following table)
- mucilage of tragacanth, 50 ml
- distilled water to 200 ml

Concentration	Amount of steroid
0.25 mg	5 mg triamcinolone
0.5 mg	10 mg triamcinolone
0.75 mg	15 mg triamcinolone
1.0 mg	20 mg triamcinolone
2.0 mg	40 mg triamcinolone

Monitor the patient for oral candidosis. Systemic absorption of this mouthwash is likely, particularly in cases of widespread oral ulceration and at high concentration of steroid.

Triamcinolone with 2 per cent chlortetracycline mouthwash

Formulary. To make 200 ml (10 ml tds), follow the instructions for triamcinolone plain but add 4 g chlortetracycline.

Monitor for oral candidosis. Systemic absorption is likely, particularly in cases of widespread oral ulceration and at high concentration of steroid.

Suggestions for further reading and reference sources

Books

- Oral Pathology: JV Soames and JC Southam, 3rd Edition, Oxford University Press (1988).
- Medical Problems in Dentistry: C Scully, RA Cawson, 4th Edition, Wright (1998).
- Oral Diseases: C Scully, S Flint, SR Porter, M Dunitz, 2nd Edition (1996).
- Colour Atlas of Oral Diseases: G Laskaris Thieme 2nd Edition (1994).
- Colour Atlas of Oral Medicine: William R Tyldesley, 2nd Edition, Mosby-Wolfe (1994).
- Essentials of Microbiology for Dental Students: T Bagg, TW MacFarlane, IR Poxton, CH Miller, AJ Smith, Oxford University Press (1999).
- Textbook of Dermatology: A Rook, DS Wilkinson, FGJ Ebling (Editor). 5th Edition (4 volumes) Blackwell Scientific Publications, Oxford (1992).

(NB Please consult the most up-to-date edition.)

Journals:

- Oral Diseases
- Oral Oncology
- Oral Medicine and Pathology
- Oral Medicine, Oral Surgery, Oral Pathology and Oral Radiology
- Critical Reviews in Oral Biology and Oral Medicine

Useful Website Addresses:

- Cochrane Collaboration – http://www.cochrane.org
- Cochrane Oral Health Group contains link to OHG abstracts without searching the whole Cochrane Library – http://www.cochrane-oral.man.ac.uk
- Clinical Evidence – http://www.clinicalevidence.com

Index

acantholysis 8
acanthosis 8
acromegaly 225
actinic cheilitis 66
acute necrotizing ulcerative gingivitis 32–3
Addison's disease 159–60
adrenaline 234
adrenocortical diseases 159–60
Albright's syndrome 225
alcohol consumption, and oral carcinoma 116
alcoholism 213–14
allergic cheilitis 66
amalgam tattoos 106
amelogenesis imperfecta 222–3
anaemias 153–6
analgesics, topical 25, 57
angina bullosa haemorrhagica 136
angioedema 168
angiomatous naevi 103
angular cheilitis 40, 63–5
angular stomatitis 40, 63–5
ankyloglossia 67
antibiotics
  oral reactions to 169–70
  topical 25–6, 57
antidepressants 209
antifungal agents 37
antiseptics, topical 25, 57
arthroscopy 196
aspirin 234
aspirin burn 169
atrophy 8
atypia 8
atypical facial pain 206–7
auriculotemporal syndrome 186
autoimmunity 169
azathioprine 27

bacterial infections 32–5
bacteriology 20
basement membrane 5
Behçet's disease 58–9
Bell's palsy 187–8
benign intraepithelial dyskeratosis 104
benign migratory glossitis 70
benzydamine 25
betel chewing, and oral carcinoma 116

betel-chewers' mucosa 115
biopsy 19–20, 87
blood disorders 153–8
blood examination 16–17
bone disorders 223–7
bruxism 195
burning mouth syndrome 207–8

C1 esterase inhibitor deficiency 168–9
calcium-channel blockers, and gingival
  overgrowth 171
Candida spp., see oral candidosis
candidal leukoplakia 114
carbamazepine 181
cervical lymphadenopathy 77–9
cheilitis granulomatosa 146–7
cheilocandidosis 67
cheilosis 40, 63–5
chickenpox 42
chlorhexidine 25
chlorphenamine 234
chlortetracycline mouthwash 239
chronic mucocutaneous candidosis syndromes
  40
chronic orofacial pain 206–10
chronic renal failure 161
ciclosporin, and gingival overgrowth 171
cleidocranial dysplasia 223–4
clinical chemistry 17
cluster headache 184–5
coated tongue 68
coeliac disease 143–4
coeliac sprue 143–4
cognitive behavioural therapy 209–10
computerized tomography 22
connective tissue diseases 136
corium 5
corticosteroids
  oral reactions to 170
  systemic 27
  topical 26, 57–8
covering agents 25, 57
coxsackievirus 44
crenated tongue 68
cretinism 160
Crohn's disease 145
Cushing's syndrome 160

Darier's disease 104
delusional symptoms 211–12
dentine, disturbances of 221–2
dentinogenesis imperfecta 223
denture granuloma 103
denture-induced stomatitis 39
dermatitis herpetiformis 134
desquamative gingivitis 9
developmental lesions 103–4
developmental white lesions 103–4
diabetes mellitus 160–1
diagnosis 22
diazepam 234
diet, and oral carcinoma 116–17
digital radiography 21–2
disc displacement with reduction 199
disc displacement without reduction 199–200
discoid lupus erythematosus 137
drug administration 232–5
drug dependency 213–14
drug reactions 169–71
dyskeratosis congenita 104
dysmorphophobia 212

eating disorders 213
enamel hypocalcification 223
enamel hypoplasia 221–2
endocrine disturbances 159–61
endocrine function 18–19
epidermolysis bullosa 134–5
epidermolysis bullosa acquisita 135
Epstein-Barr virus 43–4
epulides 101–2
erythema migrans 70
erythema multiforme 135–6
erythematous candidosis 38
erythroplakia 113
exfoliative cheilitis 66
extrapyramidal syndromes 189

facial nerve deficits 186
facial nerve supply 176–7
facial pain 175–7
facial swelling 77
fibroepithelial polyp 102
fibrous dysplasia 224–5

fixed drug eruptions 171
fluorosis 222
focal epithelial hyperplasia 103
foliate papillae, enlargement of 69
Fordyce's spots 5
Frey's syndrome 186
frictional keratosis 105
fungal infections 35–40

gastro-oesophageal reflux disorder 148–9
gastrointestinal disease 143–9
geographic tongue 70
giant cell arteritis 185–6
gigantism 225
gingival hyperplasia 170
gingival infections 31–47
glossopharyngeal neuralgia 182–3
glucagon 234
glucose 234
gluten-sensitive enteropathy 143–4
glyceryl trinitrate 234
gonorrhoea 34
gumma 33

haematology 16–17, 18
haemolytic anaemias 154–5
Hailey-Hailey disease 131
hairy leukoplakia 46
hairy tongue 68–9
halitosis 72
hamartomas 103
Heck's disease 103
herpes gingivostomatitis 41–2
herpes simplex virus 41–2
herpetiform ulceration 54
HIV, see human immunodeficiency virus
human immunodeficiency virus 45–6
  salivary gland disease 89
human papillomavirus 45
Hutchinson's incisors 34
hydrocortisone 234
hyperkeratosis 8
hyperparathyroidism 225
hyperplastic candidosis 38–9
hypersensitivity 168
hyperthyroidism 160
hypodontia 219–20
hypoparathyroidism 226
hypothyroidism 160

idiopathic oral blood blisters 136
imaging 21–2
immunobullous disease 130–5
immunodeficiency 167–8
immunological tests 17–18
inflammatory bowel disease 144–5
inflammatory overgrowths 101–3
internal derangement 198–9

investigations 15–22
iron deficiency anaemia 154

Kaposi's sarcoma 46
keratinocytes 3–4
keratohyalin granules 4
Köbner phenomenon 126

Langerhans cells 3, 5
Laugier-Hunziker syndrome 106
leukaemia 79, 156–7
leukoedema 105–6
leukopenia 157
leukoplakia 111–13
lichen planus 115, 126–30
  aetiology 126–7
  management 129–30
  oral 127–30
  skin 126
lichenoid drug eruptions 129
lichenoid reactions 129
lick eczema 67
lidocaine 25
linear IgA disease 134
lingual papillae 4
lip carcinoma 116–17
lip fissures 65–6
lips
  diseases of 63–7
  swelling 63
lupus erythematosus 137
lymph nodes, examination 78
lymphoma 46, 79

macroglossia 67
magnetic resonance imaging 22, 86
major recurrent aphthous stomatitis 53–4
masseteric hypertrophy 200–1
measles 44
median rhomboid glossitis 40, 70–1
medical emergencies 231–8
  drug administration 232–5
  emergency drugs and equipment 235
  management of 235–8
  prevention of 231–2
megaloblastic anaemias 154
melanocytes 3, 5
melanoma 107
melanotic pigmentation 106–7
Melkersson-Rosenthal syndrome 146–7, 188
menopause 159
Merkel cells 3
microbiological investigations 20–1
migraine 183–4
minor recurrent aphthous stomatitis 52–3
mixed connective tissue disease 138
monostotic fibrous dysplasia 224
Moon's molars 34

morphoea 137–8
mucocutaneous disease 125–30
mucous membrane pemphigoid 133–4
mulberry molars 34
multiple sclerosis 188–9
mumps 44
mycology 21
myelodysplastic syndromes 157

neck, swelling 77
necrotizing sialometaplasia 88
neoplasia
  oral 115–22
  salivary glands 89–90
  secondary 79
neoplasms, benign 104–5
neurological disturbances 186–9
neuropathic pain 177–83
nicotinic stomatitis 105
non-specific urethritis 35
normocytic anaemias 155
nutritional deficiencies 158
nutritional disorders 158–9
nutritional status, and oral carcinoma 116–17

odontalgia, atypical 207
oedema 8
oral candidosis 35–40
  HIV infection 45–6
oral carcinoma 115–22
  aetiology 115–17
  clinical features and diagnosis 117–18
  as genetic disease 119–21
  management 118–19
  prevention of 119
  staging 118
oral epithelial naevus 104
oral epithelium 3–5
oral mucosa 3–9
  abnormal 6–8
  age changes 6
  function 5–6
  in generalized disease 8
  infections of 31–47
  normal 3–6
  pigmentation of 106–7
  structure 3–5
oral submucous fibrosis 114–15
oral dysaesthesia 207–8
orofacial granulomatosis 145–8
orthokeratinization 4
osteoarthrosis 200
osteomalacia 226
osteoporosis 226
osteoradionecrosis 118–19

pachyonchia congenita 104
Paget's disease 226–7

palmoplantar keratoderma 104
paraesthesia 186–7
paramyxovirus 44
Paterson-Kelly syndrome 115
patient assessment 13–15
pemphigoid 132–4
pemphigus 130–2
periodontal disease, HIV infection 46
periodontium in generalized disease 8–9
perioral dermatitis 67
perlèche 40, 63–5
phaeochromocytoma 160
pigmentation disorders 106–7
pipe-smokers' palate 105
platelet abnormalities 157
Plummer-Vinson syndrome 115
polyostotic fibrous dysplasia 224–5
postherpetic neuralgia 183
precancerous conditions 114–15
precancerous lesions 111–14
   malignant transformation of 114
   management 114
pregnancy 159
prickle cell layer, *see* stratum spinosum
pseudomembranous candidosis 37–8
psychogenic orofacial problems 205–16
pyostomatitis gangrenosum 148
pyostomatitis vegetans 148

radiation mucositis 118
radiography 21, 85
Ramsay Hunt syndrome 43
recurrent aphthous stomatitis 52–8
   aetiology 54–5
   in children 54
   clinical features 52–4
   histopathology and immunopathogenesis
      55–6
   management 56–8
Reiter's syndrome 35
renal dialysis patients 161–2
renal disease 161–2
renal transplant patients 162
rheumatoid arthritis 200
rickets 226

salbutamol 234
saliva 83–4

salivary flow 84, 85
   disturbances of 90–7, 210–11
   increased 96–7
salivary glands 84
   diseases of 87–90
   examination 84–5
   imaging 85–6
sarcoidosis 88–9
scintigraphy 85–6
scrotal tongue 68
scurvy 158–9
selective serotonin re-uptake inhibitors 209
self-injurious behaviour 212–13
shingles 43
sialadenitis 87–8
sialochemistry 87
sialography 85
sialometry 85
sialosis 88
sickle-cell diseases 154–5
sideropenic dysphagia 115
Sjögren's syndrome 93–6
solar keratosis 66
speckled leukoplakia 113
squamous cell papilloma 104–5
stomatitis 148
   angular 40, 63–5
   denture-induced 39
   nicotinic 105
   recurrent aphthous 52–8
stratum spinosum 3
syphilis 33–4
syphilitic collar 33
systemic lupus erythematosus 137
systemic sclerosis 137–8

taste disturbances 71–2, 210–11
teeth, disorders of 219–23
   discoloration 221
   non-carious surface loss 220–1
   variation in eruption 220
   variation in size 220
temporal arteritis 185–6
temporomandibular disorders 193–202
   arthroscopy 196
   examination 194–5
   imaging 195–6
temporomandibular pain dysfunction syndrome
   196–8
tension-type headache 185
tetracycline 25–6

therapy 25–8
   creams and ointments 26–7
   limitations of 28
   systemic 27–8
   topical 25–6
thyroid disease 160
tobacco use, and oral carcinoma 115–16
tongue, diseases of 67–71
   atrophy of lingual epithelium 69
   developmental abnormalities 67
   enlargement of foliate papillae 69
   morphological variations 67
   traumatic irritation 69
   see also individual conditions
tongue fissures 67–8
tooth enamel, disturbances of 221–2
traumatic keratoses 105
traumatic ulceration 51–2
Treponema pallidum, see syphilis
triamcinolone mouthwash 239
trigeminal neuralgia 179–82
trismus 194
tuberculosis 35
tumour markers 121
tumours 201
tylosis 104

ulceration 51–60
   Behçet's disease 58–9
   recurrent aphthous stomatitis 52–8
   traumatic 51–2
ulcerative colitis 148
ultrasound 22, 86
urinalysis 19

varicella zoster virus 42–3
viral infections 40–6
virology 21

Wegener's granulomatosis 8–9
white sponge naevus 104

xerostomia 90–3

Firmly established as the textbook of choice on the subject, *Oral Medicine* is unique in its comprehensive coverage at a level suitable for both dentistry students and practitioners. Highly illustrated in full colour, the new edition continues to provide an introduction to oral medicine covering the principles, investigations, and therapy. It discusses infections of the oral mucosa, lips, tongue, and salivary glands as well as oral manifestations of systemic diseases in the mouth.

The fifth edition has undergone major revisions in terms of content, layout, and style, bringing the book in line with the changing dental curriculum. Case studies demonstrating oral medicine conditions have been introduced with a discussion of their differential diagnosis and management options. A number of projects have also been added with the purpose of encouraging students to consult other reference sources and to promote self-directed learning, discussion, and debate. This book will provide readers at all levels with an accurate reflection of current ideas and attitudes in this rapidly developing subject area.

From a student reviewer

'I was very impressed ... I like the idea of having the "problem cases", which is a good talking point and ideal for new developments in teaching, such as Problem Based Learning ... I was very pleased with its educational value. It's style is not too complex, but challenges the reader.'